Dr. Kaplan's Lifestyle of the Fit & Famous

Dr. Eric Scott Kaplan

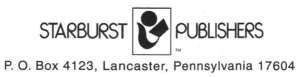
STARBURST PUBLISHERS

P. O. Box 4123, Lancaster, Pennsylvania 17604

To schedule Author appearances write:
Author Appearances, Starburst Promotions, P.O. Box 4123,
Lancaster, Pennsylvania 17604
(717) 293-0939
www.starburstpublishers.com

Credits:
Cover art by Terry Dugan Design

First Printing, February 1998 (trade edition)

ISBN: 0-914984-99-3
Library of Congress Catalog Number 97-061803
Printed in the United States of America

This book is written in memory
of my mother
Elsie Adler Kaplan

This book is dedicated to my family: my wife of fourteen years, *Bonnie,* who always supported me, consoled me, guided me and loved me. My two sons *Michael* and *Jason* who have continued to love me dispite my periodic absence, while I hibernated and wrote this book.

To my hero, my father, *Michael Kaplan,* for teaching me the values of giving, dedication, and perseverance.

To my brother, *Steve,* and his wife, *Gloria,* for their continued support, belief, and patience with me.

To my niece, *Beth,* and nephew, *Richard,* for their love.

To all my aunts, uncles and cousins, especially the *Adlers, Bernsteins, Brenners, Daniels, Garfunkels, Punyons, Siegals, Roths* and *Zucks,* for their belief in me as a child and their support of me as a doctor.

To all my friends, for being my friend.

To all my teachers, professors, coaches and mentors too numerous to name, for guiding, tolerating and unselfishly teaching me. With special thanks to *Dr. Donald Gutstein, the Bob Knight, General Patton,* of the teaching profession, for it was he who trained me and made me competent and capable of writing this book.

With special gratitude to:

Neil Chapnick
Evan Fischer
The Birnbaum family
The Brock family
The Meyer family
Dr. Ian Grassam
Dr. Jim Gregg
Ellen Hake
Dave Robie
Tom McMillen
Jim Gibson

My special thanks to *Uncle Herb Punyon* for his constant inspiration, belief and undying support. His memory lives on in these pages.

And a heart-whelmed thanks to all of my patients, for they are the nucleus of my spirit.

Comments

"The Taj Mahal of Health Books. Good luck to you—I understand the book is a winner!"

Donald J. Trump, Prominent businessman and author

"This book is unique in its common-sense approach to health. It is an exceptional guide to anyone interested in health, sports, fitness, weight loss and positive living. Dr. Kaplan's message should be part of our country's preventative health plan of action."

Tom McMillen, Co-Chairman of President's Council on Physical Fitness, Congressman, 11-year NBA veteran

"I just finished reading the first three chapters of your book, which I found very motivational and inspirational."

Gary Carter, 11-time professional baseball All-Star

"A must read book for anyone thinking of losing weight and keeping it off."

Dr. Earl L. Mindell, author of the *Vitamin Bible, Herb Bible, Food as Medicine* and *Soy Miracle*

"Dr. Kaplan's book is more than highly motivational. It is a must-read for anyone who wants to live a healthier, happier lifestyle."

Billy Cunningham, Hall of Fame NBA player, Championship NBA Coach Philadelphia 76ers, Part owner—Miami Heat

"*Dr. Kaplan's Lifestyle of the Fit & Famous* has provided a thorough approach to fitness. I would consider it mandatory reading for anyone who is serious about maintaining a healthy body and a happy disposition."

Nathaniel P. Crosby, 1981 U.S. Amateur Champion President, Jack Nicklaus Golf Company

"In a job as stressful as mine, a guide such as Dr. Kaplan's is a lifesaver."

Roger Birnbaum, Former President, Twentieth Century Fox Film Corporation

"A very interesting book—I highly recommend it."

Jeff Reardon, #2 All-Time professional baseball Save Leader

"I have found *Dr. Kaplan's Lifestyle of the Fit & Famous* extremely interesting and informative. I would not hesitate to recommend Dr. Kaplan or his book to my patients."

Larry Rosenbaum, M.D., P.A. Diplomate, American Board of Orthopedic Surgery

"If you want to get thin and win, *Dr. Kaplan's Lifestyle of the Fit & Famous* is the one to ingest and digest for immediate progress."

Mark Victor Hansen, Author—*Chicken Soup For the Soul*

Comments

"As a touring golf professional on the P.G.A. tour I have found the formulas on health and fitness provided in *Dr. Kaplan's Lifestyle of the Fit & Famous* to be like having an extra club in my bag. With the extensive travel and rigors of today's professional athlete it is most important to follow a proper exercise and diet regime. Dr Kaplan provides this and more in his easy to read and easier to follow book. It is for these reasons I would not hesitate to recommend his book to anyone."

Steve Hart, PGA Touring Professional

"After reading your book, *Dr. Kaplan's Lifestyle of the Fit & Famous,* I was very impressed with the way in which you presented technical and scientific information in a form that anyone can understand and utilize. I have used your suggestions with remarkable results. I believe your book is a must-read for all who are interested in good health."

Dr. James Gregg, D.C., F.I.C.A.
President, International Chiropractors Association

"Eric Kaplan has done a thorough job in trying to prescribe and explain the best ways to stay fit and healthy. Having been in professional baseball over 25 years, I learned that hard work and applying expert knowledge usually seems to work."

Tom Hutton, ESPN Announcer and 11-year major league baseball player

"Your weight loss book is one of the best I have ever read, let alone tried! After trying different methods of starving, dieting and 'secret weight-loss potions,' I have found yours to be the most sensible and healthiest that has ever worked for me. I definitely recommend your book and plan to give it to all my patients and friends across the country."

John A. Hofmann, D.C., F.I.C.A.
Secretary-Council on Chiropractic Education, Commission on Accreditation
Chiropractor of the year—1989

"Congratulations on the completion of your long-awaited manuscript. Your ideas are unique and thought-provoking. They work on principles that are sound. I would recommend your book to anyone seeking a natural, sensible approach to weight reduction, well being and general good health."

Fred H. Barge, D.C., Ph.C., President Barge Chiropractic Clinic, S.C.
Former President International Chiropractors Association

"*Dr. Kaplan's Lifestyle of the Fit & Famous* is an excellent guide. I would recommend it heartily."

Serge Nakache, M.D. Orthopedic Surgery

Comments

"Enjoyed reading—recommend to everyone."

Jon Sundvold, 9-year NBA Veteran—Miami Heat

"Thank you for your kind letter and your manuscript, *Dr. Kaplan's Lifestyle of the Fit & Famous—A Wellness Approach to Thinning and Winning.* It is my sincere prayer your book will be a help and blessing to many people."

Norman Vincent Peale, Noted author and speaker

"An excellent book for the man on the run . . ."

Norbert A. Schlei, Former Assistant U.S. Attorney General
(Kennedy and Johnson administrations)

"Being a professional golfer, I have read many health and fitness books. The only one that has hit home with me is *Dr. Kaplan's Lifestyle of the Fit & Famous.* I feel very privileged to have Dr. Eric Kaplan look after my health for a productive and professional career on the LPGA Tour."

Barbara Bunkowsky, LPGA Touring Golfer
Winner of Chrysler Invitational

"Congratulations on your book, *Dr. Kaplan's Lifestyle of the Fit and Famous.* It provides a different and modern approach to fitness and weight loss. With your ideas as they are presented, there is no doubt one could achieve a healthy way of life. I recommend that everyone seeking help read your book."

Buck Rodgers, Former manager—California Angels and Montreal Expos

"Wonderfully written with an understanding of a person's health and personal needs. A book 'you must read.' "

Richie Guerin, Former NBA Coach of the Year
General Manager—Atlanta Hawks

"Being an actor and stunt man for the last 14 years, I have relied upon Dr. Kaplan's chiropractic care, friendship and his book to enable me to perform at my physical and mental best."

C. James Lewis, Movie and TV regular
(Sgt. Tommy Cartrude—B.L. Stryker series)

"In simplicity there is elegance! *Dr. Kaplan's Lifestyle of the Fit & Famous* is a simple, yet spectacularly powerful book . . . for it can transform you into the person of your dreams."

Lawrence T. Markson, D.C.
President, Markson Management Services

Comments

"I have had the opportunity to review your book and found it very refreshing and enlightening. A fantastic addition to the current trend of consumer-patient awareness and their participation in a healthy lifestyle. This treasure is a must for any complete reference library."

Salvatore D. LaRusso, D.C., F.I.C.A.
President, Florida Chiropractic Society

"I would heartily recommend *Dr. Kaplan's Lifestyle of the Fit & Famous.* I found it to be highly enjoyable and very stimulating reading."

Michael I. Rose, M.D., Neurologist, Psychologist

"Enjoyed the book tremendously. I highly recommend it!"

Kevin Loughery, Coach—Miami Heat

"The nation can no longer afford the sickness model of Health Care. Dr. Kaplan has become our 'Ambassador of Wellness.'"

Ian A. Grassam, D.C., F.I.C.A., past President, Florida Chiropractic Society
Southern Regional Director, International Chiropractors Association

"You don't have to be a celebrity to live like one. This book is a real keeper. It's a must-read for not only all doctors in the United States, but every patient who values the abundant life."

David J. Kats, D.C., President, Kats Management

"A perfect message for those who want to live a full quality life. The author provides a road map to a sensible approach to personal happiness, health and success. After reading this book, you will have the blueprint to implement a program that will lead to a new level of confidence, satisfaction and a higher level of energy."

Louis Marciani, Executive Director, Amateur Athletic Union

Contents

Introduction

This book is about winning and losing. Winning the prizes of life—health, happiness, success—and losing excess weight, self-defeating ideas, and self-destructive habits.

I've often been asked how this book differs from other diet books on the market. The answer is that this book provides more than a formula for weight loss. It takes a multidimensional approach that incorporates the emotional and the physical, for the fact is, the mind and body cannot be separated.

Deprivation is not paramount to this weight-loss program. Carbohydrates and fats, rather than just calories are counted. In fact, you may actually be able to eat more than you are eating now and still lose weight.

I've been researching this subject for the past 20 years, and have used the principles both personally and professionally. This practical "how to" book will teach you how to:

> ➤ lose weight quickly without suffering from hunger
> ➤ maintain your weight loss
> ➤ mobilize your natural "fat fighters"
> ➤ determine your critical carbohydrate level
> ➤ properly combine foods
> ➤ use vitamins to help control your health and weight
> ➤ increase your energy
> ➤ restore your body to its natural state of good health
> ➤ realize your success potential
> ➤ improve your self-image
> ➤ reduce stress

Notice that maintenance is high on the list. Most diets ultimately fail because they do not teach this most important principle. Initially, most diets seem to work; if your doctor puts you on a 500 calorie diet, you will lose weight. But you'll also feel deprived, and eventually you will backslide. (How many times has this happened already?) The "diet" given in this book will enable you to dine on steak, scampi, lobster and other tasty foods while you lose weight and keep it off. You will learn the Dow Jones principle of weight control.

Why should millions of people be overweight, unhealthy, and unhappy when there is a formula to change these conditions? This formula is realistic, practical and easy to implement; virtually anyone can obtain results with these techniques.

What's more, you will not only be thinner, but more self-confident, content, and energetic. You will be able to use these techniques to improve not only your health, but your relationships with your family, friends and others.

Self conquest is the greatest of victories.

Plato

1

The Journey

Most of us were born perfect. We came into the world healthy, thin, free of fear, and brimming with potential. What happened to us? The answer can be summed up in one word: habit. Somewhere along the line we became creatures of habit, acting and reacting without conscious thought.

While some habits are helpful, a great many of them are destructive. We eat the wrong foods, drink too much, smoke, neglect to exercise, and otherwise abuse our bodies. We abuse our emotions with negative thoughts and self-defeating ideas. And we do it all automatically—it's become a habit. No wonder so many of us are dragged down by obesity, ill-health, mediocrity and unhappiness.

Before you go any further, please take a few minutes to answer the following questions.

Are you someone who:

- Has tried conventional diets and failed?
- Continues to gain weight regardless of how little you eat?
- Wants to achieve and *maintain* your ideal figure?
- Wants to be healthy?
- Wants to be happy?
- Wants to be successful?
- Loves to eat and hates to diet?

> ➤ Has lost weight only to put it back on?
> ➤ Wants to lower your cholesterol levels?
> ➤ Wants to improve your cardiovascular activity?
> ➤ Wants to lose 10 to 50 pounds?
> ➤ Wants to lose 50 to 100 pounds or more?
> ➤ Wants to increase your energy level?
> ➤ Wants to maintain your present weight without deprivation?
> ➤ Wants to eat food like steak and scampi, never feel deprived, yet lose weight and keep it off?

If your answer is "yes," then you are ready to begin a "journey." Along the way, you will find the information you need to become—and re-main—slender and healthy. I can say this with conviction, because I traveled the same road I have mapped out for you. Taking literally Saint Luke's admonition: "Physician heal thyself," I proceeded to do just that.

My adolescence was one long plague of childhood diseases. As an 18-year-old pre-med student, I was afflicted with rampant acne. At 19, my college basketball career was ended by a severe knee injury. By the time I was 30, my face had finally cleared, but I was undergoing a traumatic mid-belly crisis. Although I was dedicated to health and immersed in athletics, I found myself overweight, under par, and out of shape. I became sick and tired of being *sick and tired*. I was a man with a mission.

I began a search. But, the more health guidelines I followed that I'd read about, the more frustrated I became. I was astonished to find that the more I dieted, the more tenacious my weight problem became. I found myself—like many of my friends, patients, family and peers—caught in a nutritional whirlpool.

For as long as I can remember, I have searched for the secret to health. Always looking for that one special herb, vitamin or concept that would make me the picture of health. This curiosity has always led me to research, to find out the who, what, when and whys of health. Part of the reason I have done this is not only to obtain the highest standards of health, but also that, in turn, I could transmit health to all my patients. In today's society there is more to being a healer than just healing. It has always been my goal to not only express health but to transmit it.

Most dieters today live by the "feast or famine" principle. Skip a meal here, overindulge there. This principle, like so many others, leads to fat gain or failure. They lose minimal weight but pay a maximum price. A price so high with the discipline so stressing, they wear themselves down and eventually put their lost weight back on. Once again, failure. Unfortunately, these failures accumulate and begin to eat away at their pride, their self-image. Soon they accept these failures as a way of life, dragging themselves down to a life unfulfilled, submerged in depression.

When I began my journey on the "highway to health" I weighed 200 pounds. Today, I am 175 pounds, about my college weight. I eat well and have tremendous energy.

My favorite definition of health is the one I found in *Dorland's Medical Dictionary:* "A state of optimal mental, physical and social well being, not merely the absence of disease or infirmities." This state should be the destination of our journey.

It's inexcusable that so wealthy a country should be inhabited by so many people who are poor in health. Inexcusable, but true. Fred L. Allman Jr., M.D., points out that, "over one million American workers call in sick on any given day, with the result being more than 330 million workdays lost every year because of health-related causes."

And if you think that you know the number one health hazard facing Americans today, you may be surprised by Dr. Allman's findings.

"Physical deterioration of the body is the worst disease in the United States today. It is so prevalent that if you are 25 years of age or older then there is a 50% or more chance you are suffering from some form of disease. Deterioration may occur very slowly—so slowly, in fact, that it may go undetected for many years and not become readily apparent on physical examination by a competent physician."

The saddest part about this state of affairs is that deterioration can be slowed dramatically by a healthy lifestyle. I have often wondered why doctors have traditionally placed so little emphasis on nutritional paths to optimal health.

One thing is certain: you won't find the magic elixir of well-being in a capsule, pill or injection. Despite the billions of dollars we pay to the drug industry, doctors' offices are crammed, primarily with people looking for more medication. It is crucial for you to understand that drugs are only for the control of symptoms, and that drugs alone cannot cure disease.

My philosophy is based on the belief that the body is a self-healing organism. The power that created the body can heal the body. The most that properly prescribed drugs can do is aid our bodies' defense system against disease.

The damage that we are causing ourselves through belief in the magic of drugs is worrisome. The lesson we are teaching our children is terrifying, as Dr. Robert Mendelson illustrates in *How To Raise A Happy And Healthy Child In Spite Of Your Doctor:*

"Doctors who continually prescribe powerful drugs indoctrinate children from birth with the philosophy of a pill 'for every ill.' This may lead a child to the belief that there is a drug to treat every condition and that drugs are an appropriate response to normal feelings of frustration, depression, anxiety, inadequacy and insecurity. Doctors are directly responsible for putting millions of people on prescription drugs. They are also indirectly responsible for the plight of millions more who turn to illegal drugs because they were taught in early age that drugs can cure anything including psychological and emotional conditions that ails them."[1]

The United States has 5% of the world's population and 50% of the world's drug problem.

During our nine months in the womb we develop according to our biological clock; we grow arms, legs, etc., without the help of a doctor or any other outside interference. Then, we arrive into the world thin and healthy; rarely is an infant obese. But when we enter the world of experts, our life takes a turn, and seldom for the better. (No wonder the first thing we do is cry!)

Our life is a journey with many winding roads, enclaves and detours. It takes far more dedication and discipline to succeed on this journey than on any other journey we have embarked upon. It is a journey that leads us to making many decisions we must sit and labor over. We must consider ourselves travelers. We must sit and review the maps of life as we proceed to our final destination. We must utilize the proper information and material at our disposal to help us make these decisions.

The curse of our society, and sometimes our being, is that we must seek something we do not have. We seek wealth when we are not wealthy, we seek happiness when we are not happy, we seek health when we are not healthy. We don't live in a society which dictates our diet, mental attitude, thoughts, or goals. We exist in a free society scientifically superior to any other. So why do we continue to fail?

Our libraries are overflowing with books and periodicals on health and well-being. Yet we find ourselves continually on another road, another path searching again to find the secrets of health. We live on a ferris wheel going round and round, up and down. In God's infinite wisdom He created no two human beings the same. I cannot count how many times I'd have a patient come to me who is 75 years old, the picture of good health, only to learn in his history that he is a chronic smoker. Of course, he smoked non-filtered cigarettes for 50 years of his life.

Common sense dictates to us that smoking is not good for our health. Yet here stands a man 75 years old vibrant, healthy, active, who continues to smoke. I am sure we all know at least one person who can sit down at a table and eat to his heart's content yet never gain a pound. I have found in my journey on the "highway to health" and through my clinical experience as a chiropractic physician that no two people are the same.

These differences should be respected, but all too often they are invalidated. Just look at all of the advertising around you. Madison Avenue has decreed that we must all look like spin-offs of the faces and bodies that adorn the covers of *Vogue* and *Esquire*. (People without tight bellies, trim thighs, and small backsides need not apply.)

In spite of the fact that some people have lives that "look" healthy, burnout is the disease of the '90s. We now have automobiles that map our course, televisions with giant screens, the best stereo equipment, dishwashers, clothes washers, and refrigerators that make ice cubes for us. We have self-cleaning ovens, self-defrosting freezers, and garage doors that open with the touch of a button. Then, after a long, automated day, we are rocked to sleep in a water bed. So why are we so overwhelmed by stress that we have to invent a term like "burnout?" I believe the answer is that, while we have plenty of outside help, we have ignored the need for inside help. And this is the gap my book was written to fill.

I can't overemphasize the importance of "inner winning." In *Think And Grow Rich,*[2] author Napoleon Hill gives many case histories of successful people. Few of these people were born beautiful, rich, or incredibly talented. The one thing these individuals had in common was a burning desire to succeed. Take the story of Edward C. Barnes, who was determined to become a business associate of the great Thomas Edison.

Barnes was not a scientist, nor was he a wealthy man. And there were two obstacles to his goal: (1) He had never met Edison. (2) He lacked the train fare to New Jersey, where Edison lived.

Barnes could have given up, in which case you wouldn't be reading about him right now. Instead, he made his way to a startled but impressed Edison.

"He stood there before me looking like an ordinary tramp, but there was something in the expression of his face which conveyed the impression that he was determined to get what he had come after. I had learned from my years of experiences with men that when a man really desires a thing so deeply that he is willing to stake his entire future on the single turn of a wheel in order to get it, he is sure to win. I gave him the opportunity he asked for, because I saw he made up his mind to stand by until he succeeded."

Subsequent events proved Edison correct. Edison had perfected a new office device which was to become known as the Edison Dictating Machine. At the time he met Barnes, he was having difficulty getting his people to market the invention. His sales force simply wasn't enthusiastic. Barnes took over the job, and sold the machine so successfully that Edison gave him an exclusive contract to sell, market and distribute the Edison Dictating Machine. The rest is history.

This is only one of many success stories recounted by Hill. He also discusses the successes of such outstanding individuals as Charles Schwab, Theodore Roosevelt, and Henry Ford, who was long thought of as incompetent, unintelligent, and illiterate. These people all shared an incredible perseverance and an inner desire that kept them motivated.

You can't build a reputation on what you are going to do.
Henry Ford

2

Goal Tending

When I discuss success strategies with my patients, many of my favorite analogies are drawn from the game of golf. This sport is one of the best metaphors I know of for successful living because it contains all of the elements required for setting, tending and reaching one's goals.

I enjoy watching as well as playing golf, and my favorite event is the Pro-Ams. I find it fascinating to watch the likes of Bob Hope, former president Gerald Ford, Clint Eastwood, Tip O'Neil, Joey Bishop and Jack Lemmon give themselves over to the exhilaration of competition.

What is it about this sport that motivates already successful people to challenge themselves even further? The lure of the game is undeniable, for no less a personage than Michael Jordan, acknowledged as the best basketball player in the world, has stated one of his ambitions is to ". . . turn (golf) pro after my basketball career." And Lawrence Taylor, an all pro linebacker for the New York Giants who has had numerous bouts with drug addiction, considers golf his therapy.

I've learned that the excitement of the game comes not from getting the ball in the hole, but from the challenge of reducing the number of strokes it takes to achieve that triumph (ingrained goal setting). Life without goals is like a golf green without a flag, or a hole without a par.

The power of commitment is behind every success story, including the following:

Gail Borden—Borden's Milk & Ice Cream
An eccentric inventor and drifter, witnesses the deaths of a number of children who drank contaminated milk. He finds a way to preserve milk so that such tragedies will not recur.

George Kinney—Kinney Shoes
A widower with a young son loses his job at a department store. He dreams of becoming his own boss and scrapes together $1,500 to open his own store.

Thomas Alva Edison—Inventor of the light bulb, phonograph, motion picture, etc.
A six-year-old boy ponders ways to speed up the hatching of chicken eggs. His solution is to sit on the eggs himself. This initial glimmer of ingenuity was the precursor to the genius that later illuminated (literally) the world.

Estee Lauder—Estee Lauder Cosmetics and Skin Care Products
The little girl enjoys touching people's faces and hair, she loves to help make people more attractive. She dreams of becoming a skin care special-ist while she watches her uncle concoct creams and potions on her mother's gas stove.

Mike Ditka—Pro football player; head coach of the New Orleans Saints
Living in a government-funded housing project in Pennsylvania, he dreams of escaping the mines of his home state. He knows sports, but more important, he knows what he wants.

Burton Baskin and Irvine Robbins—Baskin-Robbins Ice Cream
Two brothers-in-law have a simple dream of starting a business together and earning $75 a week. Their marketing philosophy is likewise simple, simply brilliant: they will serve one product 31 different ways.

Robert, Edward, and James Johnson—Johnson & Johnson
Health Care Products
It's the 19th century, and many surgery patients are dying from infections caused by unsanitary conditions. A young dreamer convinces his brothers to work with him on finding a way to produce sterile bandages.

Dick Clark—*American Bandstand* host
After his older brother is shot down and killed in World War II, the teenager listens to the radio to ease his loneliness. He dreams of someday being an announcer on his own show.[1]

None of these people were overnight successes, nor should you become discouraged if you don't instantaneously produce tangible re-sults. One of the most valuable lessons I learned on the golf course was to take one hole at a time, in fact, to take one shot at a time. Many people who begin diets or health regimens become discouraged after a small setback. "I overate at a party on Saturday," or "I had a piece of cake at the office today and blew my diet." They allow one mistake to keep them from their goal and then think that the goal itself was the problem.

The best economists are intimately familiar with the workings of the Dow Jones. They know how to make the stock market run for them rather than over them. I will teach you the Dow Jones principle of weight control, which will put you in control of your metabolism. You will learn how and when to make sustenance deposits and withdrawals, to manipulate your diet as an economist manipulates stocks and bonds.

And speaking of economics, it is important to realize that you do have to pay a price for everything you want. In this case, the price is discipline. To achieve lasting good in our lives, we must have this attribute. No less a being than God made this decision, which he codified in a set of rules of life known as the Ten Commandments.

I have found this lesson the most difficult to master, but the rewards have been tremendous. I went through periods of dis-health, unhappiness and economic hardship. By increasing my capacity to withstand discipline, I increased my feelings of self-worth. As a result I became happier, more successful and more giving. In turn, I received more from my friends, my wife and my family. In response I gave more time, energy, and dedication. It's a benevolent cycle rather than a vicious one.

It was discipline that enabled me to reach my athletic goals in high school and later in college. I stand 5'8" tall, yet I played basketball despite the fact that I was told I was too short for the game. I would like to emphasize that I was not an unusually gifted athlete, but I was an unusually dedicated one. What I lacked in height, I made up for in perseverance. While not the tallest on my team, I was probably in better shape than any athlete on any team I ever competed against, and it showed on the court.

Discipline did not come naturally to me. When I played college basketball at Fairleigh Dickinson University, I developed the habit of smoking cigarettes. My uncle, Herb Punyon, warned me that cigarettes were addicting and would lower my stamina, but I was convinced of my own invincibility. I discovered that the consequences had caught up with me when I tried out for the United States Maccabea Team at age 25. As I ran up and down the court, I found myself gasping for air. Despite my strong desire to succeed, my lack of discipline prevented me from reaching the standards I had set for myself. I threw away my cigarettes that very day. But I didn't accomplish that goal or my other goals immediately. Ultimately, though, I did materialize my dreams.

One of the secrets to keeping your large goals alive is to set smaller, interim goals. If you want to lose 50 pounds, put that on your goal plan, but also make it a sub-goal to lose 10 pounds by a certain date. The excitement and self-confidence you derive from this achievement provides the feedback you need to remain on course.

Before you can make a map to your destination, you have to know where you are. Dr. Donald Gutstein, my clinic director and mentor during my internship, had a favorite quote: "The ability to recognize ignorance is the first step toward knowledge."

There are millions of people who believe they are fated to suffer from conditions ranging from obesity to poverty by forces beyond their control. Nothing could be further from the truth. God created men and women in his own image, and that image is not one of failure and lack. God created us to succeed, but it is up to us to follow his plan. "God's gift to man is life, and man's gift to God is what he does with his life."

The first time I heard that quote, it was uttered by one of the most successful health practitioners in the country, Dr. Jimmy Gregg. I had heard that Dr. Gregg has been known to treat in excess of 300 patients a day, a figure that I, as a busy physician, found difficult to believe.

Still, the reports were confirmed over and over, and it was true that people came from all over Michigan to see this man.

When, as a student, I first heard of him, he was already a legend. I set a goal to meet him, to learn from him. Then I developed my goal plan (a goal without a plan is nothing more than a wish); I decided that I would attend his next seminar.

I expected the man to have the charisma of Oral Roberts, the strength of Babe Ruth, the perseverance of Lou Gehrig, the personality of Ronald Reagan, and to stand at least 6'2" tall. I was in for a surprise. Dr. Gregg is approximately 5'6", and a good-looking man, though not as spectacularly handsome as a movie star. What is spectacular is his dedication to the principles of life, his ability to give for the sake of giving. You see, Dr. Gregg is the ultimate healer, a doctor who will treat any patient regardless of his or her ability to pay. Dr. Gregg taught me his concept of health care, and to this day I am grateful.

I learned another lesson from him on the tennis court. On one side of the net stood Jimmy Gregg, who was at least 30 pounds overweight and did not look to be in the best of shape. On the other side was the new Eric Kaplan, trim, at least semi-athletic, and very competitive. Dr. Gregg defeated me 6–1, 6–0. I later learned that he not only treated Billy Jean King, he frequently played tennis with her. The lesson here is not to judge others. We must only judge ourselves. We must learn from all people, by learning from their defeats it may lead us to our victories. "Even a clock that doesn't work is right twice a day."

I've also learned a great deal from another friend and patient, Jeff Reardon. Jeff is one of the premier relief pitchers in baseball. Presently he ranks third of the all-time saves leaders in the history of baseball. It would be easy to assume that in the four or five months that comprises the off season, he would take it easy and count his money. This is not true of Jeff, who spends the off season preparing himself for the following season.

Jeff is a man with a larger-than-life mission, which is why I enjoy spending time with him. I had the privilege of being with him during the 1987 World Series and had the pleasure of congratulating him for the fantastic success of the Twins. Did he sit back and bask in his success? Quite the opposite; not long afterward, he was talking about winning the next World Series.

Jeff wasn't born with a silver spoon in his mouth, nor did he have his victories handed to him on a silver platter. True, he has a gift, but he is not a natural phenomenon. He wasn't one of the people who signed on right out of high school. He honed his skills on the University of Massachusetts team, but after four years of college baseball he was not drafted by the pros. He entered pro ball as a free agent. The rest is Major League history.

In many ways Dr. Jimmy Gregg and Jeff Reardon are complete opposites. Their similarity lies in their understanding of the principles of goal setting. They are both dedicated and disciplined, and these common attributes explain their success in their respective professions.

There are five major health goals—one for each facet of health:

1. Proper exercise

2. Proper diet

3. Proper rest and relaxation habits

4. Positive mental attitude

5. Proper nerve supply

It is known that Babe Ruth "The Sultan of SWAT" was successful at hitting 714 lifetime runs. A total that many felt would never be equaled, a feat so spectacular that even today, years after his death, he is still a legend to every child or every person who ever enters the game of baseball. But, he also was the man who struck out a record of 1,732 times. The point here is, we as people will be remembered more for our successes than for our failures.

Another man who is remembered for his victories rather than his defeats is Abraham Lincoln. I think of Lincoln primarily as the president who brought our country through a bitter civil war, the man who ended slavery. I also knew that he did not begin life with the trappings of success. But in Dave Dean's book, *Now Is Your Time To Win,*[2] I was stunned to read the following concerning Lincoln:

"1816   Forced from home
1818   His mother died
1831   Failed in business
1832   Defeated for State Legislature
1833   Failed in business again
1834   Elected to State Legislature
1835   His sweetheart died
1836   Suffered a nervous breakdown
1838   Defeated for Speaker of State Legislature
1840   Defeated for Elector
1843   Defeated for Congress
1846   Elected to Congress
1848   Lost reelection
1854   Rejected for job of Land Officer
1855   Defeated for Senate

1856 Defeated for Vice President
1858 Defeated for Senate
1860 Elected President of the United States of America"

Here was a person with a dream so strong, no failure could dampen it. We were all taught about his greatness. Now I understand that Lincoln's greatness stemmed from his perseverance. In 28 years of politics, he had four times as many defeats as victories. Most men would have decided that life was unfair and given up. Because Lincoln remained true to his goals, he eventually won the most important race of all. In 1860, not only was he elected as President of the United States, but he went on to become one of the greatest presidents our country has ever known.

Still think your failures are of great significance? Don't dwell on the times you failed to lose weight, to quit smoking, or to make a relationship work. Concentrate on your goals, instead. If you keep your eye on the green flag instead of the sandtrap, you're halfway to winning the game.

If you find a path with no obstacles, it probably doesn't lead anywhere.

Frank A. Clark

3

Success Psychology

Relax, close your eyes, and repeat to yourself some variation of this message: "I am happy, I am healthy, I am successful, I am enthusiastic. I have never felt better than I feel today. I have my life in order. I am working to benefit myself and others. Today I am happier than ever before."

This chapter is about making this affirmation a reality. In the following pages I will teach you:

We should take lessons from the past, not regrets. Donald J. Trump, in his book *The Art Of The Deal,* says, "I try to learn from the past, but I plan for the future by focusing exclusively on the present. That's where the fun is, and if it can't be fun, what's the point?"[1]

Given Trump's ability to turn apparent failures into spectacular successes (as seen in his new book, *The Art Of The Comeback*), I think it is safe to take his advice on this point.

It's been said there are three kinds of people in the world: those who make things happen, those who let things happen, and those who wonder what happened.

Abraham Lincoln once said: "Most folks are as happy as they make up their minds to be."

You could just as easily substitute "successful" for "happy" in this sentence. If you don't feel successful, maybe it's because you don't know what success is. Many of us were given our ideas on this subject from our parents, teachers, rabbis/ministers/priests, or—worst of all—from television.

Some of us confuse success with wealth.

In 1923, some of the most "successful" financiers in the country met at the Edgewater Beach Hotel in Chicago. The eminent guests included:

> ➤ *Charles Schwab*— president of the largest steel company in America
> ➤ *Samuel Insull*— president of the largest utility company in America
> ➤ *Howard Hopson*— president of the largest gas company in America
> ➤ *Arthur Cutten*— the great wheat speculator
> ➤ *Richard Whitney*— president of the New York stock exchange
> ➤ *Albert Fall*— secretary of the Interior in president Harding's cabinet
> ➤ *Jesse Livermore*— the greatest "bear" on Wall Street
> ➤ *Ivar Kreuger*— head of the world's greatest monopoly
> ➤ *Leon Fraser*— president of the Bank of International Settlements

If money could buy happiness, these men would have been in a constant state of ecstasy. But this is where they were 25 years after the famous meeting:

> ➤ Charles Schwab went bankrupt and lived the last five years of his life on borrowed money.
> ➤ Samuel Insull died in a foreign land, a penniless fugitive from justice.
> ➤ Howard Hopson went insane.
> ➤ Arthur Cutten died insolvent in another country.
> ➤ Richard Whitney had just been released from Sing Sing prison.
> ➤ Albert Fall, having been pardoned from prison, died at home, broke.
> ➤ Jesse Livermore committed suicide.
> ➤ Ivar Kreuger committed suicide.
> ➤ Leon Fraser committed suicide.[2]

Still think you'd be willing to trade places with any one of these men? In society's terms, they had it all, but they lived unsuccessfully.

People have their own ideas about what will make them happy. You may listen to their opinions, but the ultimate decision must be yours. When I was young I wanted to be an entertainer, but my mother said, "Young Jewish boys don't become entertainers. You must go to college. You must become a doctor." I can just imagine where some of the famous Jewish entertainers would be today if they had come from my home. Would Barbra Striesand, Barry Manilow, Joey Bishop, Tony Curtis, Joan Rivers, and Steven Spielberg all be doctors?

Each of us has an innate intelligence that is constantly communicating with us. This is the voice that tells us when we are hungry, thirsty, tired, happy, lonely, excited or sad. This intelligence offers many suggestions, and it behooves us to listen to them. For this is the force that governs our whole being.

It gives us the ability to see, think, breathe, and digest our food. As you read this page, your eyes are feeding this information to your brain, which has the ability not only to absorb knowledge, but to store, interpret, and apply it. Right now, your stomach is taking food and turning it into energy, removing from your body what it cannot utilize. Your lungs are turning carbon dioxide into oxygen, and your heart is beating approximately 72 times per minute, 100,000 times per day, 700,000 times per week, and over 30 million times per year. The heart is more complex and dependable than any pump devised by humans. Modern science can imitate it, but cannot duplicate it, which is why a transplant does not function with the ease of your own organ. The heart pumps over six quarts of blood through over 96 miles of blood vessels, which is the equivalent of pumping 6,300 gallons of blood per day. And it performs this job 24 hours a day, 365 days a year, with no time off for good behavior. The minute our heart stops and takes a rest, we no longer have what is known as life.

Our body is perfect. God created us with a body far greater than anything else He could ever reward us with. God gave us a body that consists of trillions of cells, and He gave us the ability to duplicate ourselves in the amazing confines of reproduction. I have come to understand the human body as an amazing machine. Each and every one of us possesses this machine. This machine that consists of a heart, lungs, a brain, also consists of millions of pores which are constantly acting as a cooling mechanism. Our digestive system has the ability to turn simple food into healthy new blood and bones. It helps the muscles have strength, and gives the bones stability. How did this body teach the muscles and bones to work together? God has given us, within this magnificent body, a power called Innate Intelligence. This power that creates the body and operates the body has the power to heal the body. An example being, if we ever broke a bone in our arm the greatest doctor in the world can only set the bone in a cast, but the intelligence that is working 24 hours a day on an ongoing basis, acknowledges the break in the bone, it knows exactly where the break in the bone is, and it knows exactly how to re-cement or to re-ossify the weakened structure. The doctor aided us by producing the cast, and with his intelligence and ability, set the bone in the proper position, but the human body alone in its magnificence knows exactly how to mend the bone. No different than a cut on our hand. How many times have we cut ourselves and run to our mother? She puts Bactene on the cut to kill the germs, yet our body knows exactly where the wound is and it knows exactly how to heal this wound into a fresh, healthy new piece of skin.

Dr. Michael Debakey is acknowledged as one of the world's greatest heart surgeons. He can perform surgery that is little short of miraculous, but it is up to the body to perform the ultimate miracle, it must heal the wound that was created by the scalpel's knife. It must accept the correction performed by the surgeon, and prevent the body from receiving infection. Modern medicine has understood and understands how to assist the body, but the body itself, is the greatest healer the world has ever known.

Modern science has yet to come close to developing a computer as complex and creative as the human brain. As the owner of this magnificent biomachine, it is your responsibility to program it. All too often, though, we hand over the job to others, we make ourselves victims of circumstances. Say you begin the day in a great state of mind. Then your car won't start. You finally get to work and find that your secretary has called in sick. Then your boss yells at you. By the end of the day, you've been reprogrammed—and the program has plenty of bugs in it.

This is when you have to remember to take charge. To say, "I will greet every obstacle head on, face-to-face. I will turn each obstacle into a challenge and each challenge into a success."

This is not always easy to do, given the beliefs many of us were weaned on:

- No you can't.
- Don't try to be someone you are not.
- You are too big for your britches.
- A bird in the hand is worth two in the bush.
- Don't speak until spoken to.
- Don't bite off more than you can chew.
- Save for a rainy day.
- Rich people are thieves.
- A woman's place is in the home.
- The Lord giveth, the Lord taketh away.
- Men don't cry.
- Oh it's too good to be true.
- I'll believe it when I see it.
- Don't do that or God will punish you.
- It's a man's world.[3]

When I first read these lines in a text by Dr. Markson, I realized that I was raised with all these clichés. I was too young to see the inherent flaws, too dependent on the good will of the adults around me to challenge their beliefs. But in time, I learned to let go of these limiting thoughts, and you can do the same.

After all, how many of us were raised in a totally positive environment? How often did we hear that we could do whatever we wanted, be the person we dreamed of being? If you didn't hear this very often, start telling it to yourself. Regardless of how much negative programming you were subjected to, you have the ability to change.

There are two types of changes we are concerned with here. The first is physical change, to which most of you reading this book are already committed. The second, more subtle change is psychological. It involves shifting our attitudes, and releasing our fears, doubts, worries, anxieties and insecurities. I define "average" as "the best of the worst and the worst of the best." Are you willing to settle for being average?

As I said, the brain is essentially a marvelous computer. To reprogram it, you need the correct software. We'll begin with a very powerful program known as "Affirmations."

The dictionary is the only place where success comes before work.
Mark Twain

4

Affirmative Action

You've probably already learned (perhaps to your sorrow) that you are what you eat. But has it ever occurred to you that you are what you think? Just as a diet high in junk foods will distort your body, a mind full of junk thoughts will distort your goals, dreams and ambitions.

An affirmation is a positive statement about yourself or your circumstances. Affirmations enable you to program yourself to succeed by removing the fears or thoughts of failure that your subconscious has accumulated over the years. In many ways the brain is like a computer; what you get out of it depends on what you put into it. Consider these two statements:

"I respect my body and therefore eat only healthy, nourishing foods."
"I've always been overweight, it runs in my family."

Which person do you think will succeed in losing weight?

You can say affirmations aloud, repeat them silently to yourself, write them down, even sing them! The more you repeat an affirmation, the greater the power you give it, so repeat your affirmations frequently and with conviction. Believe me, you *do* have time to do this. You can say your affirmations while you shower, on your way to work (instead of cursing traffic), or while you exercise. Affirm as you cook dinner, vacuum the carpet, or mow the lawn.

A couple of other hints to help you use affirmations to their best advantage: use the present tense ("I am slender and healthy" rather than

"I will be slender and healthy") and use positive rather than negative language ("I live in harmony with my family" rather than "I no longer shout at the children").

If you doubt the power of affirmations, take a look around you. Better yet, take a look inside yourself. Have you ever known a highly successful person who was riddled with doubts and insecurities? How much of who you are today is a reflection of who you think you are?

Muhammad Ali made his affirmation into a legend. He wasn't born a great boxer. He trained, struggled, and dreamed of his triumph. And throughout his rise to the championship he affirmed: "I'm the greatest." He didn't say, "I'm almost the greatest," or "Next year I'll be the greatest." Even after he lost, he continued to affirm "I'm the greatest."

He went on the regain his title a record three times.

Successful people think successful thoughts. In *Now Is Your Time To Win,* author Dave Dean[1] provides many inspiring examples of this axiom. He tells the story of Tom Landry, who during his first season with the Dallas Cowboys ended with zero wins, eleven losses, and one tie. Yet Landry went on to become one of the most dynamic, successful football coaches of his time. What if after his first season he had thrown in the towel, or the Dallas Cowboys had thrown the towel at him? Dean also reports the triumph of Cheryl Pruitt, Miss America 1980:

"When I was five years old, I had a milkman tell me that some day I was going to be Miss America. I guess that planted a seed in my mind. I entered my first pageant when I was eighteen. It was a Miss America preliminary, Miss Chocpaw County, Mississippi. I lost. The next year I entered the Miss Mississippi State Pageant and lost again. The following year I entered the Miss Mississippi State again, and again I lost. The third year of Miss Mississippi State, which is my fourth year in the pageant, I won the university title and thought I was finally on my way, but lost at the state level. The fifth year I entered another local pageant and won. I then won Miss Mississippi and went on to a branch city and won the Miss America Pageant. But it had taken me five full years."[2]

On the other hand, consider the story of Mary Decker. She was considered a top distance runner, a strong Gold Medal contender. She had the talent and the drive. However, she often referred to herself as a "jinx." She planted this thought so deeply that it eventually bore fruit. A collision and fall ended her Olympic dreams.

In contrast, we have the story of Greg Louganis, who during the 1988 Olympics banged his head while doing a dive he had done 1,000 times before. Neither pain nor apparent "failure" altered his vision. He could have withdrawn into self-pity; the world would have sympathized. After all, continuous television replay reaffirmed his failure. Instead, he went back on the board and executed his dive to perfection. He believed in himself, now the world believes in Greg Louganis.

I encourage you to turn your personality into a success personality. To understand that the only psychology to success is the desire to succeed. You may be wondering what your personality has to do with your health. Many studies suggest that we can think our way to health—or illness. One such study, conducted by John W. Shaffer and Pirkko L. Graves at Johns Hopkins University School of Medicine, revealed that men who hide their feelings are much more likely to develop cancer than men who express their feelings.

The researchers also found that loners were 16 times more likely to get cancer than emotionally expressive men.

Rather than suppress our feelings, needs, and desires, we should express them with the confidence that they can be fulfilled:

"I am now at my optimum weight."

"I enjoy excellent health and limitless vitality."

"All of my relationships are loving and fulfilling." ·

"I love my work and always do an excellent job."

"I am now enjoying abundant prosperity."

Feel free to make up your own affirmations, using the language that feels right for your particular situation and goals—you may be surprised at the results.

In fact, results are virtually assured if you use the second word of this chapter—*action*. Affirmations are powerful, but it does take work to make them work for you.

Team your affirmations with your goals and develop a definite plan for success. Create short-term goals to build your confidence for the long-term goals. In the previous chapter, I suggested writing down your goals. I also recommend that you draw out a map or write a list of things you must do to accomplish your goals. I call these action steps.

To prevent discouragement, make your goals realistic. It's not realistic to set a weight-loss goal of 50 pounds in five weeks. It is realistic to decide that you want to lose 25 pounds in six weeks. The same is true of exercise. Don't vow to jog ten miles a week if you've never jogged before. Instead, decide that you will walk a mile or ride your bicycle two miles per day. While you should stick to your goals, don't get stuck on them. It is appropriate to modify your goals as your needs and desires change. You cannot evaluate your priorities until you are comfortable with them. So be honest with yourself, as your subconscious will always be able to detect when your conscious self is lying.

Should doubt and discouragement creep in, chase them out with your affirmations. When you find yourself lamenting, "I'll always be fat," let that thought go and replace it with, "My weight loss program brings wonderful results."

Don't limit the wonderful power of affirmations and goal setting to your weight loss. I invite you to use these marvelous tools to improve your relationships, job, finances, health, and other aspects of your life.

The law of the universe states: "You can only become what you think you are."

This is quite a bit different than the work ethic with which most of us have been raised, which tells us only: "You can be better than you are."

People who follow the work ethic equate striving with happiness, and are too often disappointed when all their hard work does not bring them joy. Remember, happiness starts from the inside out, not the outside in. Perhaps Ben Franklin said it best, "Content makes poor men rich; discontent makes rich men poor."

Work does not bring happiness, but happiness can make work a more enjoyable part of our lives.

And please don't lose faith if your goals don't immediately materialize. The need for perseverance is wonderfully illustrated in an anecdote related in *Think and Grow Rich,* by Napoleon Hill. [3]

This story concerns one R.U. Darby, who went west to make his fortune during the gold rush days. After weeks of labor, he was rewarded by the glitter of golden ore. Realizing the need for proper machinery, Darby raised money for the equipment and went to work with his crew. The first car of ore was mined and shipped, and the return proved that they had one of the richest mines in Colorado. Only a few more cars of ore were needed to clear all of Darby's debts; then it would be pure profit. But the next time the drills went into the mine, they came up empty; the vein of gold had apparently disappeared. Although the miners desperately tried to pick up the vein again, after several failures they conceded defeat. The machinery was sold to a junk man for a few dollars, and the disheartened miners took the train back home. The junk man, however, consulted a mining engineer. He was advised that the project had failed because the miners were not familiar with the fault lines. The engineer guided him to a spot just three feet from where Darby's men had stopped drilling; that is precisely where the gold was found.

The junk man mined millions of dollars in ore, because he knew enough to take one more step before giving up.

Darby's story also has a happy ending, for he learned a lesson more valuable than gold. He never forgot that he had lost a fortune because he stopped three feet too soon. As an insurance salesman, he vowed never to give up because he was told "no" by a prospective customer. Darby became one of a select group who sold over a million dollars worth of life insurance annually.

Each of us has a mental blueprint of ourselves, a blueprint that tells us who and what we are. It creates a picture of our own self-concept.

Our blueprint has been designed by the successes and failures of our lives, and it takes into account our talents, abilities, and desires. The amazing thing is how differently other people view the same picture that we have created for ourselves. Unfortunately, we are often overly concerned with how other people view our picture. I think it is common knowledge that being overweight is unhealthy, yet as a physician I notice that people are more motivated to lose weight for cosmetic reasons than for health reasons. While there is nothing wrong with wanting to improve your appearance, it is even better to lose weight because you respect your well-being and appreciate your own uniqueness and specialness.

The difference between success and failure is the action or lack of action that separates the achievers from the make believers. Consider the story of this youngster:

A little boy went into a drug store, reached for a soda carton and pulled it over to the telephone. He climbed onto the carton so that he could reach the buttons on the phone, and proceeded to punch in seven digits. I listened to the following conversation:

He said, "Lady, I want to cut your lawn."

The woman replied, "I already have someone to cut my lawn."

"Lady, I'll cut your lawn for half the price of the person who cuts your lawn now."

The woman responded that she was very satisfied with the person who was presently cutting her lawn.

The little boy found yet more perseverance and offered, "Lady, I'll even sweep your curb and your sidewalk, so on Sunday you will have the prettiest lawn in all of North Palm Beach, Florida."

Again, the woman answered in the negative.

With a smile on his face, the little boy replaced the receiver.

The druggist walked over to the boy and said, "Son, I like your attitude, I like that positive spirit. Son, I would like to offer you a job."

The little boy replied, "No thanks. *I was just checking on the job I already have.*"

It's not likely that someone with that kind of attitude will end up in the unemployment line.

Here is a very special affirmation I say when I wake up in the morning and before I retire for the night, and I feel it benefits me enormously:

I am happy, I am healthy, I am successful. God has blessed me with the gift of life, and I will not take this gift for granted. My body is functioning at 100 percent, 100 percent of the time. My body is breaking down fat and turning the food that I eat into muscle. I utilize the elements—the sun, the air, and the water—and these elements revitalize my body. They increase my life energy, and guide my body to a happier, healthier existance. I am free of stress. I do not allow stress into my consciousness. Stress is created from the inside out; it does not come from the outside in. I will not develop or cultivate stress. I am relaxed mentally and physically. I am mentally and physically prepared to enter this day to succeed. I am prepared for the obstacles and challenges that life has to offer me. I turn any and all obstacles and challenges into my successes. From these successes I grow strength and confidence. I acknowledge that the world is filled with abundance. An abundance of wealth, health, and happiness. I am part of this abundance. Today, I think only good thoughts. I say only nice things. I do only good deeds. I eat only good foods. I do not allow negative sources to enter my body. I reward my body for rewarding me with life. Today, I am happy, I am healthy. Today, I am successful. Today, I love and am loved. Today, my life is filled with abundance.

A man has to live with himself, and he should see to it that he always has good company.

C.E. Hughes

5

Thin To Win

The next time you're in a bookstore, pull out a few volumes at random and take a long look at the book jackets. It's obvious that a great deal of time, thought and money goes into the design of what may seem like the least important part of the book. But publishers, who are not in business to lose money, know that aphorisms notwithstanding, people *do* judge a book by its cover.

Once you understand this principle, you will realize the importance of your appearance. The image you present to the world speaks volumes about your character. It can say that you believe in and respect yourself, or it can shout that you couldn't care less. The old cliché stands, "You can only make a first impression *once.*" A good first impression can create lasting value, while a bad one can be a burdensome deficit.

It has been years since I have seen an obese politician, because those running for office understand that it is essential to give the people what they want. Society has dictated that thin is in, and those who want the rewards that society offers must look and feel their best.

I do not believe in counting calories. The dismal failure of so many weight loss programs is proof that this method alone does not work. Many dieters are not even quite sure just what a calorie really is.

"The calorie is a unit of heat (or energy). Just as inches are units of length, calories measure the amount of heat (and therefore energy) a particular food or drink will provide. Specifically, it is the amount of energy required to raise the temperature of one gram of water from zero to one degree centigrade. Multiplied by 1,000, you have a kilo-calorie or the calorie as you know it today." [1]

If counting these units worked, we wouldn't have so many books on the subject—one would be enough. True, if you limit yourself to 500 calories a day you will lose weight, but you'll be giving up one of life's greatest pleasures. We deserve to eat well, and we can enjoy ourselves at the table while losing weight.

The problem lies not in the *quantity* of the food that we eat, but in the *quality*. Today I weigh a slim 175 pounds, while a few years ago I was a chunky 200 pounds. I didn't achieve this by a deprivation diet. I enjoy eating. In fact, I eat more today than I did a few years ago. My successful weight loss program is based on a sound diet principle. Later on, I will go into detail about the one substance of my diet that I removed to achieve my desired weight.

Because of this principle, you can eat to your heart's content on this diet. I must note, though, that if you have any major health disorders and plan on losing a large amount of weight, you should first consult with your physician. Review the program with your doctor, and be sure to follow his or her advice.

While I am not a biochemist, health care is my specialty. Yet, although I am dedicated to this field, there was a time when I allowed myself to become unhealthy. I was devoted to the well-being of others, but neglected to look after my own well-being. I was not born with natural good looks or a perfectly toned body. I work hard to look and feel good, and I must say it is worth the effort.

When I tried to lose weight by calorie counting my efforts seemed to bring only frustration. This was before I understood that all calories are not created equal. Researchers Kekwick and Pawan demonstrated that while people can lose weight on a 1,000 calorie diet of protein or fat, they will not shed the pounds on a 1,000 calorie diet of carbohydrates.[2]

Other researchers have reached similar conclusions, and my own observations have led me to agree. Therefore, on this diet we will count carbohydrates rather than calories.

Carbohydrates can be divided into two groups:

1. Refined carbohydrates, which are found in foods such as processed cereal, white bread, pretzels, and potato chips.

2. Complex carbohydrates, which are found in fruits and vegetables.

Our primary concern here is with the first group. Though most of us have been told that sugar is fattening and detrimental to our health, few have learned that refined carbohydrates send the body the same message. When we eat sugar or refined carbohydrates, the body will signal the pancreas to release more insulin to process what we have consumed. The person who habitually takes in large amounts of sugar and/or carbohydrates will eventually begin to overreact, producing greater amounts of insulin. The excess insulin will lower the blood sugar, causing such symptoms as reduced energy and increased hunger. A diet that contains an overabundance of carbohydrates can always be identified by the degree of hunger it produces. More severe consequences may also result. As Dr. Sweelo points out:

"Avoidance of hypoglycemia is the key to prevention in diabetes mellitus. It is also the key to successful therapy and the management of a hypoglycemic phase. The overwhelmingly favorable probability should be made clear that adherence to therapy will arrest the downhill course of the diabetes and will forestall the future obligatory need for insulin for all hypoglycemic agents." [3]

Dealing as I did with hundreds of patients a week, I have noticed that the symptoms associated with hypoglycemia, or low blood sugar, are rampant in our society.

I recently received a call from a patient who was suffering from severe headaches. This slender, highly-athletic woman was only in her early thirties, but the frequency and intensity of the headaches caused her husband to suspect a brain tumor. Her X-rays and health history did not indicate this type of abnormality, but a discussion of her lifestyle was revealing. I referred her to an internist and friend with whom I work on a regular basis, and recommended that he administer a *glucose tolerance test*. Sure enough, she tested positive for hypoglycemia. We altered her diet and now she is headache free. This is just one of many similar case histories.

Many doctors concentrate on the hazards of sugar when treating hypoglycemia, not taking into account the damage that refined carbohydrates can create within the balance of the body.

As I noted, carbohydrates stimulate the production of insulin, which I call the "fattening hormone." Insulin promotes the storage of fuel. It also lowers blood sugar by converting it to a storage form of carbohydrate called glycogen, which is an animal starch, and into fat, which is known as triglyceride. Insulin also converts the other major fuels, the *fatty acids, and the ketone bodies into stored fat.*

"The most consistently found biochemical abnormality associated with obesity is an excessively high level of insulin. The very same high level of insulin is found in hypoglycemia. We can exist with minimal to no carbohydrates. Consuming little to no carbohydrates we activate the pituitary gland, which activates the fat mobilizing hormone, which aids in the breaking down of our body fats. This hormone is only activated when sugars and carbohydrates are not found in the body." [4]

I can practically hear your protests. "But I couldn't live on a diet that eliminated or drastically reduced carbohydrates." Not only could you live on such a diet, you might well be healthier and thinner. The key word here is not carbohydrates but *refined.*

"Drs. Cleave and Campbell have shown that in cultures where there are no *refined carbohydrates* in the diet, there is no diabetes. It is also often observed that where there is no diabetes there is virtually no obesity." [5]

I want to make it very clear that I am not the inventor of the modified or restricted carbohydrate diet. Many books can be found on this subject, including *The Air Force Diet, Dr. Carlton Frederick's Low Carbohydrate Diet, Dr. Yudkin's Diet, The Slinging Business, Strong Medicine, Carbohydrate Addicts Diet, Thin So Fast, Super Energy Diet, Diet Revolution,* and *Stillman's Diet.* What I have done is alter, refine, and ultimately perfect the low carbohydrate diet.

Reduced fat and carbohydrate intake is the primary principle of weight control. Would you like to lose weight simply by a switch? You can. I will teach you how to utilize the carbohydrate switch as a metabolic motivator. Imagine no longer being a slave to your metabolism. It's time to rule your own kingdom!

Many nutritionists believe that if your diet is low in carbohydrates then it must be high in protein. We must first be aware of the many benefits of protein and its importance to the growth of strong muscle. Recently it was found that protein given to chemotherapy patients gave them relief. Doctors at Duke University, in an article written in *USA Today,* gave injections to 19 patients with advanced cases of breast cancer, or melanoma, after they had undergone chemotherapy in bone marrow transplants. The result was the protein boosted the ability of the bone marrow to rejuvenate itself, without the effects and side-effects associated with chemotherapy. Dr. Arthur W. Nienhuis, Chief of Clinical Hematology, National Heart, Lung, and Blood Institute, says, "It could take two to five years before the protein is routinely used." The study builds on research by Jerome Groopman who utilized white blood cells in eight patients by using the same growth factor. Dr. Groopman also stated, "It may ultimately allow doctors to use higher doses of chemotherapy; thereby extending a patient's remission from cancer; a longer range goal would be to improve the cure rate in certain cancers." This alone must teach us something about the benefits of protein. Protein is vital, its healing properties unlimited.[6]

Refined carbohydrates and sugar, on the other hand, can cause health problems. Most overweight people are sugar or carbohydrate intolerant. They are not born this way. I cannot calculate the number of times I've heard, "I used to eat everything, Doc, and I was thin as a rail. Then one day the weight came on and on."

Carbohydrate/sugar intolerance is no different than alcohol or tobacco intolerance. All of these substances are addicting. Dr. John Yudkin points out, "We consume more sugar now in two weeks than we did in a year two centuries ago."[7] Just as alcohol abuse can lead to cirrhosis and tobacco abuse can lead to lung cancer, sugar and carbohydrate abuse can result in diabetes, heart disease, athrtosclerosis and obesity.

I often pondered the amazing variation among people. Why could that skinny person wash down a candy bar with a sugar-laden soft drink, while that overweight person had to subsist on diet soda and celery? I have come to believe that certain types of metabolism are more efficient at breaking down sugars and carbohydrates for longer periods of time.

This concept is known as the critical carbohydrate level, the level at which carbohydrates will begin to add weight to the individual.

The body must remain balanced at all times. This balance reflects itself in stability of our blood chemistry. Drugs have the ability to alter our blood chemistry. Non-prescribed drugs, such as cocaine, not only alter our blood chemistry but remove balance and stability. Len Bias of the University of Maryland (and for one day the Boston Celtics) is a prime example. After being the number one pick in the NBA draft, he went out and partied with his friends. Instead of being paid millions he paid the price of his life.

Sugar and refined carbohydrates, like drugs, affect our blood chemistry. Consumption of these substances causes the body to produce insulin to break them down. Over-consumption leads to over-production. This over-production eats away at our normal sugar balance, causing low blood sugar (hypoglycemia). Reducing our normal balance causes fatigue. The body now craves more sugar. Can you see how this vicious cycle begins?

Is hypoglycemia common?

"Dr. Georgina Fauludi and her associates in performing glucose tolerance tests on 238 obese patients in Hahnenann Hospital in Philadelphia diagnosed hypoglycemia in 101 patients or 42%, and when United Airlines tested 177 pilots, 44 had it, that is 25% or 1 out of every 4." [8]

A survey conducted by the U.S. Department of Health, Education and Welfare, *Published Data 1966-67 National Health*, indicated that some 66,000 of the approximately 134,000 people surveyed reported having hypoglycemia. This works out to almost 50%. I don't think it's an exaggeration to say that we have an epidemic of this condition on our hands.

Many respected physicians have noted that hypoglycemia is extremely common in this country. The list of authorities includes Dr. Sam Roberts, Dr. J. Frank Hurdle, Dr. John Yudkin, Dr. Carlton Fredericks, Dr. E.M. Abrahamson, and Dr. Robert Atkins.

"Exhaustion caused in treatment of hypoglycemia is probably the most common disease in the United States. I would at least estimate 50% of the work in this country is done by people who are extremely tired or exhausted and don't know it. Often they do not mention fatigue or exhaustion as a chief complaint—they have accepted it as a part of life."[9]

"Accepted it as a part of life." It's unfortunate that so many people are willing to consider mediocre or downright poor health part of the natural order of things. Compromise is fine in certain situations, but you should never compromise when it comes to your health, or you'll wind up like the hunter in the following story.

A hunter and a bear met in the woods. The frightened hunter said, "I don't want to kill you, I don't even know why I'm here. How about we make a compromise?"

A compromise was made.

The hunter ended up with a new fur coat.

The bear ended up with a *full belly*.

Carbohydrate consumption increased approximately 7,000 years ago when people first learned to till the soil. But even at this point in time these carbohydrates were still unrefined. There are different groups of carbohydrates. I am not talking about the whole grains and the whole rices that are not refined. These can be eaten in moderation. It is only through greed and economics that man began to refine carbohydrates. It has primarily been over the past century that man's diet consists primarily of sugars and carbohydrates through knowledge, education, and refining of technology. Sugar dates back to a time when it was only able to be purchased by the rich.

Diseases that were associated with sugar were primarily diseases that were seen among the rich. Sugar alone is an empty calorie, sugar in its original state comes from the cane and has some vitamins and nutrients within it. In the refining process of sugar, bread, or rice, the nutrients are now removed. I ask you—why buy cereal or bread that is vitamin-enriched? When I read the words on the label stating vitamin-enriched, it instantly educates and alerts me to the fact that this product has been refined, they have removed all the nutritional value of this product, otherwise, why enrich it? Therefore, through the great media of advertising, they must now educate us to a purpose for purchasing their product. They simply try to make us believe that it is better for us than it really is.

If the food industry promotes confusion, the diet industry has created chaos. One diet calls for you to eat only fruits and vegetables. Another is high in protein. Yet another will keep you so busy adding and subtracting food groups that it's a wonder you have time to eat. I needed a diet I could live with, so I developed one myself.

Have your blood and blood pressure checked before you go on this diet. When you have been on the diet for two months, have it checked again. If you were having a problem with hypertension, your blood pressure will almost certainly be lower on the second test. You can also anticipate improvements in your blood sugar, cholesterol, triglycerides and uric acids levels.

On my diet we will not starve ourselves; we will not count calories. We will eat, and we will eat enjoyable foods. Calorie-counting alone is a myth that has been published from diet book to diet book, from nutritional author to nutritional author. If it was easy to count calories the world would be thin. We will avoid sugars, and monitor our intake of fats and refined carbohydrates. We will not only eat to win, we will eat to be thin.

Results! Why man, I have gotten a lot of results. I know several thousand things that won't work.

Thomas Edison

6

Health's Gate

I want to commend you for reaching a milestone. The fact that you have come this far in your journey indicates that you have affirmed your commitment to your physical and emotional well-being. Health's Gate is your entry to a source of vitality that is just waiting to be tapped.

In order to gain the benefits that are available to you, you must learn and apply the rules of nutritional medicine. This is a science that aids in the treatment and prevention of illness through sound nutritional techniques rather than with drugs. You would expect this science to be high on the curriculum of every medical school, but the opposite is the case.

Dr. Alfred D. Klinger, of Department of Preventive Medicine at Rush Medical College in Chicago says, "Malnutrition in this country is responsible in large degrees for many of our present-day illnesses." He says,

"There is little or no teaching or even interest in nutrition in most medical schools. There are those in high circles of medicine who are agape at such a thing as malnutrition in the U.S. As a consequence, few doctors know about nutrition. Today, by public demand, doctors are forced to learn about nutrition. Pharmaceutical companies expound on the benefits of supplement. Often times, the consumer is more educated on supplement than their physicians. If you take interest in dietary history or understand how to prescribe a proper one or correct one they believe that is improper. Yet nutrition is the cornerstone of life. Its proper application sustains body and mind."

"Dr. Willis A. Gortner, former Professor of Biochemistry at Cornell University and Director of United States Department of Agricultures Human Nutrition

Division in Maryland said at a Science Lab Seminar, 'We can tell the farmer more about feeding his livestock than about feeding his family.' Dr. Gortner went on and stated, 'Many times patients go to a physician with symptoms and that these patients are told that they are not really sick but that they have an imaginary sickness.'" Dr. Gortner stated, "The real problem is just the opposite. Many of us have imaginary health. We think we are well when we are not because we have never really known what it feels like to be super healthy. We suffer from nutritional deficiencies that we don't even know about. We think the way we feel is natural, or that we are just getting older and it isn't true.' Dr. Gortner calls nutrition 'Internal Environmental Protection.'" [1]

One of the most important forms of "internal environmental protection" I know of are vitamins. There are physicians who scoff at the idea of vitamin therapy, which is difficult to understand in view of the evidence to the contrary. As Dr. Fredrick Hopkins and Dr. W.H. Wilson of St. Mary's Hospital in London said,

"The proof that deficiency diseases, when occurring amongst men on a ration scale deficient in necessary vitamins, can be prevented by the addition of articles containing these vitamins must be regarded as definitely established. The history of epidemics of scurvy and beriberi during the war affords conclusive evidence." [2]

Doctors have known about vitamin deficiency diseases for some time. One example is scurvy, which is caused by a lack of vitamin C. Not surprisingly, the cure for scurvy is the addition of this vitamin to the diet.

Vitamins are also utilized in the treatment of other diseases, including mental illnesses. Dr. A. Hauffer noted, "Patients are also advised to follow a good nutritional program with restriction of sucrose and sucrose-rich foods. This is found in megavitamin therapy utilizing B3 for schizophrenia." [3]

Notice that while vitamins are recommended, sucrose, one of the many names for sugar, is most emphatically not. Of all the substances that we can put into our bodies, sugar is one of the most harmful, and certainly one of the most fattening. And sugar's twin, refined carbohydrate, is not much better. Have you ever been in a hospital that has offered you vitamins to aid you in your healing? No, but they will give you artificially colored sugar (jello) for dessert. Here lies society's sickest people; we should be building them up, not sugaring them down. Even if they didn't want to accept the many benefits of vitamins, how can they reject the health warnings against sugar?

I remember how enthused I was when I read a book which advocated a high carbohydrate diet. Eat bread, eat pasta, get thin. Get real! I followed the diet with gusto, consuming all the bread and pasta I desired. My reward was a new wardrobe. I had to buy *larger* clothes.

My diet incorporates many proven nutritional principles. On my program, the individual develops an eating plan appropriate for his or her own metabolism. My clinical experience has proven to me that not only do most overweight people have a diet high in sugar, fat and carbohydrates but they suffer from carbohydrate intolerance. Quite simply, they are allergic to sugar and carbohydrates.

Many of the carbohydrates we consume are derived from vegetables rather than animal proteins. It is true that carbohydrates supply a large proportion of the metabolic fuel in the Western diet. This fuel is readily delivered because carbohydrates will break down to form glucose. But since the body has mechanisms that can produce glucose, or similar fuels that perform basically the same functions, refined carbohydrate is one nutrient that need not always be provided by the diet.

"The nonessentiality of carbohydrate is one of the biological principles that make these carbohydrate restrictive diets feasible, safe, and effective."[4]

Later, I will discuss in greater detail the difference between nutrient (complex) and non-nutrient (refined) carbohydrates. These are further broken down into acceptable and nonacceptable carbohydrates.

While the body may not require carbohydrates, it has a definite need for protein. Proteins are nitrogen-containing fuels, the principle function of which is to supply the essential building to the vital organs, muscle tissue and chemicals of the body. Proteins are basically groups of amino acids, some of which the body can manufacture on its own, and which are called nonessential amino acids. Others, which can be derived only from dietary sources, are known as essential amino acids. A diet that enables you to lose weight without hunger must be high in these essential amino acids.

Fats also have a place in this diet, for they are the major storage form of metabolic fuel. Triglycerides are a '90s buzz word, but they are important storage fats which provide two major metabolic fuels: free fatty acids and ketone bodies. These substances, when broken down and liberated, provide energy. It is my belief, and the belief of other experts in the field, that *some* fats must be provided by the diet. These are known as essential fatty acids, which cannot be manufactured or properly manufactured by the body.

Today the experts have all jumped on the low-fat diet bandwagon. However, they allow an abundance of sugars and carbohydrates. This diet will create internal havoc. As it chemically depletes your willpower, you will again find yourself overweight, frustrated and defeated.

The diet I have developed is moderate in protein, high in water, includes the proper amounts of vitamins and minerals, allows fat in moderation, and restricts refined carbohydrates and sugar.

Too many people that I see suffer from fatigue, irritability, low energy, depression, headaches, insomnia, and overall malaise. Many of these symptoms are associated with a dietary excess of sugar and/or refined carbohydrates.

When I was a child, my breakfast consisted of milk and a doughnut, Cheerios, or sugar Frosted Flakes. For lunch I might have a bologna sandwich with potato chips and Coca-Cola. Dinner was some variation of hamburgers on white buns, potatoes, frozen vegetables and, of course, dessert. Some type of sweet snack was devoured later in the evening.

Given this sugar- and carbohydrate-laden diet, it's hardly surprising that I had developed rampant acne by adolescence. I went to a dermatologist, who told me cut out chocolate and prescribed huge doses of tetracycline. My face not only worsened, but I developed stomach problems from taking antibiotics for a year. Today, antibiotics are not solely used in the treatment of acne.

Of course, the "drug" that caused my problems in the first place was sugar. Today, when we talk about a white plague sweeping over our country, we are referring to cocaine. But years ago, sugar was *the* white powder. In fact, physicians carefully added minuscule amounts of refined sugar to their prescriptions.

Maybe we don't consider sugar a drug today, but it's certainly not a nutrient. In *Body, Mind and Sugar,* Dr. E.M. Abrahamson and A.W.

Pezet note that, "A condition which blood sugar level is relatively low tends to starve the body cells, especially the brain cells."[5]

The energy that is derived from sugar is illusory, for while sugar will initially raise the blood sugar, it will ultimately level it out. Abrahamson and Pezet provide an excellent overview of how sugar reacts in the human body.

"We must understand that when all is working well the body must maintain a balance. This is maintained with fine precision under the supervision of our adrenal glands. When we consume refined sugar (sucrose), it is the next thing to being glucose, consequently it largely escapes chemical processing in our bodies. The sucrose passes directly to the intestines where it becomes predigested 'glucose.' This in turn is absorbed into the blood where the glucose level has already been established in precise balance with oxygen. The glucose level in the blood is thus drastically increased. Balance is destroyed. The body is in crisis.

"The brain registers it first, then hormones pour from the adrenal casings and marshal every chemical resource for dealing with sugar. Insulin from the endocrine 'islets' of the pancreas works specifically to hold down the glucose level in the blood, in complimentary antagonism to the adrenal hormones concerned with keeping the glucose level up. All this moves at emergency pace with predictable results. Going too fast it goes too far. The bottom drops out of blood glucose level and a second crisis comes out of the first. Pancreatic islets have to shut down; so do some departments of the adrenal casings. Other adrenal hormones must be produced to regulate the reversing of the chemical direction and bring the blood glucose up again. All this is reflected in how we feel. While the glucose is being absorbed into the blood we feel a quick pick-me-up. This pick-me-up is a surge of mortgaged energy. It is succeeded by the downs, when the bottom drops out of the blood glucose level. We become listless and tired; it requires effort to move or think until the blood glucose level is brought up again. At this point in time our poor brain is vulnerable to suspicion, hallucinations, irritability, nervousness and restlessness. The severity of the crisis on top of crisis depends on the quantity of glucose overload. If we continue taking sugar, a new double crisis is always beginning before the old one begins. This continues till we damage our adrenal glands. Thus making stress impossible to cope with."[6]

A very common disorder in our culture is diabetes, a condition in which the pancreas is no longer capable of producing insulin. There is no cure for diabetes. The person with this disease becomes dependent on the drug insulin. He or she must regulate it, may overdose from it, and is never free of it. And the association between sugar and diabetes is well-documented.

"Sir Frederick Banting, who was the co-discoverer of insulin, noticed in 1929 in Panama that, in sugar plantation owners who ate large amounts of their refined sugar, diabetes was common. He also states that, among native cane cutters who only got to chew the raw cane (not in its refined state), he saw no diabetes."[7]

The link between diabetes and sugar is not surprising, for sugar is known to upset the delicate balance of the body.

"Studies have shown sugar consumed on a daily basis produces a continuous highly acidic condition. The body in its effort to balance (to put out the fire so to speak) sends more and more minerals to rectify this imbalance. As this process continues, the body steals calcium from the bones and teeth, it does this to protect the blood. This causes bone and tooth weakening and decay. Hence a general weakening has begun."[8]

I have effectively applied the principle of reducing excess acid via diet with my ulcer patients. Ms. M is a case in point. Ms. M worked for me, and happened to mention that she was taking three or four Tagamint tablets a day for her stomach problems. After a month on my program, she was off the medication. (Of course, you must consult with your physician before discontinuing any medication.) We not only eliminated the symptoms, we treated the cause by removing sugar from her diet.

In our society, we've lost touch with our bodies that we use a substance like sugar as a reward. I'm not surprised that substance abuse is so prevalent in our culture; we simply graduate from one drug to another. The little boy who knows that, "If you are good, you can have a cookie," will learn to reward himself when he becomes a big boy. "I worked hard today—I deserve a drink." I've yet to see a candy bar wrapper that reads, "This substance may be hazardous to your health," yet there is overwhelming evidence that such a warning would be entirely appropriate.

According to Alexander G. Schauss of Washington State University, children consume on average about 274 pounds of sweeteners per year. According to the National Eating Trends Report, the average American consumes 200 snack foods per year. Not yet convinced? Consider the following:

> ➢ 3.9 billion dollars are spent annually on packaged store-bought cookies.
> ➢ Over 100 million M&M's are produced each day.
> ➢ More than 8 billion dollars worth of potato chips, pretzels, corn chips and tortilla chips are consumed annually.

Snack foods are not just high in sugars and refined carbohydrates, but fat as well. These three form a triumvirate of power. A power that destroys our will power, saps our strength, and leads us down the path to obesity and disease.

"Excess sugar eventually affects every organ in the body. Initially it is stored in the liver in the form of glucose (glycogen). Since the liver's capacity is limited, a daily intake of refined sugar (above the required amount of natural sugar) soon makes the liver expand like a balloon. When the liver is filled to its maximum capacity the excess glycogen is returned to the blood in the form of fatty acids. These are taken to every part of the body and stored in the most inactive areas, the belly, the buttocks, the breasts, and the thighs. When these comparatively harmless places are filled fatty acids are then distributed among active organs such as the heart and kidneys. These begin to slow down, finally their tissues degenerate and turn to fat. The whole body is affected by their reduced ability and an abnormal blood sugar is created. Refined sugar lacks natural minerals (which are, however, in the sugar beet or cane). Our parasympathetic nervous system is affected; and organs governed by it, such as the small brain, become inactive or paralyzed. (Normal brain function is rarely thought of as being as biological as digestion.) The circulatory and lymphatic systems are inundated and the quality of red corpuscles start to change. An over abundance of white cells occurs and the creation of tissues become slower."[9]

We want not only to lose weight, but to lose weight in certain areas: the belly, thighs, and buttocks are the main targets of most dieters. As the preceding passage indicates, excess sugar is not only stored as fat, it is stored in the most conspicuous places. It makes sense to conclude that if "sugar bringeth," the absence of sugar "taketh away."

Now, before you panic, let me reassure you that you don't have to give up sweets "cold turkey." While I am not an advocate of artificial sweeteners, I am a realist. If you are a sugarholic, then these sugar substitutes can help you to satisfy the craving until you overcome it. While artificial sweeteners are not a permanent solution, they are at least nonaddicting. Sugar, by lowering your blood sugar, makes you want more sugar. Sugar substitutes do not have this effect, and will not put you on a blood sugar roller coaster. It seems obvious that if diabetics can safely eat these sweeteners, so can a person with a sugar or carbohydrate intolerance. This book includes sweet but sugarless alternatives to help you resist the temptation to stray from the highway to health. But do keep in mind that artificial sweeteners are not 100% healthy, they're simply the lesser of two evils.

When you reduce fats, and remove sugar and carbohydrates from your diet, you are giving up a great deal, including an increased risk of: heart disease, high blood pressure, ulcers, colon diseases, allergies, alcoholism, diabetes, migraine headaches, Meniere's syndrome, schizophrenia, and other mental illnesses. And don't forget the fascinating symptoms of hypoglycemia, or low blood sugar that will disappear from your life: anxiety, fatigue, light-headedness, depression, weakness, tremors, tachycardia (rapid heartbeat), continual hunger, blurred vision, confusion, phobias, convulsions, mood swings, outbursts of temper, forgetfulness, inability to concentrate, inability to work under pressure, indecision, crying spells, prolonged sleepiness, difficulty sleeping, cramping, muscle pains, indigestion, ulcers, heartburn, and hiatial hernia. And this isn't even a complete list.

The other thing you're giving up is excess weight. I must note, however, that this is not a "quick-loss" diet. I have found that such programs tend to be followed by a "quick-gain." I have found throughout the course of my years in practice that overweight people are not healthy people. Fat to a doctor is an indication of a lack of health. When looking in the mirror, if you see yourself as being overweight, I am sure you're suffering with numerous symptoms. These symptoms are probably associated with your weight problem. It is neither normal nor acceptable to be overweight, and this overweight leads to physical and psychological problems.

Losing weight, like gaining weight, takes time. Sickness and disease don't just happen, they accumulate. The same is true of excess pounds. We cannot expect a lifetime of neglect to disintegrate by utilizing two weeks of discipline. I've had many conversations with patients that sound very much like the following:

Esther (patient): "Dr. Kaplan, in the last two weeks I have only
lost 10 pounds."

Dr. Kaplan: "How do you feel?"

Esther: "I feel good."

Dr. Kaplan: "How is your energy?"

Esther: "My energy is great."

Dr. Kaplan: "So what is the problem?"

Esther "I thought that I would have lost more weight
by now."

Losing weight, like gaining weight, takes time. On this diet, I ask you
to be patient and be prepared to lose the pounds s-l-o-w-l-y. I firmly believe
that rapid weight loss is unhealthy. The rapid loss that commonly occurs
in the initial phases of a diet is water weight. Approximately 75 percent of
the body is comprised of fluids. So there's no magic in losing water. When
I was in college, I knew of many wrestlers who wore rubber suits in the
steam room prior to weigh-in so that they could make their weight for
the match. Of course, after the weigh-in they rehydrated themselves so
that their strength would be up to tournament caliber.

My diet will work for you if you follow the Seven Principles. I've
capitalized them because, although they are simple, they are absolutely
essential.

1. You will drink plenty of water. As I will explain shortly,
   water is probably the single most important factor in both
   losing weight and keeping it off.

2. You will eliminate sugar from your diet.

3. You will eliminate refined carbohydrates from your diet.

4. You modify your fat intake.

5. You will take the proper amounts of appropriate vitamins and
   supplements.

6. You will maintain a positive attitude.

7. It is recommended that you consult your physician before
   commencing on any weight-loss routine.

You must apply these principles in order for the diet to work. You will know that the diet is working when you are losing weight and not feeling hungry. If you are hungry, excess sugar and/or carbohydrates have crept into your diet, for these substances increase your appetite.

You may not feel that you are eating excess carbohydrates, but see if the diet on the following page looks familiar to you.

BREAKFAST	CARBOHYDRATE CONTENT IN GRAMS	
6 oz. Orange Juice	19.0	grams
1 cup Cornflakes	24.7	grams
1 cup Skim Milk	13.4	grams
1 tbsp. Sugar	1.0	grams
1 cup Coffee		trace
COFFEE BREAK		
1 cup Fruit Yogurt	26.0	grams
LUNCH		
4 oz. Hamburger	0.0	grams
on a bun	20.7	grams
3 tbsp. Catsup	13.5	grams
1/2 cup Coleslaw	8.1	grams
12 oz. Diet Pepsi	18.0	grams
2 oz. Gin	0.0	grams
8 oz. glass Tonic	18.4	grams
10 Potato Chips	10.0	grams
DINNER		
1 cup Tomato Soup	15.7	grams
6 oz. Steak	0.0	grams
Baked Potato	20.8	grams
3/4 cup Peas	17.1	grams
1/2 Honeydew Melon	11.0	grams
BEDTIME SNACKS		
1 glass Skim Milk	13.4	grams
1 small Banana	21.1	grams
TOTAL (approx.)	**271.9**	**grams**

There are some experts who believe that people can maintain a reasonable weight on 60 grams of carbohydrate per day. How does that compare with the diet printed here? I believe that the critical carbohydrate level is in the range of 40–60 grams, and that when we consume more than that we experience hunger. Each person is unique, however, so you need to establish your own critical level through experimentation and ketostix.

The diet we just reviewed isn't all that high in calories, but it is loaded with carbohydrates. It is also rather high in caffeine, which can alter the metabolism by triggering the production of insulin. When the body produces insulin, it does not activate the pituitary gland, which is responsible for activating the fat mobilizing hormone. So even diet beverages should be avoided if they contain caffeine. Besides, some diet sodas contain up to 9 grams of carbohydrate per 16 ounce serving. Read the labels carefully.

Now take a look at the diet of this person, who is highly disciplined, sticks to the diet, yet can't lose weight.

	CARBOHYDRATE	
BREAKFAST	**CONTENTS IN GRAMS**	
1 6 oz. glass Orange juice	19.0	grams
1 cup Cornflakes—no sugar	24.7	grams
1 cup Coffee		trace
COFFEE BREAK		
1 Apple	20.5	grams
1 cup Coffee		trace
LUNCH		
4 oz. Hamburger—no bun	0.0	grams
3 tbsp. Catsup	13.5	grams
1 12 oz. Diet Soda	9.0	grams
SNACK		
1 Banana	21.1	grams
DINNER		
1 cup Pea soup	22.0	grams
6 oz. Steak	0.0	grams
1 Diet soda	9.0	grams
DESSERT		
1 cup Strawberries	12.0	grams
TOTAL (approx.)	**150.8**	**grams**

Here is an example of the "perfect dieter," someone who ate small portions, suppressed their appetite, and probably suffered from increased anxiety as a result of this rigid program. Yet this person went approximately 120 grams over the critical carbohydrate level. No wonder people can't lose weight; no wonder they get frustrated and give up.

Now let's create a diet that we can follow on a modified-carbohydrate regimen. Utilizing Dr. Kaplan's High Energy Modified Carbohydrate Diet, imagine the following:

Breakfast: Turkey bacon and eggs, or possibly a cheese omelet with broccoli and turkey bacon, and a cup of decaffeinated coffee.

Coffee Break: A cup of decaffeinated coffee and three ounces of cheese: American, cheddar, blue, brick, caraway, chantelle, colby, edam, gruyere, liederkranz, Monterey jack, muenster, or Roquefort (low-fat preferable).

Lunch: A cheeseburger (no bun) with some lettuce and a caffeine-free Diet Coke.

Afternoon Snack: One cup of fresh strawberries.

Before Dinner: A drink. (Not recommended on any diet plan, but here to create curiosity.) Two ounces of vodka (optional).

Dinner: Fish (6-8 ounces), and a half-cup of broccoli with melted cheese.

Dessert: A cup of herbal tea, some dietetic gelatin, and maybe a tablespoon of Cool Whip, just to be decadent.

Let's review the carbohydrate count of this "diet":

BREAKFAST	CARBOHYDRATE CONTENT IN GRAMS	
2 Eggs	8.0	grams
2 Strips turkey bacon or sausage	0.0	grams
Decaffeinated coffee	trace	
COFFEE BREAK		
3 oz. cheese (low-fat)	3.0	grams
Decaffeinated coffee	trace	
LUNCH		
Cheeseburger (no bun) Burger	0.0	grams
Cheese (low-fat)	3.0	grams

1 cup Lettuce	2.0	grams
Decaffeinated diet soda	1.0	gram

SNACK

1 cup Fresh strawberries	12.0	grams

DINNER

2 oz. Vodka		trace
6 oz. Chicken or fish	0.0	grams
1/2 cup Broccoli	4.0	grams
1 oz. Cheese (low fat)	1.0	gram
1/2 cup Cauliflower	2.0	grams
Diet gelatin	0.0	grams
1 tbsp. Cool Whip	1.0	gram
TOTAL (approx.)	**37.0**	**grams**

Although this sample menu may appear high in fat, you will lose weight following this low-carbohydrate principle. Realizing that losing weight is a reduction in fat, how is this possible? You must understand that fats alone are not the cause of obesity. The body needs and consists of fats, not carbohydrates. Our top athletes have numbers reflecting 6% body fat, never 0%. Educatedly we can use fats for flavor only, not store them on our appearance. When you combine fat with carbohydrates, the fat you consume stays in. When you void your diet of sugar and refined carbohydrates your body will use the incoming fat (and stored fat if needed) for energy. Thus, "Fat In, Fat Out."

Next day, the boss may be buying you lunch on his expense account. Why not order the lobster with drawn butter? It's more expensive than the hamburger lunch, but it's cheaper in carbohydrates. Four ounces of lobster has only .4 grams of carbohydrate, and one teaspoon of butter is just .1 gram. So by going with the lobster rather than the hamburger, you've subtracted almost 4 1/2 grams of carbohydrate from lunch. Are we having fun yet?

Now it's time for dinner. How about a crab appetizer (4 ounces = 1 gram), followed by four ounces of lamb (0 grams) and cabbage? If you get hungry later on, have a couple of teaspoons of peanut butter (3 grams). If you want to vary your snack, have a cup of popcorn with a teaspoon of butter (8.1 grams) instead of the strawberries.

After all, strawberries do contain a fruit sugar known as fructose. On my diet, even fruit is eaten in moderation while dieting. While fructose is not as harmful as refined sugar, it is still a sugar and must be broken down accordingly. Fruits should not be eaten with other foods, or consumed after 6:00 p.m. When you are inactive (as most people are in the evening), your body cannot break down sugars as it can during the day, when you are expending energy. Remember, if energy is not used, it is stored—as fat.

This sample menu is abundant in fat, yet because it is void of carbohydrates the body will not store this fat, it will break it down. A diet lower in fat will bring quicker results. The point here is that a high-carbohydrate, low-fat diet is not perfect. A low-carbohydrate, high-fat diet is not the answer either. A modified diet limiting fat and restricting refined carbohydrates is more the solution. It is the answer to "thinning and winning."

If you must have coffee with caffeine, limit yourself to no more that two cups per day. You may have as much decaffeinated coffee and herbal tea (my preference) as you desire. Of course, the most important beverage on this diet is water, the magic elixir, which I will discuss in greater detail later in the book.

Understand, that the more natural we can keep this diet, the more beneficial it will be. In the back of this text is a *Food Chart*, which lists the carbohydrate content of most foods. Use this chart, and it will save you pounds.

To arrive at any destination you must expend energy. "Health's Gate" is your privilege, your opportunity; to get there you must expend energy, make changes. Upon your arrival you will open the gates to a world of harmony and health. A world where you are in control. "Health's Gate" is within the grasp of each and every one of us. To enter it just takes commitment; reach out, reach out and be touched by someone.

If you have a scary weakness, make it work for you as a strength—and if you have a strength, don't abuse it into a weakness.

Dore Schary

7

Sugar City Revisited

You've undoubtedly visited Sugar City many times; this chapter is an opportunity to revisit it with some health experts as your guides. Sugar City is perhaps best compared to a movie set. While the facade may seem appealing and inviting, the inside is hollow and lifeless. Stay there long enough, and you may feel like a prisoner, but be assured that there is a way out.

I expected giving up sugar to be the hardest part of my personal weight loss program, but it was the easiest. I don't even miss it—and I was a sugarholic! Furthermore, I eat more food now than I did 25 pounds ago.

Sugar is addicting, habit forming, and mood altering. It is as detrimental as fat. Fat free doesn't mean sugar-free. Marla Maples has done a wonderful job of keeping her daughter, Tiffany, away from sugar. As a result, she is polite, alert, and attentive. ADD has often been treated by removing sugar and dairy products from a child's diet. The best way to drop a habit is not to hold onto it.

Sugar is a paradoxical substance: it will fatten you without nourishing you and fool you into thinking that it infuses energy when it actually drains vitality. In fact, there is evidence that sugar may be worse than no food at all. Sugar is addicting! There is no way around it. It is the most lethal substance consumed in America today. The average American consumes 130 lbs annually which amounts to 30-33 teaspoons a day. People can fast for extended periods of time without ill effects, especially if they have water. Note what happens, though, when sugar is the mainstay of a diet:

"In the course of centuries millions of tons of sugar were transported across the seas. We would make reason to believe that through its transference that these tons of sugar had eventually a vessel carrying this white treasure would become shipwrecked. One such vessel carrying this white sugar was shipwrecked in 1793. On the ship there were five surviving sailors. These sailors were marooned for nine days before being rescued, their station of health was that they were found to be in a wasted condition due to *starvation*. They subsisted by eating nothing but sugar and drinking rum."[1]

Yet another instance of sugar-induced death was recorded in 1816 by the eminent French psychologist F. Magendie. He conducted a series of experiments in which dogs were fed a diet of sugar or olive oil and water. All of the animals wasted and died, leaving Dr. Magendie to conclude that it is not possible to subsist on a diet of sugar.

Both the shipwrecked sailors and Dr. Megendie's experiment proved a point: a steady diet of sugar is more damaging than nothing at all.

Now let's consider three cases of fasting without sugar:

1. There is on record the saga of a young girl seriously injured in a plane accident who kept alive for well over a month on nothing but melted snow.

2. Two men afloat in an overturned sailboat in the Pacific survived for 72 days in the summer of 1973 with nothing but a cup of rainwater every five days, a cup of salt water, a tablespoon of peanut butter a day, and a few sardines.

3. In late 1970, a nine-year-old boy ran away from home and kept alive for ten days in the Wyoming wilderness without food, and temperatures that dropped occasionally to 40 degrees. At the end he was in remarkably good condition.[2]

You've probably heard that sugar contains only "empty" calories. I'm more inclined to say that it contains "lethal" calories. Sugar depletes the body of precious vitamins and minerals via its demands on digestion and detoxification. In my health care class, we refer to the three whites—white sugar, flour, and salt—as "white death."

One of the conditions of good health is balance. Our bodies will strive to maintain this state, and when we overload ourselves with sugar, the body will attempt to compensate.

"Sugar taken every day produces a continuously over acid condition, and more and more minerals are required deep in the body in the attempt to rectify the imbalance. Finally, in order to protect the blood, so much calcium is taken from the bones and teeth that decay and general weakening begin. Excess sugar eventually affects every organ in the body." [3]

In our affluent society, virtually everyone can afford to overindulge in sugar. This was not always the case; when refined sugar was brought from Asia to Europe by the Crusaders, it was a vice that only the rich could afford.

"It is known that Columbus brought sugarcane to the West Indies in 1493. But white sugar didn't become important before the 19th century, when Napoleon set up sugar factories in Europe. In 1850, total world sugar production was about 1.5 million tons per year. Today the world sugar production is 70 million tons, and still growing. We consume not 10 pounds a year, but 120 pounds per person." [4]

Today, every socioeconomic group can afford to abuse sugar, but it's not making our lives any sweeter. Sugar intake has been associated not only with obesity, but with high blood pressure, diabetes, coronary thrombosis, gall stones, peptic ulcer, diverticulosis, varicose veins, hemorrhoids, *E. coli* infections, dental cavities, colon cancer, hiatal hernia, gout, and elevated cholesterol levels.

This last condition is of special interest today, when so many people assume that fat is the major cholesterol culprit. Numerous studies, however, point to sugar as the real villain. Dr. Atkins reported on several studies in which cholesterol levels increased with sugar consumption, even when the intake of saturated fats was reduced. One of the many examples of this phenomenon occurred in Poland, where in only a single generation the heart attack and death rates increased alarmingly. Yet during this time, the intake of saturated fats decreased by 22 percent; sugar intake, on the other hand, increased by 366 percent. *Both the sugar intake and the death rate quadrupled.*

Other studies also link sugar with elevated cholesterol and triglycerides.

> ➤ Drs. Alfredo Lopez, Robert E. Hodges and Willard A. Krehl of the University of Iowa College of Medicine did similar studies. They compared serum cholesterol levels with diets of sixteen different countries. The results may surprise you. They found no correlation between fat in the diet and cholesterol in the blood. What they did find was a significant correlation with the amount of sugar in the diet.[5]

> ➤ In 1924, Dr. A.A. Gigon showed through his experiments that adding large quantities of sugar to an otherwise good diet causes sickness and death to a variety of animals.[6]

An increasing number of Americans are afflicted with heart disease. We know that high cholesterol levels and high blood pressure are two of the greatest risk factors for this condition. Yet most people are not aware that a diet high in sugar is related to these risk factors.

Dr. Richard Allens of the University of Maryland stated that he found that sugar caused high blood pressure in animals. And when we tested human subjects we found that all of them have high blood pressure and they ate large amounts of sugar. From Dr. Allens' data, it appears that 25% of people are particularly sugar sensitive, recording dangerously high levels of blood pressure.[7]

Although the public is primarily concerned about the effects of dietary fat, research on the harmful effects of sugar is abundant.

Dr. John Yudkin, internationally recognized nutritionist, Queen Elizabeth College in London, calls sugar, "pure, white and deadly."[8]

> ➤ Dr. Richard Allan says, "All the most carefully designed studies have consistently shown that heart disease victims consume more sucrose," and he adds, "that the epidemic of arterial sclerotic and degenerative heart disease continues to increase on a worldwide scale in direct proportion to the increased sucrose consumption."[9]

> ➤ In the 1930s a research dentist from Cleveland, Ohio, Dr. Weston A. Price, traveled all over the world—from the land of the Eskimos to the south sea islands, from Africa to New Zealand. His book, *Nutrition and Physical Generation:* a comparison of primitive and modern diets and their effects, which is all stated with hundreds of photographs, was first published in 1939.

"The work of Dr. Price took the whole world as his laboratory. His conclusion was devastating. He recorded in horrifying detail from country to country, area to area, that the people who lived under what we considered primitive condition have excellent teeth and wonderful general health.

"Their diet consists of natural unrefined foods from their own locale. As soon as refined sugared foods were imported as a result of contact with 'civilization' physical degeneration began in a way that was observable within a single generation."[10]

Many of my patients virtuously assure me that saturated fats rarely pass their lips, but that they "need" sugar for energy.

Energy? From sugar?

A diet high in sugar will make you tired, disoriented, moody, cranky and lethargic. (These are also the symptoms of hypoglycemia, or low blood sugar, but you don't have to suffer from this condition to experience the wretched effects of a blood sugar drop.) It may provide a temporary boost, but the pancreas will respond to a sugar overload with an overproduction of insulin, which lowers our blood sugar, at which point we experience a drop in energy and other hypoglycemic symptoms.

You may be tempted to relieve the discomfort with another hit of the substance that caused the symptoms in the first place, but let me tell you a cautionary tale. A man set out on a journey, taking with him only two parcels. In the first, he told a friend, was a bottle of whiskey, to be used only in case of snakebite. "What's in the second bag?" inquired his friend. "That's the snake," he replied.

When you experience the symptoms of sugar withdrawal, don't use sugar to "remedy" the problem. Give your blood sugar a natural lift with a piece of turkey, cheese, or some nuts; don't artificially "boost" it with a sweet snack. Sugar will only put you on a roller coaster of poor health. Protein will stabilize your blood sugar.

We have turned into a nation of sugar addicts—we've been taught to enjoy the stuff. And unfortunately, we're teaching our children the same unhealthy lesson. Let's consider the diet of a hypothetical little boy named Mikie. He begins his day with a bowl of sugar-coated cereal (the manufacturer has thoughtfully added the sugar, so he doesn't have to bother); his 10 o'clock snack consists of a cookie; for lunch Mikie has a peanut butter and jelly sandwich on white bread, followed by a cupcake; when he arrives home, he is rewarded for being a good boy with a doughnut from the corner bakery; Mikie's dinner tonight is spaghetti and meatballs with garlic bread, washed down with some soda. And when you're not looking, he may sneak a few Fig Newtons up to his room. It's no wonder that Mikie is ready to fall asleep in class and has energy for nothing but television when he comes home.

Mikie is a figment of my imagination, but his diet is all too real, and so are the problems that it can cause, problems that may include reduced growth rate and hyperactivity. Author Marilyn Diamond, of *Fit For Life*[11] fame reported the findings of Dr. William G. Crook, a pediatrician and allergist at the Children's Clinic in Jackson who said:

"hyperactivity was related to food allergy in about three fourths of the cases in a study of more than 100 children who were overactive. Dr. Crook observed (that) . . . children can be helped by using elimination diets to identify offending foods. He identified *milk* and *refined cane sugar* as *the leading culprits* in a list that also included corn, wheat, eggs, soy, citrus, and other items."[12]

In my home, sugar is not allowed. As a parent, I'm a realist, and I know that my children will occasionally consume sugar when they're out. The key word here is *occasionally;* addiction is a result of constant overindulgence, not moderate sampling. My kids consider sugar a treat, not a staple. Many companies now offer cookies and yogurt sweetened with fructose (fruit sugar). Though still a sugar it is much easier to metabolize than sucrose (white refine sugar).

As a parent, I also have the responsibility of setting an example, so it was especially important that I cure my own sugar addiction. In my case, the proof of the (sugar-free) pudding was in the eating. I lost 38 pounds while dining on steak and scampi. My cholesterol dropped 60 points, and my elevated triglycerides returned to the low average range. I was so pleased at how much better I looked and felt that I didn't even miss sugar and refined carbohydrates.

I admit to cheating every now and then. But I began to notice that every time I added sugar or refined carbohydrates to my diet, the feeling of well-being diminished. My weight, on the other hand, increased. When I stopped eating the offending substances, my symptoms disappeared. With this kind of built-in punishment and reward system, I became less and less tempted to stray from my dietary path.

Today, you can buy almost anything sugar-free: ice cream, cookies, candy. Although moderation is the key, artificial sweeteners may satisfy your urge for something sweet. The good news is they are not addicting, so you will diminish your intake and dependency. I keep sugar-free dark chocolate in my house for such emergencies. For an ex-addict like myself, this serves as an excellent crutch. Since artificial sweeteners have minimal effect on your blood sugar levels, you are not as apt to binge and it is not apt to cause weight gain. So, the next holiday, when everyone is bingeing on sugar, take out your sugar-free. When they loosen their belts you will be able to tighten yours.

The sugar industry is a big business, so maybe we shouldn't be surprised at the myriad and often subtle ways in which this substance finds its way into our diets. To illustrate, let's conclude this chapter with a stroll through a local supermarket, otherwise known as Sugar City. Randomly check the labels on some products, and notice how often sugar is included in the ingredient list. And it's not just in the obvious offenders like cake and candy—you may be surprised to find sugar in condiments, salad dressing and even many so-called "diet" foods.

The sugar industry is here to stay and will always remain one step ahead of us, the nutritionists. It's like the story of the two hunters:

One hunter said to the other, "Aren't you scared? What happens if we meet up with a wild bear?"

"No problem," the other hunter replied. "I have the solution right here." He took out a pair of sneakers and proceeded to put them on.

The first hunter laughed and said, "Are you kidding, do you think that you can outrun a bear?"

The second hunter replied, "No, I just have to outrun *you*."

The moral is: Don't expect the food industry—which includes the sugar industry—to look out for your health. You'll have to make your own detour past Sugar City to reach Health's Gate.

You cannot help men permanently by doing for them what they could and should do for themselves.

Abraham Lincoln

8

Insulin—ce

It's interesting to consider the similarity in sound and spelling of the hormone, insulin, and the attitude known as insolence. Webster's defines the latter as, "a haughty attitude, an insulting act." It is an insult to your body to abuse it with sugar and refined carbohydrates. Just as smokers harm their lungs and alcoholics ruin their livers, sugarholics wreak havoc on the pancreas. Insult the pancreas too much, too often, and it will fatigue and eventually fail. The medical term for this condition is diabetes, a disorder in which the pancreas is no longer capable of producing insulin.

Insulin, which is manufactured in shelves within the pancreas called the islets of langerhans, plays a vital role in metabolism. The principle function of this hormone is to act upon the carbohydrate in the blood stream, which is found in the form of glucose. The insulin delivers the glucose to the tissues of the body where it may be utilized for energy. But if there is a surplus of glucose, it is converted into stored energy, better known as *fat*. This property of insulin has caused it to be referred to as the "fattening hormone."

Remember an excess of insulin will also lower the blood sugar, thus creating a mild chemical imbalance called hypoglycemia. Insulin differs from most other hormones in that the quantity of insulin that circulates throughout the blood stream changes from minute to minute; half of the insulin that is produced is removed from the blood within seven minutes of its release. Since insulin acts upon glucose, our blood sugar is also in a constant state of flux. This is why that afternoon candy bar (which encourages the production of insulin) causes the blood sugar to fall lower than it was before you had the snack. The average person will experience a drop in energy approximately one hour after eating the sugar. A person with a sugar or carbohydrate intolerance will react sooner.

As I have emphasized, refined carbohydrates behave just like sugar, causing the pancreas to pour out insulin. Leading experts have discovered that, in addition to lowering the blood sugar, insulin can also increase the levels of triglycerides, which are implicated in the development of heart disease. This is why eminent researchers such as Dr. John Yudkin and Professor Margaret J. Alpring, of the West Virginia School of Medicine, have warned against a diet high in sugar.[1]

I am amazed that doctors will tell patients to cut back on their dietary fats, but say nothing about the hazards of sugar. As I explained earlier, when sugar and carbohydrates are eliminated, the pituitary gland will activate the fat mobilizing hormone, even when fats are included in the diet. This process essentially assists the body in breaking down fats.

"Insulin has been called the fattening hormone, that promotes the conversion of sugar (glucose) into fat by initiating the manufacture of fatty acids, that somehow prevents fat from breaking down so that it cannot be used up as the reserved source of fuel that it was meant to be."[2]

The only way to activate the fat fighters is to lower the amount of carbohydrates in the body. It is essential that we not exceed our critical carbohydrate level. You can monitor your progress with a ketosis stick, which can be purchased at any drug store. A ketone is a carbon fragment which is a by-product of the incomplete burning of fat. When you reduce your carbohydrates, your body can no longer look to them for fuel. It therefore begins burning stored triglycerides—fats—instead. This condition is known as ketosis, and should occur by the fifth day of the diet. While ketosis is not a healthy condition for a diabetic, and no one should remain in ketosis indefinitely (which is why we will reintroduce *complex* carbohydrates immediately into your diet), it is an important stage in this program, for it converts your body from a carbohydrate burning to a fat burning machine. If you are in this phase, a ketosis stick will turn purple when you dip it in your urine. Other symptoms of ketosis include weight loss and diminished hunger.

If you are hungry on this diet you are eating too much—too much carbohydrate, that is. This phenomenon is similar to that of a smoker who quits cigarettes, but then introduces nicotine back into his blood-stream—the need and desire for nicotine will become greater and greater. Well, according to my (proven) theory of "sugar relativity," as we introduce sugars and refined carbohydrates into our diets, our bodies demand more of these addictive substances. The result is increased hunger—and increased weight gain.

Overweight is also one of the risk factors for diabetes. While this condition is incurable, it is not untreatable, and weight loss can have a beneficial effect. I was gratified to receive this letter from one of my patients:

"Being on your diet and losing over 30 pounds so far has helped me in more ways than one. I'm a diabetic and because of the weight loss, my doctor has cut my medication almost in half, which is a blessing. He told me that he was proud of me and that he wanted me to keep up the good work because he has been after me for a long time to lose weight."

(Please note that this patient's *doctor* altered the medication schedule. You should always follow your physician's advice on medication.)

In fact, there are those who believe that diabetes, as well as obesity and hypoglycemia, can be altered and sometimes reversed by a diet devoid of sugar and low in carbohydrates.

"Dr. W.A. Miller, G.R. Faloona, and R.H. Unger showed the effectiveness of a low carbohydrate diet. These results were published in New England Journal of Medicine in 1970, and by Drs. E.F. Pfeiffer and H. Laube of Ulm, West Germany, who reported their data to the International Symposium of Lipid Metabolism, Obesity, and Diabetes Mellitus in 1974.

"Dr. Pfeiffer blasted starch and sugar for their effects on insulin and speculated that diabetes might not occur without them."[3]

Carbohydrates are a somewhat controversial subject in the diet industry, for while many experts recommend cutting down, there are best-selling books which encourage you to fill up on carbohydrates. One of the best known of these books is *Eat To Win,* made famous by the author's patient Martina Navratilova. There is evidence, however, that Navratilova, who won the Family Circle Cup with the help of her new trainer, Dr. Kathy Michael, has changed her eating habits.

"We have rebalanced her diet and we are working on a nutrition program (said Dr. Michael). She was eating too much fruit, which put a lot of unnecessary sugar in her system." When asked if she has cheated on her diet Navratilova laughed and said, "I know what I am suppose to eat, now with Kathy around I don't cheat."[4]

I treat many top athletes, and I'm proud to say that they excel on my program. It is true that athletes are less vulnerable to weight problems until they retire. Still, I wouldn't dream of putting them on a high-fat or high-carbohydrate diet, any more than I would consider putting 16 gallons of fuel into a gas tank with a 12 gallon capacity. Athletes burn a lot more fuel than their sedentary counterparts, but even they can't deliver at peak performance when they're flooded with sugars, fats and refined carbohydrates. Besides, sugar, like drugs, can cut short the career of an athlete by permanently wearing down the resistance of the body, making it more susceptible to injury. We've read about athletes whose cocaine habits made them feel invincible, but who ultimately proved tragically vulnerable. The same is true of a sugar habit, which makes you pay for the "high" with the "low" that follows.

As addicting as sugar is, there is no 12-step program specifically for those of us who crave the substance. As a recovered sugarholic, I get my reinforcement by viewing my slimmer physique in the mirror.

Take care to get what you like or you will be forced to like what you get.

George Bernard Shaw

9

Hormones–Nature's Fat Fighter

You have available to you a powerful and natural substance that will aid you immeasurably (and measurably!) in your weight loss program. In this chapter I'll explain how you can access this fat mobilizing hormone (FMH), so that your body will expend food as energy, instead of saving it as fat.

You will be asked to make some changes in order to produce results, and I realize that change is often met with resistance. Perhaps you will be skeptical about some of the advice offered here, but let me ask you a question: Are you reading this book because what you are doing right now is keeping you slender, healthy, and happy? If you find yourself unwilling to accept a new point of view, consider what happened to poor John Smith.

John was at the airport when his eye was caught by a sign that claimed, **"This is the world's only magic scale."**

Since it only costs 25 cents to try it out, John put in his quarter and stepped on the scale. It not only registered his correct weight, it issued him a slip that read, "Your name is John Smith, you are 47 years old, and you are taking Flight 212 to Atlanta."

Amazed, but disbelieving the evidence, John deposited another quarter, and received another slip that said, "Your name is John Smith, you are 47 years old, and you are taking Flight 212 to Atlanta."

Determined to trick this machine, John went into the men's room, where he altered his appearance with a change of clothes. He went back to the scale, dropped in another quarter, and received a slip that informed him, "Your name is still John Smith, and you are still 47 years old, but you have just missed flight 212 to Atlanta."

Don't get left behind because of an unwillingness to try something new. Many of my patients, some of whom had doubts initially, have written to thank me for introducing them to this program.

"Thank you for a diet that's easy to follow—no special recipes and no packaged foods. I lost 13 pounds and 18 1/2 inches (including 4 inches off my upper thigh) in *just one month*. It's so easy that it hardly seems possible that it's a diet!"

I can't take all the credit for this patient's success. Many of the people I treat have heard me say, "I am only as good a doctor as you are a patient." My goal is to teach you to become, if not your own doctor, then your own dietitian and your own boss. After all, *you* are the one who must carry out the basic principle of this diet—drastic reduction of sugars and refined carbohydrates—in order to achieve your weight loss goal. When you do this, you will reap the benefits available through the fat mobilizing hormone.

This hormone is a natural substance that is released by the pituitary gland and circulates in the blood stream. When sugar and carbohydrates are in short supply, FMH becomes productive, attacking deposits of fat and making them available to your body as fuel. Because FMH is releasing stored fat, you not only lose pounds, you lose them from the areas you most want to trim down.

Conversely, when the diet is high in carbohydrates, the fat mobilizing hormone cannot be found. When investigators analyzed urine samples from subjects on varying types of diets, they were able to recover FMH in samples from people who were on carbohydrate-restricted diets, but not from the samples of those on high carbohydrate diets. Of special interest was a group who were on 1,000 calorie per day diets, yet still failed to lose weight. These subjects were eating a high-carbohydrate diet, and no FMH was found in their urine samples.[1]

This program also works at breaking down the fat you don't see— cholesterol and triglycerides. Take the case of John K., one of my patients, for example. John's weight was not my only concern, for he also had elevated cholesterol and triglyceride levels. On my diet, he not only lost 25 pounds, he showed a drop of 50 points in his cholesterol.

It is important to understand that when no carbohydrates are available to the body, it must get its fuel from somewhere. So, the body sends a message that says, in effect, "Break down the fat so that I can create energy." Thanks to this process, we not only lose weight, we enjoy increased energy. Best of all, the process begins very shortly after the removal of refined carbohydrates from the diet.

"I read the work of those two brilliant English researchers Professor Kekwick and Dr. Pawan, who had shown that a fat-mobilizing substance was present in the urine when that diet had been free of carbohydrate for forty-eight hours. This and the presence of ketone bodies in the urine signified that the body was satisfying its hunger by burning its own fat as fuel."[2]

"Dr. Alfred W. Pennington, of the DuPont Company, postulated that over-weight is frequently explained by a trensic metabolic defect. He suggested a treatment for it that does not restrict calories. Dr. Pennington approved it on DuPont employees. He'd proved his treatment worked shortly after World War II when the medical division of the DuPont company gave him the job of trying to find out why low calorie diets failed with so many of their staff members. Pennington decided that overweight could be caused not by overeating but by metabolic defect, an inability of the body to utilize carbohydrates for anything except making fat. Dr. Pennington created a test diet, he found 20 staff members who volunteered to try it, the diet eliminated sugars, starches and gave proteins and fats instead. This of course is a ketogenic diet, which means the absence of carbohydrate causing ketones to be spilled over in the urine. This is a sign of the fat mobilizing hormone is circulating within the blood stream. There was no calorie counting on Dr. Pennington's diet. The basic diet allowed 3,000 calories a day, but anyone who was hungry was free to eat without limit. During the test period of 20 of his dieters reported that they felt well and were never hungry. And at the end they had lost an average of 22 pounds in an average of 3 1/2 months. Those who had high blood pressure stated happily that it had dropped parallel to the drop in weight."[3]

I was on a personal odyssey to find the hungry man's diet. After reviewing many works on the subject, I recognized the significance of the fat mobilizing hormone principle, and realized that it was possible to eat well and lose weight on a plan that did not demand excessive discipline or enforced starvation.

No refined carbohydrates means no hunger! Great news, I thought. If the absence of refined carbohydrate can switch one's body engine from being a carbohydrate burning machine to being a fat burning machine, perhaps I can eat all of the steak, chicken or fish (which is carbohydrate free) I want and lose my fat at the same time.

In my search for the perfect diet, I read everything I could find on the subject. The more I learned, the more I wanted to know. I read books and articles by Fredericks, Kedwick, Pawan, Stillman, Bloom, Atkins, and many other experts. I was the guinea pig with the world as my lab. If it advertised weight loss, I wanted to know about it. I became the Napoleon Hill of fat.

I found both differences and common denominators in the principles offered by these authors. I then took their suggestions and modified, combined or elaborated upon them. For example, Dr. Atkins put little emphasis on water and allowed unlimited fat, while Dr. Stillman put most of his emphasis on water. Both programs restricted sugar and carbohydrates. I came up with a formula that included:

1. No sugar, no refined carbohydrate

2. Eight, 8-ounce glasses of water a day

3. Modified fat intake

I was cooking, literally thinning. The more I practiced what I learned, the easier it became and the thinner I became.

I was intrigued by my program because there was no hunger on a modified carbohydrate diet. I began removing refined carbohydrates from my diet. Eventually, I included vitamins and supplements in my diet. I then introduced growth hormones (by using natural amino acids) into my program. I dramatically reduced my intake of salt, fat and refined sugar. And my fat mobilizing hormone was obviously working for me, because I was losing a great amount of weight. I also began drinking large amounts of water, and discovered that not only did it assist in weight loss, it helped clear up my skin.

Most important, I began sharing my program with my patients. I run five clinics, which see approximately 500 to 1,000 patients per week, so I had the pleasure of seeing many people obtain excellent results on the program that had worked so well for me. I received a lot of mail from happy patients.

"I would like to take this time to thank you for encouraging me to lose those unwanted pounds. So far the diet has been great. I lost 20 pounds and feel wonderful!"

I was also gratified to receive the following from my respected colleague, Dr. R. James Gregg (President of the International Chiropractic Association):

"I just wanted to take a moment to thank you for the time and energy that you put in to developing in my opinion, the greatest diet of all time. I am one of those people who have been on just about every diet known to man. Therefore, I was very skeptical when you told me that I would not be hungry, I would lose weight, and I wouldn't just be eating so called 'rabbit food.'

"In approximately 2 1/2 months, I lost 28 pounds and remained energetic during the loss. The great thing about your diet is that I don't really consider it a diet, more a way of life. This is truly a plan that can be followed for the rest of your life."

The health program was also popular with my celebrity patients. ESPN announcer and former major league baseball player Tom Hutton offered the following testimonial:

"Eric Kaplan has done a thorough job in trying to prescribe and explain the best ways to stay fit and healthy. Having been in professional baseball over 25 years, hard work and applying expert knowledge usually seems to work. Eric Kaplan supplies the knowledge, now it's up to you to do the work."

One of the bonuses of my diet was that, in addition to looking better, I was feeling much better. My self-confidence seemed to rise with every pound lost and my energy increased. This new found self-assurance was noticed by others. I was happily surprised when I was asked to sit on the board of advisors at Bear Lakes Country Club. The membership of this prestigious club includes the likes of Jack Nicklaus,

Greg Norman, United States Amateur winner Nathaniel Crosby, British Open winner Mark Calcavecchia, 11-time baseball All-Star Gary Carter, John Havlicek and Bob Cousy of the Boston Celtics, Richie Guerin of the New York Knicks, Perry Como, Joe Namath, Jeff Reardon, and numerous other successful and powerful people. Within the same week, I was invited to be on the board of trustees of Temple Judea, the temple to which I belong. Then I was asked by my homeowner's association to serve on the board of directors. And although I was off sugar, it was icing on the cake when Florida National Bank and then Governors Bank invited me to sit on their board of advisors.

I attributed my sudden popularity to my weight loss, increased stamina, and more positive attitude. You see, I started to believe in the philosophy of "plan your life and live your plan." More important, I started to practice it. I began to understand that success comes from the inside out, not from the outside in. And my life illustrated this shift in attitude. I began to read great books about great people—and to watch less television. I now wrote my goals down, so that they would be anchored and not drift away. I also came to realize that I was a sugarholic, an important revelation to me.

We're appalled when someone puts white powder up his nose, but we go so far as to encourage people to use the white powder that goes in the mouth. Yet both substances are addictive, unhealthy and ultimately unsatisfying.

The fat mobilizing hormone is our metabolic switch, and we turn it on by turning off to sugars and carbohydrates. Whether you do this or not is up to you, but I can offer a word of advice on how to do it:

The best way to break a habit is to drop it.
　　　　　　　　　　　　　　Leo Aikman

If you must make a mistake, make a new one each time.
Dale Carnegie

10

Beverage Blues

On Friday the 13th, 1988, Barbara Walters hosted a special episode of *20/20* that included a report on Beech-Nut industries. The program revealed that the apple juice sold by the company was far from being "pure apple juice." It was not, in fact, apple juice at all—this famous product contained no apples! The imitation fruit juice was criticized by the media, and dubbed a "chemical cocktail." A chemist who worked for Beech-Nut revealed that the beverage contained fructose and glucose; in other words, sugar. Beech-Nut, in the biggest economic court case in Justice Department History, eventually paid two million dollars in fines.

I'm not surprised that our children graduate from the nipple to the needle. Their well-meaning parents are the first ones to introduce them to an addictive substance—sugar—in the form of baby formula or "pure" fruit juice. "According to Elijah Muhammad the Black Moslem prophet, bottle babies end up loving the bottle and hating their mamas."[1]

A strong statement, to be sure, but the fact is many of our children subsist on a diet of non-foods such as Sugar Frosted Flakes, sandwiches on white bread (smothered with catsup and other sugary condiments), and pasta made with refined flour; then we have the ubiquitous cookie, offered as a reward for good behavior.

It's hardly surprising that so many of these children turn to alcohol. They learned early to satisfy their thirst with sugar-filled, non-nutritious beverages.

"Figures suggest that 25% of the sugar consumed in the United States reaches the American gullet in the form of soft drinks of all kinds. Between 1962 and 1972 coffee drinking dropped as did the consumption of milk, while the consumption of soft drinks almost doubled in excess of 30 gallons per person per year from 1972 as against 16.2 gallons for 1962."[2]

In 1951, Dr. McCay, who was in charge of nutritional research for the U.S. Navy during World War II, made some startling revelations about Coca-Cola before a Congressional Committee.

"I was amazed to learn," he testified, "that the beverage contained substantial amounts of phosphoric acid. At the Naval Medical Research we put human teeth in cola beverage and found they softened and started to dissolve within a short period." When the Congressmen gaped, the doctor went on: "The acidity of cola beverages is about the same as vinegar. The sugar content masks the acidity, and children little realize they are drinking a strange mixture of phosphoric acid, sugar, caffeine, coloring and flavored matter." A Congressman asked the doctor what government had charge of passing on the contents of soft drinks. "So far as I know no one has passed upon it or pays any attention to it," the doctor replied.

Another Congressman asked if the doctor had made any tests of the effect of cola beverages on metal and iron. While the doctor said he hadn't, the Congressman volunteered: "A friend of mine told me once that he dropped three ten-penny nails into one of the cola bottles, and within 48 hours the nails had completely dissolved." "Sure," the doctor answered, "phosphoric acid there would dissolve iron or limestone. You might drop it on the steps and it would erode the steps coming up here."[3]

Our addiction to soft drinks begins in the cradle and ends in the grave. One of the most important weight-loss suggestions I can make is: *Drink plenty of water.* Make this refreshing, calorie-free, carbohydrate-free liquid your primary beverage; drink at least eight, eight ounce glasses per day. Water cleanses the body, and enables the kidneys to function. Water is the real thing.

In a published report, Dr. Donald Robertson, M.D. says, "Water also suppresses the appetite and water assists the body in its mobilization of stored fat. Studies have shown that a decrease in water intake will cause fat deposits to increase, while an increase in water intake can reduce fat deposits."

Dr. Robertson goes on to say that the kidneys cannot function properly without enough water and if they don't work to capacity some of their load is dumped onto the liver. One of the liver's primary functions is to metabolize stored fat into usable energy for the body, if the liver has to do some of the kidney's work it can't operate at full throttle. As a result, it metabolizes less fat, more fat remains stored in the body and weight loss stops. Drinking water is the best treatment for fluid retention. When the body gets less water, it perceives it as a threat to survival and begins to hold onto every drop. Water is stored in extracellular spaces (outside the cells). This shows up in swollen feet, legs and hands.

Diuretics offer a temporary solution at best. They force out stored water along with some essential nutrients. Again the body perceives a threat and will replace the lost water at the first opportunity. Thus, the condition quickly returns. The best way to overcome the problem of water retention is to give your body what it needs—plenty of water. Only then will the stored water be released.

If you have a constant problem with water retention, excess salt may be to blame. Your body will tolerate sodium only in certain concentration. The more salt you eat, the more water your system retains to dilute it. But getting rid of unneeded salt is easy—just drink more water. As it is forced through the kidneys it takes away excess sodium. The overweight person needs more water than the thin one. Larger people have larger metabolic loads. Since we know that water is the key to fat metabolism, it follows that the overweight person needs more water.

Water helps to maintain proper muscle tone by giving muscles their natural ability to contract and by preventing dehydration. It also helps to prevent sagging skin that usually follows weight loss. Shrinking cells are buoyed by water, which plumps the skin and leaves it clear, healthy and resilient.

Water helps rid the body of waste. During weight loss, the body has a lot more waste to get rid of—all that metabolized fat must be shed. Again, adequate water helps flush out the waste.

Water can help relieve constipation. When the body gets too little water, it siphons what it needs from internal sources. The colon is one primary source. Result? Constipation. But, when a person drinks enough water, normal bowel function usually returns.

So far we've discovered some remarkable truths about water and weight loss:

1. The body will not function properly without enough water and can't metabolize stored fat efficiently.

2. Retained water stores up as excess weight.

3. To rid excess water you must drink more water.

4. Drinking water is essential to weight loss.

How much water is enough? On the average a person should drink eight, eight ounce glasses every day, approximately two quarts. However, the overweight person needs one additional glass for every twenty-five pounds of excess weight. The amount you drink also should be increased if you exercise briskly or if the weather is hot and dry. Water should preferably be cold, it is absorbed into the system more quickly than warm water. And some evidence suggests that drinking cold water can actually help burn calories. . . . When the body gets the water it needs to function optimately the fluids are perfectly balanced. When this happens you have reached a breakthrough point. What does this mean?

1. Endocrine function improves.

2. Water retention is alleviated as stored water is lost.

3. More fat is used as fuel because the liver is free to metabolize stored fat.

4. Natural thirst returns.

5. There is a loss of hunger almost overnight.

If you stop drinking enough water your body fluids will be thrown out of balance again, and you may experience fluid retention, unexplained weight gain, and loss of thirst.

Dr. Stillman is one of the pioneers of the water diet, and I had the pleasure of meeting him shortly after I graduated from college. During our conversation he said, in effect, "You can lead a horse to water, but you can't make him drink."

At this point in my life, weight loss was not a goal of mine; I was still at my college weight of 163 pounds and had a 32-inch waist. Nonetheless, I found Dr. Stillman to be a fascinating and informative gentleman. We played Blackjack for hours, and while I lost a small fortune, I was more than repaid by his company. This was not a great night for my economic status, but it was well worth the price!

We went out to eat, and it was clear that Dr. Stillman believed in and practiced his system. In the course of the evening, I also had the pleasure of meeting his niece. When I noted that she was not thin, the trim Dr. Stillman, who always seemed to have a glass of water in his hand, said simply, "I haven't seen her drink her water tonight." This brought me to the realization that, if we are to achieve weight reduction, we must not only follow the pioneers of the weight loss industry, we must follow the pioneers who live by their own rules.

To sum up some of the principles we have learned so far: William Duffy, author of *Sugar Blues,* avoids sugar like the white plague; Dr. Atkins diet is low in sugars and refined carbohydrates, as is Carlton Fredericks' diet; Dr. Stillman's diet requires us to drink large amounts of water. The Pritikin diet is low in fats.

Are you beginning to see a pattern? I know that when I combined these principles I felt like the person who first mixed peanut butter with jelly.

And I didn't just read about these rules, I used them in my own life. Practical experience tells me that consumption of large amounts of water does suppress the appetite. Research confirms that water helps the body through the period of ketosis by flushing out the extra ketones created by the lack of refined carbohydrate and the production of fat mobilizing hormone. The result is that we will have a fat burning metabolism, not a carbohydrate burning one. By burning fat, not storing it, fat becomes our ally, not our enemy.

A successful man is one who can lay a firm foundation with the bricks that others throw at him.

Sidney Greenburg

11

Preparatory Phase

The preparatory phase of this diet is crucial to the success of your weight loss program, for during this four-day period, you will unleash the fat-burning power of your body. The purpose of this phase is to create within your body a perfect chemical balance, called homeostasis, which will enable you to derive optimum benefits from the program. By following the instructions in this chapter, you will turn on your metabolic switch, thus motivating your body to expend the fat it has been hoarding. The results will delight you: you will experience rapid weight loss, a surge of energy (remember, fat is stored energy), and a sharp reduction in hunger.

The key to this phase is, of course, the reducion of fats and the elimination of refined carbohydrates. Carbohydrates—the right kind in the correct amounts—will be reintroduced in later phases of the diet. Some other restrictions will apply, but the one thing you need not restrict is the amount of food you eat.

You may eat allowable foods as often as you wish.

During the preparatory phase, you may have unlimited amounts of chicken, turkey, fish or lean beef. I recommend broiling or barbecuing your food, and don't use breading or butter in the cooking process (lemon juice or Pam are good substitutes). Fried foods must be avoided, and you should remove skin from your meat.

You may have all the green vegetables you desire, with the exception of peas, but they must be eaten raw, as cooked vegetables do contain additional carbohydrates.

For the first four days, use only olive oil and (apple cider) vinegar or a low-calorie fat-free Italian dressing on your salads.

You are also allowed one egg per day for the first four days. In addition, you should have one orange per day, to be eaten in the morning, to ensure that your potassium level is maintained. Active people and larger people may have a second fruit; a small apple is recommended. I also recommend that you take a good multivitamin with each meal.

Absolutely no other foods are permitted during the preparatory phase. This means no fruit juices, no cooked vegetables, and, of course, no bread, pasta, or dairy products. Condiments containing salt or sugar must also be eliminated. Therefore, you must not use mustard, mayonnaise, relish or catsup during the preparatory phase.

Your primary beverage during this phase (and other phases) of the diet will be water. You may drink mineral water, distilled water, or designer water, such as Perrier, if you want to treat yourself. Other allowed beverages include:

> - Up to 24 ounces per day of decaffeinated, low carbohydrate diet soda
> - Sodium free club soda
> - Coffee—up to four cups of the decaffeinated variety, and up to two cups of coffee, or tea, with caffeine
> - Parsley tea and herbal tea, unlimited amounts

A greater variety of foods will be introduced in later phases of the diet, but even this preparatory phase is far from stringent. Just think, you can wake up to a breakfast of scrambled eggs, an orange, and a cup of coffee. For lunch, you can have a lean hamburger, steak, or chicken with a nice large green salad. Dinner might consist of fresh fish and an appetizer of raw vegetables.

The preparatory phase is specifically designed for those individuals who wish to lose weight. If this is not your goal, you can skip ahead to Phase 3 of the diet; many of my underweight patients were able to gain weight by following the instructions. Keep in mind that the ideal is a condition of homeostasis, or perfect balance; if you do not stress your body it will help you find your perfect weight.

To further motivate you, let me summarize the advantages of this program:

1. It is simple to follow. You are allowed plenty to eat; it is probably one of the least restrictive of all reducing diets.

2. It reduces hunger. This is a real plus for people who have addictive eating patterns.

3. It makes your metabolism work for you, not against you. Not only will you lose weight, you will lose it in the areas you most want to reduce. And you don't have to count calories to get your results.

4. It will have a favorable effect on your blood fats and blood sugar.

5. It has a diuretic—i.e., water eliminating effect. This is very helpful to people suffering from edema or high blood pressure.

6. It will increase your energy level, making you a happier, healthier, more productive person.

7. Because the proteins on this diet are easier to digest than refined carbohydrates, people with stomach disorders will benefit. It is also very helpful for individuals with overactive intestines, for example, those who suffer from colitis.

8. Most important, this diet will make you thin to win, producing maximum results in a minimum amount of time.

If you think this diet is easy, let me assure you that you're right! When I was formulating this plan, I thought of the complaint of the golf pro Dallas A., who was working toward his tour card on the Pro Golfers Association (PGA). One day while I was out with him, he remarked on how difficult it is to count calories when you have to eat out at every meal. When you don't have to count calories, eating out can be a pleasure rather than an exercise in arithmetic.

How difficult is it to order fresh fruit or a salad at any restaurant? How complicated is it to select a shrimp cocktail from a menu, or order a cheeseburger and ask the waiter to hold the roll? You can even eat at Wendy's (salad bar), McDonald's (McLean 97% fat-free hamburgers) or Burger King (grilled chicken) if you wish. If you want an afternoon pick-me-up, you can eat an orange and a couple of pieces of low-fat cheese (although not during the preparatory phase). True, you can't combine refined carbohydrates and proteins on this diet, but isn't it easier to remember this rule than to remember exactly how many calories there are in a scoop of cottage cheese?

Low-carbohydrate diets have been criticized, but most good ideas have been. (It was once very unpopular to suggest that the earth was round.)

This diet is as much a high salad diet as it is a low-carbohydrate diet. This diet modifies carbohydrates. You can eat all the salad your heart desires. These green vegetables are known as complex carbohydrates (the good carbohydrates). It is our desire to eliminate the bad carbohydrates (refined), eliminate sugar and modify fat intake. By doing this we will balance our blood sugar. We will utilize our stored fat and any injested fat will be used for energy. Any diet that allows sugar and restricts fats, proteins, carbohydrates, etc., is a fad diet. This is not a fad diet, but a lifestyle! The body needs a balance of food sources. We must do more than eliminate, we must modify, coordinate and control our eating habits.

I believe that as a reader of this book, you are a seeker, not a critic. You are seeking a diet that you can realistically follow for a lifetime, and therefore you require a program that is effective, easy to follow, and nonrestrictive. A large body of evidence indicates that low-carbohydrate diet is just what you have been looking for.

In doing research of carbohydrate diets, high-protein, low-carbohydrate diets, Dr. U.A. Roberts of Wrzburg, West Germany, studied patients on 1,000 calorie diets of two different compositions, the following diets were used:

> ➤ High-carbohydrate diets, 170g., and low fat 11g.
> ➤ Low-carbohydrate, 25g., and higher fat 75g.

The study that was conducted lasted over a month and at the end the low-carbohydrate group had lost an average of 30.8 pounds and the high-carbohydrate group consuming the same number of calories had lost only 21.6 pounds. The daily weight loss was 20% greater among those on the low carbohydrate formula. Imagine the results if we cut our fat intake to 40 grams.

Similar studies were done at Cornell University. Dr. Charlotte Young and her associates compared 30g., 60g., and 104g., carbohydrate diets of 1,800 calories. Among their data a body composition studies demonstrating that whereas 25% of the weight loss on 104g. diet is non-fat tissue only 5% is non-fat tissue on the 30g. diet. In nine weeks, the 104g. dieters lost 17.5 pounds of body fat, whereas the 30g. dieters lost 30.7 pounds.[1]

In yet another study reported on in *Nutritional Breakthrough*, subjects were put on a 2,870 calorie regimen similar to the Atkins diet, consisting of 260 grams of protein, 190 grams of fat, and 12 grams of carbohydrate. The investigators found that 16 of the 17 subjects lost between 0.66 and 6.4 pounds per week. But when they were switched to a high-carbohydrate diet *containing the same number of calories* more often than not there was a weight gain.

Wouldn't it be great to lose weight and to trim fat from those especially stubborn areas? What would you be willing to do for a flat tummy and thin thighs?

Begin the preparatory phase tomorrow, and you'll be on your way to having what you want. Just follow the instructions, keep a positive attitude, and enjoy your meals!

Success is a journey, not a destination.

Ben Sweetland

12

Dr. Kaplan's Low Stress, High Energy Diet

On Dr. Kaplan's Low Stress, High Energy Diet, you won't have the experience of trudging uphill. Just as we become more fatigued when we walk up a steep incline as opposed to a level path, we tire more easily when we overload our bodies with sugar and refined carbohydrates. Because these substances are eliminated in this eating plan, you no longer have to cope with the stress induced by blood sugar highs and lows. Your body is therefore more at ease and capable of providing you with greater energy.

This program eliminates stress on the digestive system and metabolism by eliminating excess. The principle behind this is based on four basic food qualities:

1. Quantity

2. Quality

3. Nutritional concentration

4. Digestibility

One method of avoiding excess is to evaluate food according to these criteria. And, of course, you must also know precisely what "excess" means in this context. For purposes of this diet, I define a dietary excess as a stomach overload, a digestive overload, or the ingestion of foreign substances.

Stomach overload occurs when more food is eaten than the body can efficiently utilize. When this excess food is digested and absorbed into the bloodstream, it will cause a systemic overload. This in turn creates stress which affects the glandular system, because one of the primary functions of the glands is to regulate the internal environment. I've already discussed some of the diseases associated with this type of overload. Diabetes, hardening of the arteries, and gout are among the conditions linked with this type of excess. Keep in mind that too much quantity in the diet is as bad as too little quality.

Digestive overload results from taking in more food than can be broken down into simpler substances and absorbed (digested). This excess is carried, undigested, into the intestinal tract. These undigested food particles are foci of toxic end products by bacterial action. The fat particles become rancid, the carbohydrates ferment, and the proteins putrefy; some of these toxic end products are actually poisons. To keep your body from becoming a repository for toxic waste, it is important to combine your foods properly. The body, via the fat mobilizing hormone, is capable of breaking down proteins and fats when they are not mixed with refined carbohydrates and sugars. One of the worst things we can do is eat dessert after a large meal. Eating sugars right after a meal of proteins and fats turns *off* the *metabolic switch,* and this alone can create a digestive overload. I'm realistic enough not to expect you to eliminate desserts altogether, but I strongly recommend that you follow these two rules at all times:

1. Wait at least one hour after your meal before eating sugars.

2. Implement moderation.

Moderation is the key to any successful diet. Even though my diet allows you to eat your fill of permitted foods, you must take care to avoid digestive overload. When toxic end products accumulate in the digestive tract, we have a condition called intestinal toxemia, perhaps more widely know as a "tummy ache." This condition is often seen in children after a day at the circus, where they have eaten indiscriminately of hot dogs, popcorn, cotton candy, peanuts, soda, ice cream, and other assorted goodies. It is also frequently seen in adults shortly after Thanksgiving dinner.

Occasional overeating is not what causes people to develop a weight problem, however. I have many patients who insist that their weight problems result from overindulgence on weekends. I've frequently had patients tell me, "Doc, I gained five pounds this weekend."

This seems unlikely in view of the fact that one pound represents 3,500 calories; in order to gain five pounds, a person must consume five times this amount, or 17,500 calories. Not very realistic, I'm afraid. I have figured that I put on two pounds per year, starting when I graduated from college. So, it was easy to understand how I could put on 30 pounds in 15 years. Two pounds per year averages out to a little over an ounce a month. Weight accumulates slowly. If you eat an extra 100 calories per day you will gain 10 pounds in one year or 30 pounds in three years. Start your diet today, take your diet one day at a time.

"Inch by inch, it's a cinch."

If we must be careful to avoid digestive overload, we must be ultracautious when it comes to foreign substances, such as drugs, smog, substances found in the water supply, industrial poisons, food preservatives and refined products. When we introduce foreign substances into our bodies, our defense mechanisms rise to our aid. These mechanisms include the kidneys, liver and glands, all of which do their best to expel the invaders—they can only do so much, however. I recommend therefore, that you:

> ➤ Try to keep your diet as natural as possible.
> ➤ Drink plenty of water to help your body rid itself of foreign
>   substances.

Vegetables meet the four criteria listed at the beginning of the chapter. It is difficult to exceed the appropriate quantity by eating vegetables. Also, the nutritional quality is high, although you should wash vegetables well to remove any contaminating insecticides (foreign substances). Vegetables are not a concentrated food, especially when they are eaten raw. You should also be aware that raw vegetables seldom cause the gas and discomfort associated with cooked vegetables. Finally, vegetables are usually easy to digest, although radishes, cucumbers and a few other vegetables cause distress to some people. (If you have a problem digesting any type of food, be sure to mention this to your doctor.) In short, vegetables are a wonderful food, and should be a staple of your diet. Although cooked vegetables are allowed in Phase 2 of the diet, raw is the preferred form.

Animal food sources are generally high in nutritional quality, although we must take care to avoid the preservatives, such as nitrates and nitrites, which are frequently added to these foods. Also, while animal foods are rich sources of minerals, proteins, and fats, in high concentrations they can be the foci of toxic end products, so it is important to practice moderation. Because these foods are generally easy to digest, it is easy to find yourself overeating; this is particularly true of muscle meat such as beef steak. I recommend that men eat no more than 10-12 ounces at each sitting, and women no more than 8-10 ounces.

Fruit, which is a healthy food and an important source of roughage, should nonetheless be eaten in moderation, for it does contain sugar. Also, as mentioned earlier, fruit should not be eaten after 6:00 p.m. Fruit juice is not permitted on my diet, for this beverage is a highly concentrated source of fruit sugar. (How many oranges go into that glass of juice?)

Fruit sugars are easily absorbed, requiring practically no digestion. But when sugars are combined with other foods, especially animal foods, the digestive process is compromised. Therefore, fruits should not be eaten with other foods.

This diet allows for certain types of fats and oils. However, the hydrogenated types, such as margarine, shortenings, commercial mayonnaise, coconut oil, and hardened peanut butter are absolutely forbidden. Also not allowed are animal fats, such as lard. The exception to this rule is fresh butter, which has a low carbohydrate content and is easily digested. Butter can add zing to foods such as vegetables, and I feel it is very important not to allow your diet to become boring. Make your food tasty with imaginative use of butter, salad dressing, and home-made mayonnaise, but use these products in moderation. The best fats and oils are the cold pressed (not chemically extracted) types, including olive oil (which recent studies have shown can lower your cholesterol level), sesame oil, sunflower oil, and safflower oil. Heat is the enemy of all fats, and prolonged heating (associated with frying) is detrimental because the unsaturated fatty acids of even the best oils in the raw state become saturated and rancid.

If you have any doubts about whether you are following the diet plan, consult the following rules:

Rule #1: For the first week, eat only the permitted foods—there are no exceptions. If you cannot find the food on your permitted list, this means that it's refined carbohydrate, fat or alcohol content is too high for you at this point.

Rule #2: Drink eight, eight-ounce glasses of water per day. This will not only aid in suppressing your appetite, it will improve endocrine function, alleviate fluid retention, and help the liver to metabolize stored fat. Plus, it will help maintain proper muscle tone and relieve constipation.

Rule #3: Eat whenever you are hungry, but do not eat except when you are hungry (boredom, frustration, and anger are not hunger, so don't eat to appease these emotions). Remember, diets low in sugars and refined carbohydrates do not promote constant hunger. Conversely, individuals with poor appetites will notice an improvement when concentrated foods such as sugars are restricted. (This is especially true of children.)

Rule #4: Eat foods in their natural, unprocessed forms whenever possible. Fruit, as I mentioned, should be consumed whole, not in the form of fruit juice. Bread made with refined flour should be avoided. (Breads are allowed in either Phase 2 or 3, depending on your metabolism.)

Rule #5: Never eat sweets with other foods. Sugars and proteins must never be combined. This goes not only for desserts, but for fruits as well.

Rule #6: Eat foods from animal sources in moderation.

Rule #7: Eat raw foods with every meal. The best choice is salad. Raw green vegetables behave almost like a zero carbohydrate food, so you can eat them in abundance. Some vegetables, however, are high in carbohydrates. One onion, for example, may contain over 9 grams of carbohydrate, while one cup of spinach has only about 1 gram. A half cup of carrots consists of 5 grams of carbohydrates, whereas one cup of lettuce contains only 2 grams. Tomatoes have been found to promote the digestion of foods from animal sources. It is therefore recommended that you eat a ripe tomato—fresh, not canned—with meat products.

Rule #8: Eat small meals, but do not skip meals. I have found that when people do not eat at one meal, they not only slow down their metabolism, they tend to consume more at the next sitting. In so doing, they make themselves vulnerable to a digestive overload. This problem can be avoided by eating many small meals rather than a few large meals. Feel free to snack, provided you eat only the permitted foods.

Rule #9: In line with the above, make sure that you eat breakfast every day. This meal gets our metabolism off to a good start. If you have trouble eating this meal, or are the type to skip meals in general, I will be happy to provide you with information on Dr. Kaplan's meal supplement. This protein, fiber and vitamin enriched drink can be used in place of a meal. It is low in carbohydrates, and very effective during weight loss. For details, please write to: Dr. Eric Kaplan, 648 U.S. Hwy 1, North Palm Beach, FL 33418.

Rule #10: Take the proper supplements in the morning and evening. These will be discussed in greater detail in later chapters.

Rule #11: Avoid all sugars and refined carbohydrates. When I say no sugar, I mean absolutely *no sugar.* Read labels carefully, as sugar can be found where you least expect it, in preparations such as lozenges, chewable vitamins, and even laxatives. If you're taking a medication that contains sugar, please ask your physician if he or she can suggest a sugarless substitute. (But do not stop taking medication without your physician's approval.)

Rule #12: Caffeine, although not forbidden, should be restricted as much as possible. Drink no more than two cups of coffee-containing caffeine per day.

Rule #13: Consider alcohol a carbohydrate, and treat it accordingly. Alcohol interferes with the fat mobilizing hormone, and must be restricted; none is permitted during Phase 1 or 2.

Rule #14: Exercise! Later in the book, we will review this important part of your weight loss/health improvement program.

Rule #15: Consult your physician before embarking on this program. Have a urine test, a basic CBC, a complete blood profile, and a blood pressure check. Have another series of tests done when you have reached your goals, and compare with the first tests: you'll find that the internal results are as impressive as the external results.

Apart from these rules, which you'll find surprisingly easy to follow, you can live it up. A "diet" consisting of turkey bacon or sausage and eggs or fresh fruit for breakfast, blackened chicken with a green salad and seafood appetizer for lunch, eight ounces of veal or fish with another green salad and broccoli for dinner, and a dietetic gelatin for dessert consists of only 10 grams of carbohydrates. So turn on that metabolic switch and let those fat fighters loose.

It may help you to consult the following guidelines when planning your meals.

Meats

Most meats are legal. Steak, hamburger, corned beef, veal, lamb chops and tongue are all permitted. The only meats not allowed are pork or those with fillers or additives, for they may contain too much or too many refined carbohydrates. You will therefore want to avoid packaged cold cuts, meatballs, sausage, and hot dogs. For best results, stay with leaner cuts of meat. Bacon when allowed must be cooked crisply. Meats such as pork which will be allowed later in the diet should never be eaten twice in the same day, two days in a row, or more than three times per week.

Fowl

Chicken, duckling, and turkey are legal. Eat to your heart's content. Do, however, be sure to remove the skin. Turkey sausage and bacon are low in fat and are tasty breakfast treats.

Fish

Most fish is legal. This includes canned tuna or salmon, lox, crab, and shrimp. You should never eat crab two days in a row, however. Also, swordfish, scallops and crab should be eaten no more than twice a week, as they are high in sodium, and they should not be eaten on the same day as beef. Not recommended: clams, mussels, or oysters. They are allowed later in the diet, but not during Phase 1. Use fresh or fresh frozen fish.

Salads

It is recommended that you eat two salads per day. The best dressings are olive oil and vinegar. Low-fat dressings may be used. Legal salad materials include celery, cabbage, chives, cucumber, lettuce, peppers, olives (green or black), and shallots or scallions (instead of onions). Avoid pickles—which are high in sodium—and parsley, radishes and water cress. Permitted salad garnishes include crumbled crisp bacon, grated cheese, minced hard boiled egg yolk, and mushrooms.

Vegetables

The list of permitted vegetables on this diet includes:

Asparagus	Avocado	Olives (green/black)
Bamboo shoots	Onions	Bean sprouts
Peppers	Beet greens	Pumpkin
Broccoli	Rhubarb	Cabbage
Sauerkraut	Cauliflower	Snow pea pods
Chard	Spinach	Collard greens
String beans	Wax beans	Dandelion greens
Summer squash	Eggplant	Tomato
Kale	Turnip greens	Mushrooms
Turnips	Mustard greens	Water chestnuts
Okra	Zucchini squash	

Although some of these vegetables are higher in carbohydrates than other foods on the diet, they do not contain *refined* carbohydrates, and thus should be a staple on your eating plan. Again, raw green vegetables can be eaten in abundance. Later in the diet you will be allowed cooked vegetables, but do not overcook as this depletes the vitamin content.

Condiments

Lite Salt, pepper, garlic, paprika, basil, horseradish, vinegar (apple cider), artificial sweeteners, juice of one fresh lemon, any combination spice, fresh or dried herbs that does not include sugar. No catsup.

Beverages

Eight, eight-ounce glasses of water per day, 24 ounces of diet soda (watch the caffeine and carbohydrate content), unrestricted amounts of beef or chicken broth, herbal tea and decaffeinated coffee. No more than two cups of caffeine-containing coffee per day.

No beverages should be substituted for water!

Fruits

Limit yourself to one or two servings per day when reducing. Consult the four phases of the diet to determine your legal fruit consumption. A "serving" consists of one of the following:

Apples—1 small
Apricots—3 medium
Blueberries—1/4 cup
Cantaloupe—1/4 medium-sized
Cherries—9 medium
Grapefruit—1/2 medium
Grapes—10 small
Oranges—1 small
Peaches—1 small
Pineapple—1/2 cup
Strawberries—1/2 cup
Watermelon—1 cup, diced

I recommend that you have no more than one serving per day of fruit for the first week. After the second week, you will be allowed two servings, depending on weight reduction. I do not recommend eating three servings until you reach maintenance, unless you exercise actively or are trying to lose less than 20 pounds. This will be reviewed later in the book.

Starches

After the second or third week, review Phases 2 through 4 to determine when starches can be introduced into you diet. The person who needs to lose a moderate amount of weight may have two servings per day; one serving is plenty for the person who has a considerable amount to lose. A "serving" consists of the following:

Diet bread (Fresh Horizons, Less, Measure Up)—1 slice
Melba toast (unseasoned)—1 slice
Bread sticks (Diet Stella Doro)—1/2 stick
Akmak Cracker—1/4 board
Rice cakes (unsalted)—1/2 cake
Miller's Bran—2 tablespoons

Fats

Butter (but not margarine), the oils mentioned earlier in the chapter, and home-made mayonnaise (you will find a recipe in this book) are permitted in moderation.

Dairy Products

You may eat eggs, prepared however you like, but do not consume more than two per day, or more than six per week. A maximum of four teaspoons of heavy cream per day may be used in coffee. Cream is lower in carbohydrates than milk, which is not permitted. Cheese spreads, such as cream cheese, are initially not allowed. After Phase 1, cottage cheese is allowed, provided it is 1% low fat. Light and Lively is a good brand, but avoid the Weight Watcher's variety as it is high in sodium. After phase 1, four ounces of low-fat hard cheese is permitted per day.

Snacks and Appetizers

Low-fat cheese (see above), chicken drumsticks and wings, hard boiled or deviled eggs, meatballs (with no bread filler), smoked salmon, tuna, sardines, shrimp, steak tartar, raw vegetables, sugar- and carbo-hydrate-free jello, and chicken salad are examples of allowable snacks. Later in the diet nuts will be permitted.

High-Fat and High-Carbohydrate Foods

Foods that must be avoided include bananas, beans (except green or wax), bread and bread products (such as bread crumbs), cake, candy, cashews, catsup, cereal (all types), cookies, corn, cornstarch, corn sweeteners, crackers, dates, figs, white flour, dried fruit, honey, ice cream, frozen yogurt, jam, jelly, macaroni, pancakes, pasta, peas, potatoes, raisins, rice, sugar, sweet pickles and relish, sweetened any-thing, syrup (except artificially sweetened, low carbohydrate types), yams, and yogurt. This isn't a complete list, but these are among the worst offenders. For more information, consult the food chart. (Here you can notice the marriage of fats and carbohydrates. By reducing your sweet intake you will reduce your fat intake.)

Desserts

Diet gelatin. Make sure that the product you select has no carbohydrates. In later phases of the diet, Cool Whip, which contains less than 1 gram of carbohydrate, will be permitted on special occasions.

Sweeteners

Artificial sweeteners such as saccharine and NutraSweet are allowed, but it is recommended that you limit your consumption to no more than two packets per day. Also, make sure the brand you are using contains no more than 1 gram of carbohydrate. I am not an advocate of these sweeteners, as I believe that they may be hazardous to your health, but I believe that the body can handle moderate amounts of these substances better than it can refined sugar. Most important, using artificial sweeteners can help you overcome your sugar addiction permanently. I know that sugarless hard candy helped me with my cravings, because it satisfied my need for a sweet taste. My patients who use artificial sweeteners tend to find that they gradually reduce their intake of the substances. This is because artificial sweeteners, unlike sugar, are nonaddictive. These substances helped me break my addiction without feeling deprived. For children I recommend fructose substitutes like Frookies which offer a more natural and digestible dessert. Still, these products should be used sparingly—they're not health foods.

Gum

You may have up to three sticks of sugarless gum per day. I recommend one stick after each meal. Most of these gums contain 1 gram of carbohydrate.

Just how hard is it to follow this diet? I think I'll let one of my patients speak for me.

"I have only great things to say about Dr. Kaplan's diet. I lost 33 pounds and kept it off. I have tried every kind of diet, but this is one I can live with for life!"

Make the most of yourself, for that is all there is of you.
                                                    R.W. Emerson

13

Unlocking the Power Within

The last several chapters have dealt primarily with nutrition and weight loss principles. Now let's shift the emphasis from what goes into your stomach to what goes on in your head. Your attitude is extremely important in this program, for without the cooperation of your subconscious, your conscious mind will not be able to make a success of this diet—or any other undertaking.

This chapter is therefore designed to help you enlist the assistance of your subconscious. If we can master this often hidden but powerful part of our minds, we can unleash our stored potential.

The key to this process is autosuggestion, a technique which we use all the time, but frequently to our detriment. Whenever you tell yourself that you can't do something, your subconscious takes you seriously, and does everything in its power to sabotage your conscious efforts.

Many of these destructive thoughts originated in childhood, when adults scolded us for doing something "wrong." We became frightened, and made a decision not to take that kind of risk again. Now that we are adults ourselves, we often begin a project with negative expectations, thus ensuring failure before we even begin. If there is ever a way to eliminate destructive thoughts from entering our subconscious then success would always be within our grasp. If we can master this tool, failure would be a thing of the past.

I am asking you to put aside these thoughts of failure and lack, and replace them with positive, vital images. Use your imagination—it's more powerful than you may realize. Try this simple experiment. Close your eyes and picture a lemon. Imagine the sharp, citrus smell. Now imagine yourself biting into it; feel the tart, juicy pulp on your tongue.

Are you drooling yet? The lemon is not real, but your subconscious doesn't know that.

Now use that same power of imagination to picture yourself at your ideal weight. Your imagination is the tool that carves the way. Imagine yourself buying clothes two sizes smaller, admire your new reflection in the mirror. Hear yourself telling your friends that you've never looked or felt better. Say it out loud.

Write down your favorite goals and affirmations and place them where you will see them frequently—the bathroom mirror is a good spot. Say your affirmations frequently and with conviction, until you make them a part of yourself.

Now create an image of what success means to you, and then write down the attributes needed to make this image a reality. Do your ideas differ from those you held before you started this book? Now take your image further, to the outer limits of what you believe possible. See yourself not where you are, but where you want to be. Imagine what it would be like to have no limitations in life. Think of how far you could go if you knew that your past could not hold you back. Now realize that these images can become tangible, that the only limitations you have are those which you placed on yourself.

I know from personal experience that this is true. You are reading one of my dreams right now. I had a great desire to become a writer, and I used affirmations, imagery and the other techniques I am sharing with you to help myself realize this dream.

Perhaps you are telling yourself that I started out with certain advantages, an education, for example. Well, my education was also once only an idea, and in any case I had no formal training in writing. And what is true for me is true for everyone who ever lived. Successful men and women enter the world as naked babies; they do not leave the womb wearing a three-piece suit or reading *The Wall Street Journal*. They learned the secrets of success and—just as important—used them in their own lives.

Whatever you desire you can acquire. Don't let obstacles get in your way—use them as stepping stones to success. And don't promise yourself that you will "try" to reach your goals, because that attitude will only hinder you. In the successful movie *The Empires Strikes Back,* Yoda, the Jedi teacher, explains to Luke Skywalker how to use the Force, the greatest power in the universe. He says to his prize student, "Luke, there is no try, there is either do or not do."

If faith can move mountains, it can also enable you to scale a mountain. Don't be afraid to aim for the top, or be tempted to rest on a comfortable plateau. Maybe weight loss is your mountain; don't hesitate to go for it. Dr Kaplan's Low-Stress High-Energy Diet works if you are willing to work with it.

You are an infinite source of energy, so there is no reason for you to settle for a limited existence. Give of yourself in any way imaginable. Life will become something that you experience, rather than something that you have become a passenger in. You can follow a rainbow that never ends, but leads to an infinite combination of colors that culminate in one bright light.

Your dreams are not illusions, but your fears are. In the phrase made famous by Franklin Delanor Roosevelt, "We have nothing to fear but fear itself." In *Think And Grow Rich,* Napoleon Hill claimed, "Confront your fears and you can make them disappear." It's true. Our fears of failure are especially destructive and unnecessary.

Napoleon Hill interviewed Thomas Alva Edison, who provided an enlightening perspective on what most of us call "failure."

Hill asked the great inventor, "Mr. Edison, what have you got to say about the fact that you've failed thousands of times in your attempts to create the light bulb?" Edison replied, "I beg your pardon. I've never failed even once. I've had thousands of learning experiments that didn't work. I had to run through enough learning experiments to find a way that did work."[1]

I am sure that we have all felt the fear of failure one time in our life. What begins with a conservative attitude of playing it safe soon enlarges within itself to become a total obsession with fear and failure. By focusing on our successes and not on our fears with the aid of imagination one can overcome these hurdles in one fell swoop. Think of what you are most afraid of. Picture it until you can feel the emotions. Are you experiencing anxiety? Good. Now push that picture aside and imagine yourself in the same situation, but triumphing over your fears. It feels different, doesn't it? You create your own emotional responses, so why not create the ones that are most pleasant?

I should note that "success" is not a selfish enterprise. We must still reach out to others, to give as well as take. And you will find that the more you give, the more others give to you.

In order to achieve our goals we need to develop certain qualities. Great men and women have common traits, and it makes sense to model ourselves on individuals who have accomplished what they set out to do.

Leadership Qualities

People who are successful in business and in life are leaders rather than followers. Leadership is a quality made up of a number of attributes, including:

1. Courage

2. Self-control

3. A sense of right and wrong

4. Decisiveness

5. Giving more than necessary

6. A pleasing personality

7. Sympathy and understanding

8. Willingness to accept responsibility

9. Attention to detail

10. A spirit of cooperation

Consider how prominent these attributes are in your own life. Maybe you would like to eat a candy bar. If you lack self-control, chances are you will eat that candy bar. But if you are willing to deny yourself a small, transitory pleasure, you will eventually achieve enormous, long-lasting satisfaction.

Leaders take action. My goal is to help you turn positive thinking into positive doing. Don't wait until tomorrow; take action steps **now!**

> Don't wait until conditions are perfect. They never are.

> Expect difficulties, and then use your creativity to overcome them.

> Don't be stopped by past failures. Today is the first day of the rest of your life.

> Plan your life and live your plan.

> Set goals.

> Determine how you will reach those goals.

> Use your affirmations, visualization, and other techniques discussed in this book.

Perseverence

The secret to perseverance is persistence. This may sound like circular reasoning, but the fact is that successful people refuse to succumb to setbacks. They put themselves on the line for their dreams, and they do it over and over again. They know that they must take risks and that there are no guarantees, but they also know that they have more to gain than they have to lose. People who are successful are people who dare to be successful.

In life we have the doers and the talkers. Talkers are usually characterized by their lack of enthusiasm, their lack of commitment to their work, their lives and themselves.

Doers, by definition, are the people who get things done. Talkers nourish every failure until it becomes powerful enough to overcome their hopes of success. Doers learn from their failures, then let them go. Talkers spend a lot of time wishing that things were different. Doers make them different. Nothing in this world is for free. Success takes work. But then, so does failure. If you want to be one of the doers instead of one of the talkers, you must develop certain characteristics.

Willpower—By focusing on your goals instead of your distractions, you will be able to persevere in the face of obstacles and temptations. Use your imagination to see yourself as you want to be, and you will also develop your willpower.

Self-esteem—Understand that you are in control of your destiny, and not vice versa. This belief provides you with the courage to follow through on your plans.

Purpose—Vague ideas bring vague results. You must know why you are here, what you want, and what you are willing to do to achieve it.

Answer the following questions to see where you rate on the Purpose Scale:

A. Do you fail to clearly define your goals? Do you procrastinate?

B. Do you waiver when making decisions?

C. Do you settle for second best?

D. Do you care who you are?

E. Do you blame others for your mistakes rather than accept responsibility for them?

F. Are your desires weak, shallow, and lifeless?

G. Are you motivated to achieve your goals?

H. Do you quit at the first sign of defeat?

I. Do you have specific plans for your success?

J. Do you wish for things to happen rather than make them happen?

K. Do you lack ambition?

L. Do you look for short cuts?

M. Are you stopped by criticism?

If your answers don't satisfy you, then you need to work on the areas in which you are weak. Don't just do the minimum. **Go the extra mile!** In order to succeed in anything, you must give it all you have, and then give some more. This is as true for a diet as it is for a business plan. My formula will work, provided you bring to it the necessary commitment and perseverance.

Keep in mind that you have nothing to lose but your past history of failure. There are risks in this approach, but there are far greater risks involved in doing nothing. And there are no rewards involved when you do nothing, but ask anyone who has ever persisted in reaching a goal whether the effort was worth it.

Yes, there may be times when you feel discouraged. This is a normal emotion, not your enemy. Through these times of emotional weakness, look to your allies. Through discipline, controlling your emotions, stating your affirmations, and utilizing your imagination, you will shed pounds and thus will increase your success level. Allow your awareness and desire to become a result rather than a mere image. Look to yourself for courage and look to others for additional help. We are all here to help each other in loving and sharing. What better success could there be than the offering of these to another?

The highest reward for a man's toil is not what he gets for it, but what he becomes of it.

John Ruskin

14

Health Food Phenomenon

Have you ever wondered why supermarkets, which seem to stock just about everything from gourmet coffee to microwave dinners, tend to have only one small aisle for what they call "health foods?" I may be naive, but it seems to me that all foods should be "health foods"—i.e., good for you. And if we label certain foods as health foods, it stands to reason that everything else is unhealthy. Which unfortunately is not far from the truth.

I suppose my diet could be called a "health" diet, since it enables you not only to lose weight, but to eat nutritiously. It is a comprehensive plan providing all of the necessary food groups.

As I mentioned, one of the staples of this diet is protein, which comes from a Greek word that translates as "of prime importance." After water, protein is the most abundant substance in the body and it is the building blocks of cells. The government R.D.A. (recommended daily allowance) for protein is eight tenths of a gram per kilogram of body weight. For example, a 150 pound person (approximately 68 kilograms) requires 54 grams of protein per day. When you consider that one ounce of red meat contains 7 grams of protein and a cup of skim milk has 8 grams, you can see that it takes a fair amount of this food to meet the R.D.A.

However, guidelines are just that. Individual needs for protein and other nutrients vary greatly. Proteins are digested with the help of the enzyme pepsin, which functions best in the presence of hydrochloric acid. Some of us produce ten times as much of this substance as others; some people produce virtually none at all. These variations explain why some people are satisfied with as little as 4 ounces of protein a day, while others might need 20 ounces.

This is also true of amino acids, which are the building blocks of protein. One person might require 100 mg of arginine, for example, while another needs 500 mg daily.

The same individual variation principle holds true for your critical carbohydrate level. Dr. Carlton Fredericks has stated that the critical carbohydrate level could be 60 mg daily, while Dr. Atkins recommends keeping it at 40 mg per day. To determine *your* critical carbohydrate level, use ketostix.

Your limits may be very different from someone else's. The insulin-producing islets in the pancreas vary tremendously from person to person. Some individuals have as many as 1,000,000, while others have as few as 100,000. It is because of this difference that the ability to handle sugars and starches varies so radically. The person with a minimal number of islets will produce less insulin, and therefore is more easily overtaxed by sugar consumption.

After years of being challenged by excessive sugar intake, the pancreas can become overactive, burning sugar so rapidly that the brain and the nervous system become starved for fuel. This condition is known as hypoglycemia, or low blood sugar. When the abused pancreas is finally exhausted, the hypoglycemia is replaced by the disorder known as diabetes. We now know that hypoglycemia is the precursor of diabetes. It has also been determined that people who have difficulty utilizing sugar can develop blood chemistry changes that lead to atherosclerosis, better known as hardening of the arteries. Where do all these problems begin? They begin with breakfast.

The all-too-typical American breakfast consists of coffee, with which we wash down danish pastries, cookies, doughnuts and white bread in all its guises—toast, rolls, bagels, etc. We start off our day with foods that are denatured, overprocessed, oversalted, oversweetened, overconcentrated, overcooked, overrated, scraped, and denuded of all natural vitamins and minerals. Many parents believe that they start their children off with a good breakfast. However, by "good" they mean "cereal" in a form that is refined, processed, and high in sugar and carbohydrates. Dr. Carlton Fredericks had a few things to say about this breakfast staple.

"If you were in the habit of feeding a family the average packaged cold breakfast cereal, you should be interested in the following account of a visit to one of this country's celebrated breakfast food factories. Although the cereal described here is Corn Flakes, the procedure is essentially the same for all cold cereals not specifically labeled (whole grain). First I saw machinery removing the outer coat, then the germ (in other words, the life) then corn. This, my guide explained, was to prevent their corn flakes from 'rancidity and spoilage.' He said they sent the discarded husks to 'fox farms and other places where they feed animals.' What was left of the corn at this point was an unlifelike powder as befits any corpse. Masses of this corpse-like substance (I refuse to call it corn) were put in large pressure cookers, heated to a temperature of 250 degrees and held at that temperature for 2 1/2 hours when it was ready to be mixed with artificial flavoring and coloring to make it look and taste like the corpse it really was. The entire mass was then cooled until it reached the stage at which it was ready to be run through machines to flake it. At this point it began a journey on endless belts that passed through heaters where it reached a temperature of 450 Healthdegrees, thus assuring loss or deterioration of nutritional elements that might have survived up to this point. The process set the flakes to prevent them from sticking together. Now it was ready for packaging in wax paper lined cartons. This, said the guide, would keep their product 'as fresh as a daisy.' The factory was sending out 65 car loads of this foodless pack and other breakfast foods everyday to be eaten by human beings. A tank car full of corn germ oil left every month for the pharmaceutical houses the little foxes got the rest of it."[1]

Despite all the concern over "lifestyle" disorders such as heart disease, there is evidence that few of us are watching what we eat. A Lewis Poll conducted for *Prevention* magazine revealed that 42% of those surveyed try hard to limit high cholesterol foods, down from 46% the previous year. Only 54%, down from 57%, indicated that they try to limit their salt intake. Also, 54% try to avoid fat, compared to 56% the previous year, while only 59% (down from 63%) attempt to make sure they get enough vitamins and minerals. As Thomas Duybdahl of *Prevention* noted, "People know more about nutrition now than ever, but they are not acting on what they know."

The frustration here lies in the nearsightedness of every facet of the health fraternity. Statistics show our concern for fats and cholesterol. The sugar problem remains intellectually ignored. As we have decreased our fat consumption, we have increased our sugar consumption (as have our children). There is a sugar-cholesterol connection. Until we sever this tie we will continue to bully fat alone, ignoring one of the leaders of this vicious gang, **sugar.** Sugar is a prime culprit of poor health. Sugar lowers our discipline, weakens our tissue and intoxifies our brain. Yet it comes in so many disguises. This is not a low-carbohydrate diet, nor a low-fat diet. This is a no-*sugar* diet. Any diet that allows sugar would be both frustrating and ineffective. Over time it will slowly and silently alter your blood chemistry. This will result in continued cravings for sugar or refined carbohydrates. You will put back the unwanted pounds. Sugar is the real "silent killer."

One day a new patient, Mrs. M., told me of her frustration with cholesterol problems. "Dr. Kaplan, I eat no eggs, no fats, no cholesterol-rich foods. However, yesterday my blood results came back and my cholesterol was 260." I asked her if she ate a lot of sweets. She said, "Well, I do like a good dessert. Yes, I guess so."

Why, with all the information we have available to us, are people continuing to eat so poorly? Is it ignorance? Confusion? Or is it simple frustration that stems from the inability to readily find wholesome, natural foods? So many of our foods are loaded with preservatives and chemicals that have been linked with cancer in laboratory animals. Our water is polluted, our meats are dosed with hormones, our chickens are fed on antibiotics, our fish have been contaminated with mercury. Our fruits and vegetables are dusted with pesticides. Even "pure" maple syrup has been known to contain formaldehyde. Today, Europe will no longer import our meats because of all the hormones, etc., found in them. Many patients report weight loss on their visits, I wonder could the hormones we use to fatten our animals fatten us? Think about it. We consume frozen and packaged foods that contain nothing but calories, and drink beverages that are nothing but a cocktail of chemicals, caffeine, and sugar. No wonder manufacturers of remedies for headache, stomachache, heartburn, and indigestion are so eager to purchase advertising time.

Our menus have not become holistic, they have become futuristic. Our menus are now chemicalized, bringing us an assortment of thousands of food additives, brought to us at such a fast level it is almost impossible for the average nutritionist to keep up with each and every one of them. Our diet is predicated upon habit, conditioning, folklore, advertising, impulse, mood, price, convenience, myth, desire, quantity, taking little into account the nutritional values and quality. And we ask ourselves, are we self-destructive? There really is no set answer to this question: Is this a good diet? For each of us as individuals develop individual needs. Therefore, you must know a great deal about your individual self and what foods your body can tolerate and what you have an intolerance toward.

Given all the unnatural substances we expect our bodies to cope with, it is no wonder that so many of us suffer from food allergies. The human body was not designed to ingest these chemicals, and it responds by producing the unpleasant symptoms we know as allergies. (An excellent book on this subject is *The Food Depression Connection* by June Roth.)

It is also important to realize that some people have a true allergy to sugar and refined carbohydrates. Yet in the course of my studies on allergies, I don't recall mention of this widespread condition. A primary symptom of carbohydrate allergy is being overweight. For these people, indulgence in carbohydrates results in overproduction of insulin, resulting in a lowering of the blood sugar, which creates an array of symptoms, including a craving for the very substance to which they are allergic. The person who is allergic to sugar and refined carbohydrates is no different than the person who sneezes in the presence of a dog, or breaks out in a rash when wearing a wool jacket. If this allergy goes undetected, the result, as I mentioned earlier, may be diabetes. Do you have to develop this disease in order to realize that you are sugar and refined carbohydrate intolerant?

As a child I was brought up with a pet, and I have known numerous people that have pets, it is amazing that we have the knowledge not to feed sugar to our animals. Sure we can feed them dog food, cat food, etc., which contains more additives and artifacts than is probably known to the average chemical lab. Yet, our simple knowledge of life, health, and sugar dictates to us not to offer this vile substance (sugar) to our animals. We must face the facts that some of us are better and more protective of our animals than we are to ourselves and to our children.

I frequently implore my patients not to dig their own graves with a knife and fork. If we listen to our innate intelligence, we will not ingest foods that are harmful to us. I urge you to tell your physician, family and friends that you are now going to change your eating habits for the better. Enlist their support, but remember that you are the final judge of your own well-being.

As a teenager, I was a smoker. The little voice in my head frequently reminded me that this was a harmful habit. When I didn't listen, I developed a chronic cough and other irritating symptoms. When I finally quit, not only did my health improve, my self-esteem soared. I was beginning to understand that my mind controls my body and not vice versa.

You can also decide to improve your life. A good place to start is with your shopping list. The next time you go to the supermarket, follow these eleven guidelines:

1. Read the labels very, very carefully.

2. Purchase only complex carbohydrates.

3. Be on the lookout for high sodium content. The names this substance goes under include sodium chloride, monosodium glutamate, baking soda, baking powder, sodium, and, of course, salt. If you are especially fond of salty foods, you should be aware that researchers at the University of Pennsylvania found that long-term reduction of this substance alters the taste for salt.

4. Avoid chemical additives. Canned goods, processed meat, many types of sausage, bacon, cold cuts, hot dogs, lunch spreads,dry cereals, soft drinks, packaged desserts, and precooked foods are likely to contain numerous additives. Even meats marked Grade A are no longer additive free. The Food and Drug Administration has reported that nearly 80% of

our meat comes from animals fed with tetracycline or other antibiotics

5. Don't plan on frying your foods. I recommend poaching, broiling, baking, roasting, steaming, or barbecuing.

6. Make your own salad dressing, using olive oil, apple cider vinegar, and an assortment of natural spices.

7. Select whole grain foods. Oatmeal made from rolled oats (please skip the instant) is probably higher in protein than any other grain. The rolling of the oats is probably the least damaging method of grain processing.

8. Learn the many names of sugar. Leave on the shelf foods containing corn syrup, fructose, sucrose, glucose, lactose, maltose, molasses, and maple syrup.

9. Assume nothing. Foods that you least suspect of containing sugar may be loaded with it. Peanut butter is a prime example. Although you can purchase the natural kind, the type you find in the supermarket is likely to be very high in sugar. Other products that have a great amount of sugar include cranberry juice, mayonnaise, catsup, spaghetti sauce and soup.

10. Wash your food carefully. I recommend scrubbing fruits, meats and vegetables before consuming them. This way we get more of the vitamins and less of the pesticides.

11. Remember that your diet begins in the supermarket. You can't eat what you don't buy.

This last point is very important, for our food shopping habits can have a significant impact on our health. With 50% of all Americans at risk for heart disease, diabetes, hypertension, and cancer, it makes sense to shop with care. The link between food intake and health has been well established.

"In 1977, George McGovern headed a congressional committee that investigated the American diet. The McGovern committee studied the relationship between this diet and the nation's major killers, heart disease, cancers of the colon and breast, stroke, high blood pressure, obesity, diabetes, arteriosclerosis, and cirrhosis of the liver. They estimated that if the Americans modified their rich diets there would be an 80% drop in the number of obese people, a 25% drop in deaths from heart disease, a 50% drop in deaths from diabetes, and 1% annual increase in longevity."[2]

At this point, we've pretty well covered the nutrition destroyers: processing, refining, contaminants, etc. In the next chapters I'll discuss the nutrition enhancers—vitamins. These substances can help our bodies overcome the toxins provided by so many of our "foods." Vitamins can help us put more vitality into our diets. Vitamins can add years to our lives and life to our years.

Why not go out on a limb? Isn't that where the fruit is?
                                                                    Frank Scully

15

Vitamania

On September 22, 1997, a cover story in *USA Today* stated, "Why Can't Doctors Just Say NO!" It was subtitled, "An Increasingly Drug Dependent America." Total prescriptions for some drugs in 1996: antibiotics—282,631,000; tranquilizers and anti-anxiety—76,370,000; sleeping pills and sedatives—23,681,000; anti-obesity—23,596,000. It is time we followed our neighbors. We have a choice, a natural choice, called vitamins.

Stuart Berger, M.D., author of *How To Be Your Own Nutritionist,* has recommended that people not become the patients of doctors who do not believe in or have knowledge of vitamins and nutrition. I am 100% in agreement with this advice. Vitamins are vital to our health and well-being, and are an essential element in my diet.

To my patients and peers, who frequently ask questions such as, "Are supplement users healthier than nonusers?" and "Do vitamins really work?" my answer is a resounding "Yes." Then there are those who insist that, "My medical doctor (or my other chiropractor, osteopath, dermatologist, or podiatrist) doesn't believe in vitamins." My response to these individuals is, "Then have your doctor give you his or her evidence in support of this theory."

There is abundant evidence that generous intake of vitamins, minerals and other nutrients aid the body in protecting itself against numerous disorders, including osteoporosis, cancer, heart disease, hypertension, insomnia, irritability, and a host of other ills.

Vitamins are health enhancers. They provide us with the edge we need to fight back against the hazards of such harmful substances as sugar, pesticides, antibiotics, food coloring, nitrites, nitrates, hormones, and preservatives.

Consider all the people who take vitamin and mineral supplements. Are they doing it because they don't always eat right? Because they believe supplements help them to remain healthy? Because they think that there are not sufficient nutrients in food? Because they believe that supplements help them to feel better and more energetic? According to a 1982 *Good Housekeeping* survey it is all of the above.

Let me emphasize that vitamins are not intended to replace a balanced diet, but to supplement it. Nor should vitamins be confused with medicine. They are derived from food sources, and are a concentrated form of the nutrients we require.

Our food itself should provide us with these nutrients, but the refining process has stripped many of our foods of their goodness.

Often, upon advising a patient with a cold to take vitamin C, I've been told, "Doc, I drink plenty of orange juice." Unfortunately, the orange juice they drink has been cooked, processed and pasteurized, to the point where the nutrients have been drastically reduced.

Ten years ago, few doctors, if any prescribed vitamins. Then the drug industry caught wind of this new wave. A health wave that could generate millions of dollars. The travesty of what they did is no different than that of bread. Instead of keeping bread in its whole form, its pure form, they refined it. They refined it until it reached its simplest level—white bread. This wasn't the good whole wheat bread that grandma made on the farm. This same drug industry utilized this concept with vitamins, they refined, then synthetically produced them. The drug industry turned a natural supplement into a chemical concoction.

Vitamins in their purest form are derived from food, or natural sources. The purest form of vitamins should be those produced from their most natural state.

Europe does double blind studies to prove their efficacy. Their insurance pays for vitamins, but most U.S. providers don't.

Some diseases resulting from vitamin deficiencies, such as scurvy, produce dramatic symptoms. But how many people go to their doctors looking for help with vague yet distressing maladies? The physician dutifully orders a full battery of tests, only to inform the patient that the results are negative and the cause of the symptoms still unknown. I've had numerous patients say to me, "Dr. Kaplan, I've been everywhere. No one has been able to find my problem. No one has been able to help me."

In many cases, these patients are helped by proper nutrition and supplement use. This is because the problem can often be traced to a marginal, or subclinical, deficiency which may not show up on a conventional test. Yet the symptoms these deficiencies cause are very real. According to nutrition expert D.I. Thurnham, "Marginal vitamin deficiencies may have different effects on the body's metabolism which depends on the stage of life and demands facing its normal development. Growth restrictions, degenerative changes in tissues, fetal abnormalities, interference with milk production or composition, increased susceptibility to infection, altered response to dietary constituents, diminished work ability are among the possible effects of chronic marginal restrictions in the diet.

"These deficiencies don't develop suddenly; bad health, like good health, is a cumulative process.

"Certainly you cannot assume that a person who isn't getting his recommended dietary allowance (RDA) of a specific nutrient is in a state of marginal depletion, since it takes time for such a state to occur. But it is clear that the diets of large segments of the population are not meeting the RDA for certain vitamins and minerals. And such nutritional shortfalls can eventually lead to marginal status."[1]

The results of a survey reported in the *Journal of the American Dietetic Association* indicated that less than 60% of dietitians and only 47 to 54% of other Americans use nutritional supplements. Survey co-author Bonnie Worthington-Roberts, Ph.D., noted that,

"The attitude of 20 years ago, 'if you eat right you don't need dietary supplements,' still prevails among most, but some dietitians today recognize that they themselves don't always get what they need, especially if they are dieting."[2]

I was taught by Dr. Donald Gutstein, a mentor during my student days, "never to treat a person as a people."

In other words, no two individuals are exactly the same, and this must be taken into account when prescribing anything, including vitamins.

I believe that everyone can benefit from taking supplements. Especially children.

As the father of two perfect children, I am naturally concerned with their nutritional habits and energy levels. I am also, as every parent must be, a realist. As Linden Smith, M.D., pediatrician and author of *Dr. Smith's Diet Plan For Teenagers* and *Feed Your Kids Right,* has noted,

"Everyone who has any kids knows that they don't eat right everyday. Even though we'd like them to, it's unrealistic to expect it. You should look at the overall diet. It is okay if your child doesn't get the RDA every day, is he getting it every week?"

A study conducted at the University of Washington, Seattle, and reported in *The Journal of the American Dietetic Association* found some problems in the nutrient levels of a group of healthy children aged 3 1/2 to 9. While certain nutrient levels were adequate, some of the children showed intakes below 70% for folate and B-6.

Dr. Smith noted that zinc, a trace element that aids normal growth, tends to be low in the average child's diet. "But it's iron more than any other nutrient that is most commonly in short supply."[3]

Dr. Smith is not alone in this opinion. Alvin N. Eden, M.D., a pediatrician and associate clinical professor of pediatrics at the State University of New York Downstate Medical Center says,

"Iron is a very neglected area. I think there is a large group of children out there who are iron deficient without being anemic. For this reason I think it is important for parents to consider giving their children an iron supplement. In fact, the most important thing I tell parents is to think iron."[4]

As a parent, you must consider an all too common scenario: Vitamin-deficient boy meets vitamin-deficient girl; they fall in love, marry, and inevitably produce a vitamin-deficient child.

Dr. Smith strongly suggests giving children multivitamin supplements— "for insurance, not as a food substitute. It is good to remember that the RDA is only a *minimum* and an *estimate* at that." He also reminds us: "And keep in mind that every child is different. How each person absorbs nutrients and their degree of wellness can vary." Sound familiar?

Some people may need additional supplements if they are at risk for certain degenerative diseases. If you have a tendency toward osteoporosis, for example, common sense tells you that you require more than the bare minimum of calcium. If I were at risk for this condition, I'd want to take the maximum daily requirement.

A person who does not get sufficient vitamins from childhood on can develop subtle, but ultimately profound, health problems. According to Dr. David Ostreicherdds, professor of nutrition at Bridgeport University,

"If you are not getting enough vitamins A and C you might not know until 20 years later when you develop cancer. If you are eating a diet high in saturated fats and salt, the staples of most convenience foods, you might not know until you've had your first heart attack at age 50."[5]

Diet is something that surrounds us, food is something that consumes us. The same people that make the decisions that rule this country are ruled by a chemical environment that may be deficient. James S. Goodwin, M.D., and his colleagues at the University of New Mexico School of Medicine have investigated the possibility that marginal deficiencies can impair the thinking of men and women 60 and older. "We know that institutionalized elderly people have been shown to improve mentally when supplemented with vitamins."[6]

Furthermore, Douglas Hineberger, M.D., an expert on the nutritional needs of hospitalized patients, says that nutritional deficiencies can dramatically affect the well-being of elderly patients.

"Vitamin A and C are important in wound healing, especially from patients recovering from surgery. Lung and urinary tract infections are common in the elderly and it is possible that vitamin C would have a role here. For instance, C plays a part in the function of white blood cells (scavenger cells) and also acidifies the urine to inhibit infection in the bladder.

"Finding deficiency is most implicated in decreased mental capacity often seen in nursing home residents. The confusion and meandering thoughts in the elderly are frequently attributed to Alzheimer's Disease or the effects of just sitting around all day but it can also be caused by a thiamin deficiency."[7]

Women also have special needs that may not be met by a conventional diet. According to the National Academy of Sciences, "Iron is one nutrient that women need more than men, and that menstruating women require almost twice as much iron as men (18 mg compared to 10 mg) and pregnant women, they need 30-60 mg of iron each day."[8]

Cecilia Davis, former president of the Nationwide Dietitian's Referral Service, notes that, "Women absorb only about 6 mg of iron per 1,000 calories of food in a typical diet. They would need to eat about 3,000 calories a day to meet their iron RDA. If you eat that much so many women need supplemental iron." Dr. Davis contends that teenage girls are in even worse shape. "I'd say 80% could be iron deficient. Some eat as few as 1,000 calories a day and their food preferences are poor in iron."[9]

Then there are athletes, who demand far more from their bodies than the average person. Dr. Paul Zabetakis, a research physician at the Institute of Sports Medicine and Athletic Trauma in New York, says that, "Both men and women may sometimes become iron depleted during strenuous athletic training."[10]

The adage about an ounce of prevention being worth a pound of cure has never been more true than it is today. People are beginning to understand that it is far more economical, not only financially, but emotionally as well, to preserve their health rather than cure disease. In a recent study, investigators found that, of the people examined, 62% of those who did not take vitamins suffered from some deficiency. But only 10% of those who used supplements were found to have deficiencies.

I do not claim that vitamins alone can keep an individual free of disease. Many factors, especially proper nutrition, positive mental attitude, proper nerve supply, and appropriate exercise, are required if we are to become healthy. Vitamins help to keep us on the right road.

One of the questions I hear most frequently is, "How do I choose a multivitamin?" It's no wonder that people are confused. The average grocery store offers shelves of vitamins, ranging from chewable Flintstones to multicolored "megavitamins." Then of course we have the single vitamins, A, B complex, C, E, etc.

My own preference is to take one pill rather than several separate vitamins. One-A-Day is the right slogan, it just belongs to the wrong pill. Choosing the multiple vitamin that is right for you requires comparison shopping. Read the labels and compare the nutrients in the capsule with the U.S. Recommended Daily Allowances (review the table in the back of the book).

Your objective is a multiple vitamin that contains at least 100% of all the RDAs. It is important to realize that some vitamin manufacturers add inadequate amounts of certain nutrients just so they can put them on the label. Select a multiple vitamin and mineral supplement that contains sufficient amounts of calcium, magnesium, and the B-complex vitamins. I also recommend that you purchase natural vitamins, not the processed or refined type. The best vitamins, as I said, are those derived from natural sources. Because the chemically produced vitamins are cheaper to produce, they are cheaper to buy. But it does not pay to pinch pennies when it comes to your health.

Most important, don't be fooled by appearances. I have a favorite story that illustrates this point.

Moses and Jesus Christ were on the first tee when an old man walked over and asked if he could join their golf game. Moses and Jesus smiled at each other, then assured the man that he was welcome to play.

Moses hit the ball first. His ball went toward the water hazard, but the waters parted before the ball could get wet, and it hit the now dry surface and rolled onto the green.

Jesus smiled at Moses and said, "Nice shot." Then he stepped up to the tee and struck his first ball. Once again, the ball landed in the water hazard, but instead of dropping to the depths, the ball walked across the water until it reached the green.

Now Moses complimented Jesus. "Nice shot," he said.

Finally, it was the old man's turn. He approached the tee, and swung at the ball with all his might. But he barely grazed it and it just dribbled off the tee.

Moses and Jesus exchanged a smile. Then, a squirrel appeared. It picked up the ball in its mouth and proceeded to run down the fairway. Suddenly, a giant bird plunged from the sky and picked up the squirrel. Then a roar of thunder came forth, and a bolt of lightning shot from the sky, striking the bird. The bird screamed in pain, dropping the squirrel to the ground. Upon impact, the squirrel spit out the ball, which landed at the very edge of the hole. Finally, a great gust of wind came from nowhere, and gently directed the ball into the hole.

Moses looked at Jesus, and Jesus looked at the old man and said, "Nice shot, DAD."

Because food is the ultimate source of vitamins, it is important to get the most from what you eat. Overeating is not the way to do this. Karen Pinto, Ph.D., assistant professor of nutrition and medicine at Cornell University Medical College, says,

"If you stop and think how some people eat a large amount of proteins and carbohydrates at one meal, they really swamp their systems with this influx of nutrients all at one time, and many of those nutrients won't be absorbed. That's because it's easier for the gastrointestinal tract to absorb nutrients from small amounts of food over a small period of time."[11]

And what you eat is as important as how you eat. A 20-year, ongoing Japanese study, one of the largest of its kind, has found that people who eat green and/or yellow vegetables every day have a decreased risk of lung, stomach and other cancers. This study also indicates that the damage caused by bad habits, such as spurning vegetables or smoking, for example, is reversible. Former smokers who eat their green and yellow vegetables on a daily basis also experienced a reduction in lung cancer risk, and there was more than a 25% reduction in the number of deaths from stomach cancers.[12]

In addition, a Harvard study of more than 1,200 elderly masters residents found that those who report the highest consumption of carrots, squash, tomatoes, salads or leafy greens, dried fruits, fresh strawberries, or melon, broccoli or brussels sprouts had a decreased risk of cancer.[13] These foods all contain vitamin A, which is known to fight disorders ranging from cancer to stress.[14]

Eli Seifter, Ph.D., professor of biochemistry and surgery at Albert Einstein College of Medicine, New York, says that,

"Cancer and cancer therapy are very stressful to the body, and those very stresses promote cancer growth. The result is an increased breakdown of body tissue, weight loss, a suppressed immune system and an increased production of hormones, such as adrenaline, which are associated with stress."

Dr. Seifter found that vitamin A reduced the physical symptoms of stress in mice who were stressed through partial body restraint. "It shrank the size of the stretched enlarged adrenal gland and enlarged the thymus otherwise shrunk by stress," he reported. Dr. Seifter believes that stress reduction can give cancer patients a real edge in fighting their disease.[15]

We spend so much energy searching for the perfect drug that we have forgotten the perfect plant form which remedies are derived. Digitalis, once used widely as a heart medicine, is derived from the herb foxglove. Penicillin is extracted from mold. And the list goes on and on. Why reinvent the round wheel? My friend Andy Brock owns a real estate company named KISS, after the famous acronym Keep It Simple Stupid. Don't look for a magic potion, just stick with the basics—sound nutrition and adequate supplementation. Understand that health comes from within, and work with the body's natural healing powers. Vitamins can support us in remaining healthy and in losing weight.

Nutrition in the '90s is being influenced by a convergence of trends in health care. Business, government and consumer driven trends are moving us from a sickness care system to one of wellness care. Vitamins have been used in the sickness model for many years, primarily to treat the symptoms of sickness diagnosed by a physician. The wellness model is based on a proactive philosophy utilizing nutrition and other methods to stay well.

The vitamin revelation of this decade is found in antioxidant formulas. Antioxidants are linked to their possible role in slowing down the aging process, reducing risks of heart disease and certain cancers, while assisting the body in combating the effects of environmental and nutritional pollution.

Prominent doctors, scientists and researchers have clearly demonstrated antioxidants ability to search out toxic materials known as "free radicals" in the body and neutralize their harmful effects. By removing these toxic "free radicals" we maintain happier, healthier cells.

One fine company that has positioned itself as a leader in nutrition is Douglas Laboratories in Pittsburgh, PA. Since vitamins are not regulated in our country, the quality of the supplement is vital. Douglas Laboratories meets and often exceeds USP standards, has its 100,000 sq. ft. Facilities inspected by the F.D.A., and is approved as a nutritional supplement manufacturer by the Canadian Health Organization and the Commission of the European Communities.

Douglas Laboratories provides the supplements for many of my offices as well as my own family. Many of the celebrities who have endorsed my book utilize their products also. Douglas has thousands of doctors nationally who integrate their product line into their practices. Supplements should be doctor supervised, and Douglas' doctors are continually updated on all nutritional trends. For a doctor in your area, call Douglas Laboratories at 1-888-Doug-Lab (368-4522).

The evidence indicates that the value of vitamins is no longer a matter for debate. Vitamins have been found to increase our productivity and energy levels. Vitamins are giving us stronger, healthier children, a natural means to combat disease, and a weapon against aging. What magic potion could do more?

I will study and get ready and perhaps my chance will come.
                                                    Abraham Lincoln

16

The Vitamin Alphabet Health's ABC's

In my opinion, a well-educated patient is more likely to be a healthy patient. Since vitamins are an essential part of your diet, I feel that you should have an idea of the what these supplements can do for you and which foods are the richest sources of these nutrients.

Vitamin A

1. Helps counteract night blindness

2. Assists your immune system

3. Builds resistance to respiratory infections

4. Helps promote healthy skin

5. Helps reduce age spots

6. Assists in the treatment of acne, impetigo, boils, carbuncles, and open ulcers when applied externally

7. Helps promote the growth of:
   A. Skin
   B. Strong bones
   C. Hair
   D. Teeth
   E. Gums

The standard daily dose of this vitamin is 10,000 to 25,000 units. Consult a physician before taking doses over 25,000 units.

It is important not to become deficient in this vitamin.

"Dr. John B. Bieri, of the National Institute of Health, Biochemist said that vitamin A deficiency is probably the most common world wide vitamin problem. Some studies indicate that as much as 30% of the population had below average concentrations of vitamin A. Vitamin A is essential to normal growth and to the health of the mucus membranes of the skin. It is necessary to prevent night blindness. In this regard its dosage can be regulated."[1]

"Dr. Eli Seifter has described vitamin A as a powerful agent against viruses, greatly enhancing the body's immune response."[2]

The best source of this vitamin is beta-carotene, which is actually a vitamin A precursor. While vitamin A itself can be toxic if taken in dosages greater than 50,000 I.U., beta- carotene has no known toxicity. As Frank L. Meyskens, Jr., M.D., of the Larry Smith Cancer Center of the University of Arizona, points out, "With an overdose of Beta-carotene, on the other hand, all you do is turn yellow."[3]

Best Food Sources Of Beta-Carotene (Vitamin A)

FOOD	Portion	Vitamin A (I.U.)
Apricots	1	24,877
Asparagus, cooked, sliced	1/2 cup	746
Avocado	1	1,230
Beans, green, cooked, sliced	1/2 cup	413
Broccoli, cooked	1 spear	2,537
Broccoli, cooked, chopped	1/2 cup	1,099
Cantaloupe	1/4	4,304
Carrots, raw	1	20,253
Carrots, cooked, sliced	1/2 cup	19,150
Kale, cooked, chopped	1/2 cup	4,810
Lettuce, iceberg	1/4 head	445
Lettuce, loose-leaf, shredded	1/2 cup	532
Nectarines	1	1,001
Okra, cooked, sliced	1/2 cup	460
Papaya	1	6,122
Peaches	1	465

FOOD	Portion	Vitamin A (I.U.)
Peas, green, cooked	1/2 cup	478
Spinach, cooked	1/2 cup	7,370
Squash, winter, butternut, cooked, cubed	1/2 cup	7,141
Sweet potato, baked	1	24,877
Tangerines	1	773
Tomatoes, raw	1	1,530
Turnip greens, cooked, chopped	1/2	3,959
Watermelon	1/16	1,762

> Note: A complete listing of sources for the charts in this chapter can be found in the extended bibliography.

Vitamin A value reflects the amount of vitamin A derived from the yellow, orange and green pigments, including beta-carotene, that are found in fruits and vegetables.

B-Complex Vitamins

"The B's work in the body to help convert proteins, carbohydrates, and fats into fuel. The brain helps synthesize the mood controlling chemicals." [4]

This is why a deficiency of vitamin B often manifests itself as extreme muscle weakness, and as psychiatric problems ranging from mild irritability to full-blown psychosis.

"Doctors Abraham Hoffer and Humphrey Osmond in Saskatchewan, Canada, cannot shake from their minds the similarity between the psychosis of pellegra, a niacin deficient disease and schizophrenia. In 1952 they treated their first schizophrenic patient with vitamin B3. Fortunately for the world today; their results were dramatically successful." [5]

B1 Thiamine

"Thiamine was the first of the B vitamins to be discovered when it was isolated in 1911 from the rice polishing that prevents Berry-Berry. It is essential to the functioning of the central nervous system. When it is deficient there can be numbness in the arms and legs or a tingly burning sensation, powers of concentration, memory, mood and perception may be affected. Fatigue and depression can be caused." [6]

Thiamine deficiency, though rare in this country, still claims victims. People whose calorie intake is highly restricted and who drink alcohol as a substitute for eating, are prone to this deficiency.

In a study conducted by the National Institute of Mental Health, researchers induced thiamine deficiencies in a group of rhesus monkeys. The animals exhibited the typical symptoms of human thiamine deficiency, including nerve damage. The researchers found that these symptoms were reversible with the administration of thiamine supplements. Like other B vitamins, thiamine is lost in the milling of wheat or the polishing of rice.[7]

Derick Lonsdale, M.D., a former pediatrician who is now practicing preventive medicine, found (not surprisingly) that many teens ate large amounts of junk food, especially sweet soft drinks, candy, and other high carbohydrate foods with little nutritive value. Since thiamine is *essential in the metabolism of carbohydrates,* those who have a diet high in carbohydrates require more of this vitamin. Since the teens were not receiving an adequate supply, Dr. Lonsdale found that,

"These children displayed behavioral characteristics that we have come to accept as normal. They complained of headaches, abdominal and chest pains, and sleeping problems. They were irritable and some were aggressive and hard to handle. What they were was nutritionally disoriented. A blood test showed them to be deficient in the common form of thiamine. We changed their diets and gave them thiamine supplements. Of the ten we retested all showed normal behavior."[8]

At New York's famous Bellevue Hospital Center, Lewis R. Goldfrank, M.D. and his emergency room staff are using thiamine in the treatment of unconscious patients. Dr. Goldfrank says, "Since thiamine is needed to metabolize sugar you simply cannot give glucose and expect to get a high energy yield unless thiamine is present."[9]

B2 Rivoflavin

Riboflavin, which is plentiful in dairy products, should be part of an active person's diet. This nutrient is easily lost in the body; in fact, you can literally sweat riboflavin away. Researchers at Cornell University discovered that very active women require about double the RDA of 1.2 mg of riboflavin. Deficient levels of riboflavin are found in the plasma of many rheumatoid arthritis patients. Those suffering from depression may also be deficient in riboflavin.[10]

B6 Pyroxidine

This supplement is very important to my weight loss program. Pyroxidine plays a vital role in fat and cholesterol metabolism, and also helps us to assimilate protein. In addition, it is necessary for the absorption of vitamin B12 and for the production of hydrochloric acid and magnesium. Pyroxidine can be used to correct a common type of nutritional anemia. It is also a natural diuretic, and so helps prevent water retention.

Scientists at Virginia Polytech Institute believe that, without B6, the brain is unable to produce an adequate supply of the mood-controlling neurotransmitter serotonin. Therefore, that vitamin B6 deficiency has been linked with depression by these and other researchers.[11]

Even more dramatic were the findings of researchers at Kobe University, in Japan. When they administered high doses of B6 to 19 children suffering from uncontrollable seizures, 17 of them improved; in fact, three of the youngsters experienced complete relief from the problem. And it took only 2 to 14 days for the B6 to have an impact on the patients.

Vitamin B12

This vitamin, along with folic acid, helps in the production of red blood cells in the bone marrow. Without it, red cell production diminishes, and pernicious anemia will result.

Vitamin B12 may also have important implications for cancer patients. Sister M. Eymard Poydock, Ph.D. and associates at Mercyhurst College, Pennsylvania, reported remarkable results with B12 and C supplements. The found that the vitamins increased the survival rates of mice with leukemia and several forms of malignant tumors. Dr. Poydock reported, "Even in the early stages we see no increase in malignant cells. After the seventh treatment, no tumor cells at all are present. The tumor cells just disintegrate, it is very exciting." [12]

B12, known as the cobalt-containing vitamin, is part of the coenzyme involved in the metabolism of proteins, fats, and carbohydrates. It is also instrumental in the formation of the sheath of nerve fibers, and its deficiency produces a form of neuritis.

Because this vitamin is sometimes difficult to absorb when taken orally, it is customarily given by injection. However, it is not easy to become deficient in B12, for it is stored rather efficiently in the body.

Vitamin B12 is not readily available through all vegetable foods; it is mostly found in animal proteins, which is why vegetarians are more prone to B12 deficiencies. Birth control pills can cause B12 loss, as can large amounts of vitamin C.[13]

B15 Pangamic Acid

This water-soluble vitamin is, like vitamin E, an antioxidant. It was brought to world attention by the Russians, who were thrilled with the results they obtained. Pangamic acid has been utilized in extending the cell life span, reducing craving for liquor, increasing recovery from fatigue, and lowering cholesterol levels. Soviet studies also indicate that B15:

- Protects against pollutants
- Aids in protein synthesis
- Stimulates immune response
- Wards off hangovers
- Relieves the symptoms of angia asthma

Research in the United States has been limited so far.[14]

B17 Laetrile

This is one of the most controversial vitamins, for it has been both touted as a cancer remedy and denounced as a placebo. As of this writing, it is considered unacceptable as a cancer treatment in most of the United States, although its use is legal in 24 states. In Mexico, it is widely used as a cancer treatment. Laetrile, which is extracted from fruit seeds (especially apricot kernals) is also known for its effectiveness in the treatment of sickle cell anemia.[15]

Biotin

Biotin, a water soluble member of the B-complex family, is fragile in certain ways. For example, eating raw egg whites will destroy this vitamin. It acts as a coenzyme in a wide variety of body functions, including energy production and the maintaining of healthy skin and hair (it is used as a baldness preventative).

Biotin also assists in the functioning of the sweat glands, nerves, bone marrow, and sex glands. In addition, it is essential to the normal metabolism of fats and proteins. Biotin is used to alleviate muscle pains, eczema and dermatitis.[16]

Choline

Choline is another important B vitamin. It is vital in any weight loss program, as it is a fat emulsifier. It works with Inositol to utilize fats and cholesterol. Fish, liver, eggs, green leafy vegetables, yeast, and wheat are all good sources of choline.

Current research indicates that this substance may help preserve the ability of the brain to reason, learn and remember. For example, investigators at Ohio State University found that mice fed a diet heavy in choline-rich lecithin or phosphatidylcholine, one of the ingredients in lecithin, demonstrated far better memory powers than mice on a regular diet. When investigator Dr. Ron Pervis examined the brain cells of these mice he found that they showed fewer of the expected signs of aging. Dr. Pervis believes that lecithin may have similar effects in humans, although this is yet to be verified.[17]

Choline, which is water soluble, is synthesized in the liver in limited quantities. It functions as a fat stabilizing agent.[18]

Problems associated with choline deficiency include fatty degeneration of the liver, nerve degeneration, high blood pressure, atherosclerosis, and high cholesterol. Increased intake of this nutrient is recommended for alcoholics and diabetics. It is also useful to dieters, especially those with elevated cholesterol.

Folate

As I mentioned, folate, in conjunction with B12, forms red blood cells. It also plays a role in cell division, protein synthesis, and of amino and nucleic acids. Folic acid is necessary for metabolism of RNA and DNA; it is crucial to blood formation and genetic code transmission. It also enables newborns to build up resistance to infection. In addition, folic acid is important to a healthy pregnancy, as a deficiency may result in spinalbifida, premature birth, maternal toxemia, premature separation of the placenta from uterus and habitual miscarriage.[19]

Research indicates that if the body is unable to properly utilize folate, chromosome damage may result. And as Richard Branda, M.D., professor of medicine at the University of Vermont points out, "Many researchers believe that chromosome damage is an important part of the process that causes malignancy."[20]

Folic acid deficiencies are widespread, and many people who suffer from this particular lack do not respond to vitamin therapy. A Canadian survey found folate deficiency to be the single most prevalent nutritional deficiency. Another survey, conducted in the United States, showed a similar pattern.[21]

A number of factors can be responsible for a folic acid deficiency. Cooking or canning can destroy 50 to 95% of this nutrient. Alcohol consumption can also create a deficiency, and alcoholics often have difficulty absorbing folic acid, B1 and B6. Folic acid deficiency can also be caused by pregnancy, birth control pills, the aging process, and many drugs.

Symptoms of folic acid deficiency include weakness, fatigue, breathlessness, irritability, sleeplessness, forgetfulness, and mental confusion.

Inositol

This water-soluble member of the B-complex family is frequently lost in the refining process. When whole wheat is refined into flour, approximately 87% of the inositol may be processed away, and it is not restored through enrichment.[22]

Inositol is not considered a true vitamin, as the body is capable of manufacturing it in limited amounts. It functions as a fat mobilizing agent and a mild anti-anxiety agent. This nutrient also helps maintain healthy hair and controls blood cholesterol levels.[23]

Niacin

Dr. Atkins said that niacin is "The vitamin that began the megavitamin movement."[24]

The functions of this nutrient are certainly varied as well as vital. As I noted earlier, this nutrient has been successfully used in the treatment of schizophrenia. And this is only one of its many applications.

Investigators at the Eppley Institute for Research of Cancer at the University of Nebraska used nicotinamide, a form of the B vitamin niacin, to counteract the toxic effects of a drug used to induce pancreatic cancer in hamsters. Niacin is known to be an antitoxin, but the investigators were nonetheless surprised that the animals developed no pancreatic tumors at all.[25]

Niacin is also utilized for the reduction of blood cholesterol and triglycerides. Ravi Subbiah, Ph.D., of the Lipid Research Center of the University of Cincinnati Medical Center, noted that, "Niacin has an added bonus. It also reduces blood cholesterol and triglycerides, though at large doses, making it potentially useful as therapy for heart disease."

Similar results were reported by Paul Kana, Ph.D., of the Neuro Medical Research Institute. His survey of over 1,000 heart attack survivors revealed that the group given niacin had a death rate 11% lower than the group given placebo.[26]

Niacin does produce an uncomfortable side-effect, known as the "niacin flush." The dilation process caused by this nutrient produces heat and itching of the face, neck and shoulder. These unpleasant symptoms can be avoided by using time release capsules.

Niacin is a staple in my diet program. I recommend 400 mg three times a day for anyone who consumes animal or dairy products. Dr. Siegel, my associate of 7 1/2 years, and a great help with the vitamin portion of our practice says, "Niacin helps keep our plumbing clear."

PABA—Para Aminobenzoic Acid

Para aminobenzoic acid, a member of the B-complex family, is a great natural energy booster. I recommend starting with a dose of 1 gram per day; this can be increased if your energy level remains low. I recommend PABA for patients on high protein, modified low-carbohydrate diets.

Whenever a person does not achieve energy from a standard vitamin-mineral regimen, addition of PABA given in doses of 1000 mg will sometimes remove the fatigue of the patient.

Although many of the functions of PABA in humans remain unknown, it has been shown to have a role in protein synthesis and red blood cell production in animals. A PABA deficiency in animals has been linked with premature graying of hair, and at least one study indicates that PABA can be used to retard graying hair in humans.

Liver, eggs, molasses, brewer's yeast, and wheat germ are the richest sources of PABA.[27]

In recent years, PABA has become widely recognized for its usefulness in providing protection against sunburn and alleviating the pain of burns. Many people use PABA to keep the skin healthy and smooth, and it has been claimed that it can help delay wrinkling. Eczema may result from a PABA deficiency.

Panathenic Acid

This water-soluble B-complex vitamin is usually found in supplements in the form of calcium pantothenate.

Panathenic acid functions as a coenzyme, and plays a vital role in energy production, production of anti-stress hormones, control of fat metabolism, formation of antibodies, maintenance of healthy nerves, and drug detoxification.

It is also used therapeutically for patients suffering from rheumatoid arthritis. Panathenic acid has also been found useful in helping people to withstand stress.

The B-complex vitamins are essential to our health, and a crucial part of this diet. If you want to find out just how important they are, skip a few meals or splurge on sugars and refined carbohydrates. In no time at all, you will find yourself listless, moody, and tired.

According to Jack Cooperman, Ph.D., director of nutrition at New York Medical College, a subclinical or marginal vitamin deficiency is first signaled by a low level of B vitamins.

The B vitamins help convert proteins, carbohydrates, and fat into fuel. The after-work athlete, the erratic eater and the dedicated dieter run the risk of marginal deficits because they do not replace the B-vitamins as rapidly as they utilize them.[28]

Best Food Sources Of B Vitamins

FOOD	Portion	Thiamine (mg)	Riboflavin (mg)	Niacin (mg)	B6 (mg)	B12 (mg)	Folate (mcg)
Beef, round, full cut, separable, lean only, cooked	3 oz.	0.086	0.195	0.430	2.50	3.540	9
Beef kidneys, simmered	3 oz.	0.162	3.450	0.440	43.60	5.110	83
Beef liver, braised	3 oz.	0.167	3.480	0.770	60.35	9.110	185
Brewer's Yeast	1 tbsp.	1.250	0.340	0.200	0.00	3.000	313
Brown rice, raw	1/4 cup	0.170	0.030	0.280	0.00	2.350	8
Chicken, light meat, cooked	3 oz.	0.060	0.100	0.510	0.29	10.560	3
Chicken liver, cooked	3 oz.	0.130	1.490	0.500	16.49	3.780	654
Chick peas, boiled	1/2 cup	0.095	0.052	0.114	0.00	0.431	141
Egg, hard cooked	1	0.040	0.140	0.060	0.66	0.030	24
Kidney beans, all types, boiled	1/2 cup	0.141	0.051	0.106	0.00	0.509	114
Milk, whole	1 cup	0.090	0.400	0.100	0.87	0.210	12
Navy beans, boiled	1/2 cup	0.184	0.056	0.149	0.00	0.483	127
Peanuts, all types, dry roasted	1/4 cup	0.000	0.035	0.093	0.00	4.930	53
Rye flour	1/4 cup	0.200	0.070	0.100	0.00	0.880	17
Salmon steak, cooked	3 oz.	0.150	0.060	0.640	2.95	8.400	18
Soybeans, boiled	1/2 cup	0.133	0.245	0.201	0.00	.034	46
Sunflower seeds, dry	1/4 cup	0.820	0.090	0.450	0.00	0.162	85
Swiss cheese	2 oz.	0.010	0.210	0.050	0.95	0.050	4
Wheat germ, toasted	1 tbsp.	0.120	0.060	0.070	0.00	0.400	25
Whole wheat flour	1/4 cup	0.170	0.040	0.100	0.00	1.300	16

Vitamin C

Vitamin C is also a water-soluble vitamin. Because humans, unlike most animals, do not produce the enzyme needed to synthesize vitamin C, we must obtain this vitamin from our diets or from supplements.

The therapeutic properties of vitamin C were first discovered when citrus fruits (a rich source of C) were used to treat scurvy. This versatile vitamin has also been used to treat iron deficiency anemia, respiratory distress, bleeding gums, colds and influenza, high blood cholesterol levels, alcoholism and many other ailments.

Vitamin C is an antioxidant, and its wide range of functions make it essential in the promotion of iron absorption from food, maintenance of healthy collagen (providing resistance to infection), control of cholesterol levels, activation of folic acid, production of anti-stress hormones, production of brain and nerves substances, and maintenance of healthy bones, teeth, blood system, and sex organs.[29]

Perhaps most widely known as a remedy for the common cold and a form of cancer therapy, this vitamin is a one of the great natural healers.

Dr. Irving Stone and Dr. Linus Pauling advise taking approximately 2,000 mg or more of this vitamin daily, and recommended high doses for treating colds. Investigators have reported that treatment with C tremendously reduced the symptoms of the common cold, producing excellent results in hundreds of subjects.

The anti-tumor properties of vitamin C have also caused excitement in the research world. According to Seymour Romnex, M.D., "We tested at Bronx Municipal Hospital, a lot of people are intrigued by the prospect that vitamin C might have anti-tumor properties, and there are reasonable scientific studies that support that idea."[30]

Heart disease also appears responsive to vitamin C therapy. According to Anthony Verlangieri, Ph.D., of the University of Mississippi, "Vitamin C deficiency causes atherosclerosis. True cholesterol does clog arteries. But cholesterol is really a Johnny Come Lately, and a cardiovascular bad guy who takes advantage of an already bad situation caused by vitamin C deficiency."[31]

Investigators at the Institute of Human Research in Czechoslovakia administered vitamin C to middle-aged men and women, and found that cholesterol levels were significantly reduced, while triglyceride values dropped to almost half of their pre-therapy levels.

Robert H. Davis, Ph.D., professor of physiology at the Pennsylvania College of Pediatric Medicine, has also explored the use of vitamin C and aloe—two natural substances that have few, if any, side-effects—in the treatment of arthritis.[32]

In a prize-winning study, Dr. Davis and his students combined vitamin C, aloe and ribonucleic acid (RNA)—a cellular building block believed to reduce inflammation—in an ointment which they applied to the arthritic hind paws of laboratory rats. They reported that joint tissue swelling was reduced both in the early stage of the disease and after the arthritis had progressed for several days.

I recommend a minimum of 2 g. of C daily for all of my patients. It should be noted, however, that the need for vitamin C can be affected by many factors, including ingestion of preserved foods and exposure to environmental toxins. Smoking is very destructive to vitamin C. One cigarette destroys 25 to 100 mg of C, which means that someone who smokes a pack a day would run a minimum deficit of 500 mg.[33]

Best Food Sources Of Vitamin C

FOOD	Portion	Vitamin C (mg)
Banana	1	11
Blackberries	1/2 cup	15
Blueberries	1/2 cup	9
Broccoli, raw, chopped	1/2 cup	41
Brussel sprouts, raw	4	65
Cabbage, raw, chopped	1/2 cup	17
Cantaloupe	1/4	56
Cauliflower, raw, chopped	1/2 cup	36
Cherries, sweet	1/2 cup	5
Grapefruit	1/2	39
Grapefruit juice, freshly squeezed	1 cup	94
Green peppers, raw, chopped	1/2 cup	64
Guava	1/2	83
Kiwi	1 medium	75
Lemon	1 wedge	21
Mung bean sprouts	1/4 cup	3
Orange	1	70
Orange juice, freshly squeezed	1 cup	124
Papaya	1/2 medium	94
Potato, baked	1	26
Raspberries	1/2 cup	15
Snap beans, green, boiled	1/2 cup	6
Spinach, raw, chopped	1/2 cup	8
Strawberries	1/2 cup	42

FOOD	Portion	Vitamin C (mg)
Tangerine	1	25
Tomato, raw	1	22
Tomato juice	1 cup	45
Turnip greens, cooked, chopped	1/2 cup	20
Watermelon	1/16	47

Vitamin D

With sufficient sun exposure, dietary sources are not required to ensure an adequate amount of this fat-soluble vitamin. However, in the absence of sufficient sunlight, a deficiency can be caused by inadequate intake of meat, poultry, fish, and dairy products.[34]

In children, a deficiency can lead to rickets, while adults may develop osteomalacia. Symptoms of a vitamin D deficiency include unnatural limb posture, excessive sweating of the head, knock knees or bow legs, bone pain, muscular weakness, muscular spasms, and brittle, easily broken bones.

Vitamin D is used in the treatment of such ailments as rickets, osteomalacia, osteoporosis and rheumatoid arthritis.[35]

It also appears to have applications in cancer therapy. Vitamin D is converted by the liver and kidneys into its active form, calcitriol, a hormone that regulates calcium in the body. Japanese researchers have found that this hormone suppresses leukemia cells by converting them to noncancerous cells. Hector DeLuca, Ph.D., professor of biochemistry at the University of Wisconsin commented on these findings.

"Where this will go therapeutically isn't clear at this stage. In the long run, someday we may be able to control some types of leukemia. This may also have applications for controlling other types of malignancies."[36]

I was particularly interested in vitamin D because of the implications for my own diet. Dr. Deluca's own research suggested that a vitamin D deficiency may lead to problems with glucose metabolism and ultimately with insulin secretion.

"Part of the fall off in glucose tolerance that occurs in many older people could be due to a lack of vitamin D, so if we prevent the deficiency of calcitriol, perhaps we can control some cases of diabetes."[37]

Best Food Sources Of Vitamin D

FOOD	Portion	Vitamin D (I.U.)
Cod-liver oil	2 tsp.	675
Halibut-liver oil	2 tsp.	9,636
Herring, grilled	3 oz.	850
Mackerel, fried	3 oz.	717
Mackerel, raw	3 oz.	595
Milk, 1% fat	1 cup	102
Salmon, Pacific, steamed	3 oz.	425
Sardines, canned in oil, drained	3 oz.	255
Tuna, canned in oil, drained	3 oz.	197

Vitamin E

This fat-soluble vitamin is also known as D-alpha tocopherol. Because the claims for vitamin E have been so varied and dramatic—everything from clearing of ateriosclorotic valves to restoral of sexual potency has been attributed to this vitamin—it is no wonder that the Harvard Medical School Health Letter referred to it as "a recreational drug."

Vitamin E functions as an antioxidant; it reduces the oxygen needs of muscles, acts as an anti-clotting agent, and serves as a blood vessel dilator.[38]

Vitamin E protects blood vessels, protects polyunsaturated oils, amino acids, and vitamin A, and protects against thrombosis, atherosclerosis, and thrombophlebitis. It keeps cholesterol levels in the safe range, acts with selenium, and promotes the ability of white blood cells to resist infection.

What more could one ask of a vitamin? Well, there's a lot more. Vitamin E has been used in the treatment of intermittent claudication, cerebral and coronary thrombosis, varicose veins, menstrual problems, low fertility, skin ulcers, diabetic gangrene, nerve, joint and muscular complaints, hemolytic anemia in newborns, sickle cell anemia, and cystic breast disease, as well as breast cancer.[39]

Externally, vitamin E has been used to treat scar tissue, stretch marks, sunburn, burns and scalds.[40]

Because vitamin E increases the supply of oxygen to our cells, it is very important in my diet as a source of stamina and energy.

Peter T. Pugliese, M.D., vice-president of research and development at the Xienta Institute for Skin Research, Pennsylvania, says, "Much more research must be done, but right now it appears that vitamin E has much more of a biological effect than any of us ever dreamed of."[41]

James Litton, Jr., Ph.D., former assistant professor of biology at St. Mary's College, University of Notre Dame, Indiana, has offered a hypothesis to explain the varied applications of this vitamin.

"What E probably does is maintain the integrity of individual cell membranes. If we relate aging to the degradation of cell membranes, then, the theory is, if we maintain their integrity we live longer.

"Vitamin E helps prevent platelet aggregation, the 'clumping' that occurs when red blood cells stick together like stacks of poker chips according to research by R.V. Panganamala, Ph.D., of the department of physiological chemistry at Ohio State University School of Medicine. While such clumping is essential in the event of a cut, if it occurs in an intact blood vessel, it can trigger a heart attack or stroke.

"There must be a proper ratio of thromboxane to prostacyclin for blood to flow without clumping. When the ratio gets out of balance, clumping is much more likely to occur. Vitamin E keeps these two substances in optimum balance."[42]

Vitamin E may be especially essential for people who drink alcohol. Helmet Redetzki, Ph.D, professor of pharmacology at Louisiana State University School of Medicine, found that in rats, even a single intoxicating dose of alcohol hurts heart muscle cells.

"We know that E-deficient animals suffer more heart damage from drinking than animals fed adequate vitamin E. Alcoholics often have lower blood levels of vitamin E so they may be particularly prone to this kind of heart damage."[43]

A vitamin E deficiency can be caused by the malabsorption of fats, consistent use of liquid paraffin, gastric or intestinal surgery, alcoholism, cirrhosis of the liver, obstructive jaundice, cystic fibrosis, celiac disease, excessive intake of polyunsaturated oil (lacking E), and excessive oxygen (for example, use of an oxygen tent). Vitamin E deficiency in children may cause irritability, water retention, and hemolytic anemia. Adults may suffer from lack of vitality, lethargy, apathy, concentration impairment, irritability, decreased sexual interest, and muscle weakness.

The best natural sources of vitamin E include wheat germ, soy beans, vegetable oils, broccoli, brussel sprouts, leafy greens, spinach, enriched flour, whole wheat, whole grain cereals, and eggs.[44]

Best Food Sources Of Vitamin E

FOOD	Portion	Vitamin E (I.U.)
Almonds, whole, dried, unblanched	1/4 cup	26.8
Cod-liver oil	1 tbsp.	3.9
Corn oil	1 tbsp.	2.9
Corn oil margarine	1 tbsp.	2.7
Hazelnuts, dried, unblanched, chopped	1/4 cup	10.2
Lobster, boiled	3 oz.	2.3
Peanuts, shelled, dried	1/4 cup	6.0
Peanut butter	2 tbsp.	3.8
Pecans, halved, dried	1/4 cup	1.3
Safflower oil	1 tbsp.	8.2
Salmon steak, broiled	3 oz.	2.0
Soybean oil, hydrogenated	1 tbsp.	2.0
Sunflower oil	1 tbsp.	10.9
Sunflower seeds	1/4 cup	26.8
Wheat germ, raw	1/2 cup	12.8

As you can see, your vitamin needs are determined in part by your lifestyle. If you drink alcohol, vitamin E is helpful; smokers require extra vitamin C; people who are on a diet or under stress should make sure they get adequate B vitamins. Check with your physician or nutritionist to determine your optimal dosage.

I believe that vitamin therapy is significantly underrated. If a disease can be treated with a vitamin, isn't that preferable to using a chemical remedy? (Which is not to say that you should refuse medication prescribed by your physician; these treatments do have their place.)

Cynics have disputed the efficacy of vitamins simply because vitamin advocates have fallen victim to the human condition. The death of Adelle Davis, author of Let's Eat Right To Keep Fit and other famous health books, caused an outcry. If she was so healthy, argued the skeptics, why did she die? This type of reasoning is absurd. We all die eventually; the question is, what is the quality of our life like while we are on this planet?

Unfortunately, today's physicians have little or no training in nutrition. This is a shame, because one of the functions of a healer is to educate patients. (In fact, the word "physician" means "teacher" in Greek.) I wrote this book to provide people with the information they need to make the most of what they have. Genetics, environment, upbringing, and other factors have a lot to do with how long and how well we will live. But through the application of sound principles such as the ones discussed in this chapter, we can significantly improve our lives.

I have a strong personal stake in these techniques. In 1988, my father went through two major operations, a quadruple bypass and removal of an abdominal aneurysm. He was surrounded by the cream of the medical community: the best surgeons, cardiologists and internists.

I will be forever grateful to these people. However, during his 20-day stay in the hospital, my father was not given vitamin E to promote the healing of scars; he was not given vitamin C to build up his cells; he was not given zinc to increase the power of his immune system.

On the other hand, he was given numerous medications. Certainly, this medicine was necessary and effective and I am not suggesting that vitamins could have replaced the drugs. But vitamins could have been given in conjunction with the medication, and I am convinced they would have accelerated my father's recovery.

I assure you, it is a rare day in my office when vitamins are not recommended to a patient. Thomas Edison once said that, "The doctor of the future will give no medicine, he will interest his patients in the care of the human frame, in diet, and in the cause and prevention of disease."

This future can't come fast enough for me.

Even if you are on the right track, you'll get run over if you just sit there.
Oliver Wendell Holmes[1]

17

Mining for Minerals

Your food supplements should contain more than vitamins. Minerals are also essential to a well-balanced diet, and they are an important part of my program. The most vital minerals, and the sources from which to best obtain them, are covered here. You may be in for a few surprises if you thought that your diet was providing you with the minerals you need.

Calcium

When most people think "calcium" they also think "milk." But the advisability of eating and drinking dairy products is controversial. Not that you would ever guess it from the American diet; more dairy products are consumed in the United States than in the rest of the world combined. According to a survey by Gross's *Journal of California,* only 6% of Americans do not consume milk in some form. Yet the overall level of health in this country is not impressive.

"If dairy products are such good foods and we in America eat more than the rest of the world combined, then it would stand to reason that we should be experiencing the highest level of health as well. As a matter of fact, the American worker leads the world in degenerative diseases, according to Richard Ockeela, Director of Program Development of the President's Council of Physical Fitness reported in the Los Angeles Times in April 1981."[1]

Earl Mindell's *Vitamin Bible* reports that, "American men rank 13th in world health, American women sixth." Even more astonishing in this country of dairy devotees is the fact that, "Eighty percent of American women are calcium deficient."

Calcium deficiency can have serious consequences. In children the consequences of a calcium shortage may include rickets, which is characterized by excessive sweating of the head, sleeping problems, constant head movements, slowness in sitting, crawling, walking, bow legs, knock knees, and pigeon breast.[2] Calcium deficiency in adults has been associated with osteoporosis, high blood pressure, osteomalacia, bone pain, muscle weakness, delayed healing of fractures, and tetany (twitches and spasms).

Deficiencies can be caused by low dietary intake, lack of vitamin B, an increase in the intake of whole cut bran, phosphates, animal fats, and oxalic acid. Oral contraceptives and corticosteroid drugs have also been linked with calcium deficiencies. Poor calcium absorption can be due to a lack of stomach acid, celiac disease, lactose intolerance, drug use, and pregnancy.

Calcium functions as an antioxidant, and promotes iron absorption from food, maintains healthy collagen, provides resistance to infection, controls blood cholesterol levels, and produces anti-stress hormones.[3]

Therapeutically, calcium is used to treat scurvy, iron deficiency anemia, respiratory disease, bleeding gums, cold and influenza, cancer, high blood cholesterol levels, alcoholism, arthritis, and leg cramps.[4] Calcium is essential to the blood clotting process, and to nerve and muscle function.

Calcium also appears to influence blood pressure, an important consideration in a country in which hypertension is so widespread. Investigators at Cornell University Medical School reported that,

"In one of the first research studies to actually test the power of calcium supplement against hypertension in humans the researchers gave 26 mildly hypertensive patients 2,000mg of raw calcium for six months. The result was a modest but consistent drop in pressure from an average of 161 over 94 at the start of the study to 154 over 89 six months later."[5]

Lawrence Resnick, M.D., who headed the research team, noted that patients who started with lower levels of calcium in their blood showed the greatest decrease in pressure.

"In some cases diastolic pressures dropped 10 to 20%. Patients with higher calcium levels, however, weren't helped at all by the calcium supplements. So the nutrient can benefit some but not all hypertensives."

Dr. Resnick theorizes that supplemental calcium alters the hormones that help regulate blood pressure.

Given the importance of calcium, and the myth that milk is a good source of this mineral, it can be difficult to wean people from dairy products. (I'll discuss the subject of milk and milk products at greater length in "The Dairy News.") Many of my patients are aghast at the very idea of reducing their intake of these products. "But doctor, where will I get my calcium? Where will my children get their calcium?"

Calcium can be obtained from nuts, legumes, root vegetables, eggs, cereals, fruits, whole grain flour, green leafy vegetables (an excellent source), sesame seeds (which contain as much calcium as any food on the planet), tofu, and fish, as well as from dairy products.

In fact, a person whose diet is high in milk, cheese, yogurt, ice cream, etc., may develop significant circulatory and structural problems. Furthermore, they are consuming large amounts of unnecessary carbohydrates, which is why these people are often overweight and sluggish.

So, the next time you think calcium, think of something else besides milk.

Best Food Sources Of Calcium

FOOD	Portion	Calcium (mg)
Almonds	1/4 cup	100
American cheese	2 oz.	348
Blackstrap molasses	1 tbsp.	137
Brick cheese	2 oz.	382
Broccoli, cooked	1/2 cup	89
Broccoli, raw	1 cup	42
Buttermilk	1 cup	285
Cheddar cheese	2 oz.	408
Colby cheese	2 oz.	388
Collards, cooked	1/2 cup	74

FOOD	Portion	Calcium (mg)
Dandelion greens, cooked	1/2 cup	74
Ice cream	1 cup	176
Ice milk	1 cup	176
Ice milk, soft serve	1 cup	274
Kale, cooked	1/2 cup	47
Limburger cheese	2 oz.	282
Milk, skim	1 cup	302
Milk, whole	1 cup	291
Monterey Jack cheese	2 oz.	424
Mozzarella cheese	2 oz.	294
Muenster cheese	2 oz.	406
Mustard greens, cooked	1/2 cup	52
Navy beans, cooked	1/2 cup	64
Parmesan cheese	1 tbsp.	86
Pizza, cheese	1/8 of 14" pie	144
Provolone cheese	2 oz.	428
Ricotta cheese, part-skim	1/2 cup	337
Salmon, sockeye, drained solids	3 oz.	271
Sardines	3 oz.	372
Scallops, steamed	3 oz.	98
Shrimp, raw	3 oz.	54
Soy flour, defatted	1/4 cup	60
Soybeans, cooked	1/2 cup	88
Swiss cheese	2 oz.	544
Tofu, raw, coagulated with nigari	3 oz.	174
Tofu, raw, firm,coagulated with calcium sulfate	3 oz.	581
Yogurt, low-fat	1 cup	415

> Note: a complete listing of sources for the charts found in chapter 17 can be found in the extended bibliography.

Zinc

This trace mineral is vital to the functioning of the immune system, which is our natural defense against diseases.

"Over a hundred years ago scientists discovered an interesting phenomenon. They found that as people grew older their organ weights changed. They discovered that the lungs, the liver, and brain, weighed slightly less in an

80-year-old than they do in a 20-year-old. They further concluded that the thymus gland actually shrank to a mere fraction of its original size. Twenty years ago this phenomenon became a significant scientific fact. It was at this time that scientists learned the function of the thymus, a flat pinkish gray two-lobed gland that nestles behind the sternum and lungs high in the chest. A gland that is essential to distribute and nourish white blood cells, which we commonly call lymphocytes, which aid the body against disease. It is the thymus gland that produces the T-lymphocytes, which when a foreign invader enters our body (like a virus cancer cell) they can be stimulated into larger active cells that react with the invader and work on killing it. These T-lymphocytes act like Pac-Man, like scavengers that literally gobble up the enemy that try to invade our body."[6]

The body is a self-healing organism; the power that created the body has the power to heal the body. Within our bodies is a defense system far more miraculous than any antibiotic ever invented. Unfortunately, however, the immune system does tend to wane with the years.

According to Ranjit Kumar Chandra, M.D., of the Department of Immunology at the Dr. Charles Janeway Child Health Center in New Foundland, "There is at least a distinct possibility that some illnesses and abnormalities we are seeing in the immune system in the elderly may now be part of the normal aging process, that there are environmental factors, particularly, that may have a causal role to play."[7]

Yet another factor associated with problems in immune defenses is zinc deficiency. Robert Good, M.D., Ph.D., chairman of the pediatrics department at the University of South Florida, conducted field work among malnourished children. He and his associates found that malnutrition was accompanied by a profound decline in immune function. It is surprising is that neither protein nor calorie deprivation was responsible for this decline—lack of zinc was the cause. Dr. Good noted that other researchers have found that it is possible to correct the immunological dysfunction in these cases simply my administering zinc to the children.[8]

Zinc deficiencies have been associated with lack of physical, mental, and sexual development (which can be reversed in pre-puberty children by increasing zinc intake), as well as growth failure, impaired sense of taste, and poor appetite (also reversible with zinc intake). Eczema, hair loss, apathy, defects of the reproductive organs (particularly the testes), decreased growth rate, post-natal depression, congenital abnormalities in newborns, impaired sense of smell, white spots on the nails, and susceptibility to infection may also be associated with zinc deficiencies.

Therapeutic uses include treatment of acne, eczema, psoriasis, prostate problems, mild mental problems, schizophrenia, elevated blood fats, hyperactivity in children, the common cold (zinc gluta-mate), and anorexia nervosa.

Zinc is also associated with growth insulin activity, which makes this mineral a vital part of my high energy diet. Zinc is necessary for the metabolic functions of the pituitary, adrenals, ovaries, and testes, and plays a role in maintaining healthy liver function. It is important in the development of the skeleton, nervous system, and brain of the fetus. Zinc interacts with calcium in bone mineralization. It also serves as a kind of overseer in the maintenance of the enzyme systems. It is essential for protein synthesis which governs the contractility of muscles.[9] Zinc also accelerates the healing rate of internal and external wounds.

The best natural sources of zinc include oysters, liver, dry brewers yeast, shellfish, meats (especially round steak, lamb chops, pork loin), hard cheese, canned fish, whole wheat bread, eggs, legumes, whole grain cereals, rice, green leafy vegetables, potatoes, pumpkin seeds, and ground mustard.

Best Food Sources Of Zinc

FOOD	Portion	Zinc (mg)
Beef, ground, lean, broiled, medium	1/3 cup	7.12
Beef liver, braised	3 oz.	5.16
Beef, round, full cut, separable lean only, broiled	3 oz.	3.98
Black-eyed peas, cooked	1/2 cup	1.50
Brazil nuts, dried	1/4	1.60
Calve's liver, cooked	3 oz.	5.20
Cashews, dry-roasted	1/4 cup	1.90
Cheddar cheese	2 oz.	1.80
Chick peas, boiled	1/2 cup	1.25
Chicken, dark-meat, cooked	3 oz.	2.40
Chicken heart, cooked	3 oz.	6.00

FOOD	Portion	Zinc (mg)
Chicken, light-meat, cooked	3 oz.	1.10
Chicken liver, cooked	3 oz.	3.70
Clams, raw meat only	3 oz.	1.34
Filberts, dried	1/4 cup	0.70
Lamb, lean, cooked	3 oz.	4.20
Lentils, boiled	1/2 cup	1.26
Oats, regular, cooked	1/2 cup	0.60
Oysters, raw, meat only	1/3 cup	7.12
Peanuts, all types, dry-roasted	1/4 cup	1.20
Peas, cooked	1/2 cup	1.00
Pumpkin seeds, roasted	1/4 cup	4.20
Sunflower seeds, dry roasted	1/4 cup	1.70
Swiss cheese	2 oz.	2.20
Tuna, canned in oil, drained	1/2 cup	4.01
Tuna, light, canned in water	1/2 cup	0.70
Turkey, light-meat, cooked	3 oz.	1.70
Turkey, dark-meat, cooked	3 oz.	3.80

Potassium

Potassium is essential because it works with sodium to regulate the body's water balance and normalize heart rhythms. Potassium works inside the cells, whereas sodium works outside them. Nerve and muscle functions suffer when sodium potassium balance is off kilter. Many dieters and heavy exercisers are afflicted with muscle cramps, spasms and fatigue because of sodium potassium imbalance.

The eight major functions of potassium are:

1. maintaining a normal balance of water, within body cells as the major positively charged ion within these cells.

2. as an essential activator of a number of enzymes, particularly those concerned with energy production.

3. to help stabilize the internal structure of body cells.

4. in assisting specialized cell particles to synthesize proteins.

5. in nerve impulse transmission in conjunction with sodium.

6. to increase the excitability of the heart and skeleton muscle to make them more receptive to nerve impulses.

7. in preserving the acid-alkali balance of the body in conjunction with bicarbonate, phosphate and protein, as well as sodium, calcium, and magnesium.

8. in stimulating the normal movements of the intestinal tract.[10]

Potassium can promote clear thinking by sending oxygen to the brain, help dispose of body waste, and assist in reducing blood pressure. Potassium has also been used in the treatment of allergies. It is significant that people suffering from mental or physical stress can also have a potassium deficiency.

The best food sources of potassium are citrus fruits, cantaloupe, tomatoes, watercress, green leafy vegetables, mint leaves, sunflower seeds, bananas, and potatoes.[11]

Heavy coffee drinkers may be interested to learn that the very beverage they are drinking to fight fatigue may be contributing to it; regular coffee drinking can deplete the body's potassium reserves, causing deficiency-related fatigue.

Heavy alcohol and sugar intake are also associated with potassium shortages. If your diet is heavy in sugar, then you are probably losing potassium while retaining water. This water retention will show up as extra pounds on the scale. And if you take a diuretic to counteract the water retention, you will lose even more potassium. My professional experience has taught me that most people who take diuretics are overweight and hypertensive. A proper diet with ample water and without sugar, salt, and refined carbohydrates, will correct the underlying problem, and you won't have to depend on diuretics.

On a modified carbohydrate diet such as this one, it is possible for potassium levels to fall. That is why I recommend an orange a day, large amounts of green leafy vegetables, and vitamin supplements. I believe that 100 to 200 mg of potassium a day—in association with a good multi-vitamin—is ample.

Dieting can also be a risk for the person with low potassium reserves—e.g., someone who is taking diuretics. If you are on any medication, you must consult with your physician before embarking on any diet program.

If you suffer from fatigue or muscle weakness while on this diet (or any diet, for that matter), please consult your physician; these symptoms could signal a potassium deficiency. However, I believe that if you avail yourself of the unlimited quantities of leafy green vegetables on this diet, the chances of a deficiency are remote.

Best Food Sources Of Potassium

FOOD	Portion	Potassium (mg)
Apricots, dried	1/4 cup	448
Apricots, fresh	3	313
Avocado	1/2	602
Banana	1	471
Beef liver, pan fried	3 oz.	309
Broccoli, cooked*	1/2 cup	127
Buttermilk	1 cup	371
Cantaloupe	1/4 medium	413
Chicken, light meat, roasted	3 oz.	210
Cod, baked	3 oz.	345
Flounder, baked	3 oz.	498
Great Northern beans, cooked	1/2 cup	344
Haddock, fried	3 oz.	297
Leg of lamb, trimmed of fat, cooked	3 oz.	274
Orange juice	1 cup	496
Perch, fried	3 oz.	243
Pork, trimmed of fat, cooked	3 oz.	283
Potato, baked	1 medium	844
Raisins	1/2 cup	545
Round steak, trimmed of fat, broiled	3 oz.	352
Salmon fillet, cooked*	3 oz.	378
Sardines, Atlantic, drained solids*	3 oz.	501
Sirloin, trimmed of fat, broiled	3 oz.	342
Skim milk*	1 cup	406
Squash, winter, cooked	1/2 cup	445
Sweet potato, baked	1 medium	397
Tomato, raw	1	279

FOOD	Portion	Potassium (mg)
Tuna, drained solids	3 oz.	225
Turkey, light meat, roasted	3 oz.	259
Whole milk*	1 cup	370

*—Also high in calcium.

Iron

A great many people obtained their information about this essential trace element from the many television commercials on the subject. You know, the ones that talk about "iron-poor blood" and the fatigue resulting from it. Because iron-packed red blood cells carry energy-giving oxygen to every part of the body, there is a grain of truth in these advertisements. But the full picture is larger than the one on the television screen.

We are beginning to view iron deficiency as a disorder of the whole body, a problem that can affect the immune system, body temperature, and even learning and concentration. We are also learning that what we once considered an adequate amount of iron may not be optimum. Symptoms may develop even from mild iron deficiency that has not reached the point of outright anemia.

A great deal of research has been conducted on iron and immunity. One investigator, Jose I. Santos, M.D., assistant professor of pediatrics and pathology at Boston University School of Medicine, has noted that,

"Phagocytes, white blood cells that serve as the body's primary defense mechanism against bacterial infections, depend on iron containing enzymes to do their job.

"These cells engulf bacteria as it creates a variety of corrosive substances known as oxidants must digest the invading microbe once it is engulfed. Phagocytes need plenty of oxygen to produce peroxides and iron brings it to them.

"Certainly iron deficiency is going to directly impede this process."[12]

Frank Oski, M.D., professor of pediatrics at Johns Hopkins University School of Medicine, has found a high risk of iron deficiency in infants aged nine months to two years.

This occurs because the infant has used up the body stores of iron and is weaned from iron-rich breast milk to *iron-poor cow's milk* at this time. Dr. Oski found that iron deficiencies range from 10 to 25% in infants from affluent families, and are as high as 50% in infants from lower socioeconomic groups.[13] Once again, dairy products do not supply adequate amounts of an important mineral. Nor is iron deficiency confined to infants. Studies have shown that this condition affects 5% of children 5 to 8, 2.6% of all adolescents, and 25% of all pregnant teenagers. A screening of Yale University women under age 21 revealed that 18% were mildly iron deficient.[14]

Two thirds of the iron present in the body is in hemoglobin, the oxygen-carrying pigment of red blood cells. The remainder is stored in the liver, spleen, bone marrow, and muscles. Iron functions as an oxygen carrier in hemoglobin and myoglobin, which acts as an oxygen reservoir in muscles. In body cells it acts to transfer oxygen in cytochromus. Iron is also essential in the development of resistance to infection.

Iron is utilized therapeutically in the treatment of iron-deficiency anemia, generalized itching, and impaired mental performance in the young.

Iron-deficiency anemia is a widespread condition.

"The ultimate test of deficiency is blood hemoglobin content, which should be within the range of 12-16 grams for 100 mg of blood. A level less than 12 grams is considered anemic. In the United States an estimated 20 million people are iron deficient. 35-50% of women show signs of iron deficiency anemia, and 60% or more of infants and pregnant women are affected."[15]

The symptoms of this disorder include tiredness, lack of stamina, breathlessness, giddiness, headaches, insomnia, and palpitations.

Best Food Sources Of Iron

FOOD	Portion	Iron (mg)
Almonds, dried, unblanched	1/4 cup	1.3
Apricots, dried, sulfured, cooked	1/4 cup	1.0
Beef, ground, extra lean, broiled	3 oz.	2.0
Beef liver, fried	3 oz.	5.3
Beef, rump roast, lean, cooked	3 oz.	3.1
Beef, sirloin, broiled	3 oz.	2.9
Beet greens	1/2 cup	1.4

FOOD	Portion	Iron (mg)
Blackstrap molasses	1 tbsp.	3.2
Broccoli, cooked	1 spear	2.1
Broccoli, raw	1 spear	1.3
Brussel sprouts, cooked	1/2 cup	0.9
Cashews, dry-roasted	1/4 cup	2.1
Chicken, dark-meat, cooked without skin	3 oz.	1.1
Chicken, light-meat, cooked without skin	3 oz.	0.9
Chicken liver, cooked	3 oz.	7.2
Cod, cooked	3 oz.	0.9
Crab, pieces, steamed	1/2 cup	6.0
Endive, raw	1/2 cup	0.2
Haddock, raw	3 oz.	0.6
Lima beans, large, boiled	1/2 cup	2.1
Lobster, broiled	1/2 cup	1.5
Peanuts, dried	1/4 cup	1.2
Peas, cooked	1/2 cup	1.2
Pistachios, dried	1/4 cup	2.2
Potato, baked	1	2.8
Prunes, dried, cooked	1/2 cup	1.2
Raisins, seedless, packed	1/4 cup	0.8
Scallops, steamed	3 oz.	2.5
Sesame seeds, whole, dried	1 tbsp.	1.3
Soybeans, boiled	1/2 cup	4.4
Soybeans, dry-roasted	1/4 cup	1.7
Spinach, cooked	1/2 cup	3.2
Spinach, raw, chopped	1/2 cup	0.8
Sunflower seeds, dried	1/4 cup	2.4
Swiss chard, cooked	1/2 cup	2.0
Tuna, canned in water	3 oz.	1.4
Turkey, dark-meat, cooked without skin	3 oz.	2.0
Turkey, light-meat, cooked without skin	3 oz.	1.1

Copper

When I was working on this section, my son walked into the room and questioned me on the progress of the book. I explained that I was writing about the vitamin copper. He replied, "Dad, copper isn't a vitamin, they make pennies out of copper." His remark made me realize how many people find it difficult to understand that something we consider small change can be so vital to our health.

Actually, my son was partly right: copper is not a vitamin, but a trace element essential for humans, animals and many plants. Copper is necessary for the development and maintenance of nerves, blood vessels, and bones. When we are deficient in copper we absorb more from the food we eat and excrete less. Not good for weight loss.

Copper performs its functions as an integral part of more than a dozen of the proteins classified as enzymes. Because the copper is cloaked in these large protein molecules, we are protected from the toxic effects it would produce if it were allowed to roam free.

As a co-factor with enzymes, copper is involved in producing skin pigments (those needed for skin healing), protection against toxic agents, and serves in nerve impulses to the brain. Copper is involved in blood formation, aids iron absorption and incorporation into hemoglobin, helps promote the development of healthy bones, and has a role in infection resistance. It also may decrease the risk of coronary heart disease.

Joseph R. Prohaska, Ph.D., associate professor of biochemistry at the University of Minnesota School of Medicine, provides a graphic picture of copper deficiency.

"Our best evidence for copper's role in humans comes from children who have menkes disease. Menkes is a fatal genetic disease of abnormal copper metabolism in which the children die at two or three years of age.

"What happens to children with menkes disease is almost exactly what we see in copper deficient experimental animals. Some of their brain cells die, some degenerate, and in some there is delay in the process of myelination, the formation of an insulating sheath around the neurons (the characteristic cell of the brain). These children also have abnormal blood vessels, they are twisted and have a tendency to rupture if blood pressure gets too high. The children's bones are weakened, too."[16]

Copper deficiency in infants can be responsible for failure to thrive, pallor, diarrhea, depigmentation of the hair and skin, and permanent dilated veins and skin. In adults, deficiencies can cause anemia, water retention, irritability, brittle bones, hair depigmentation, poor hair texture, and loss of the sense of taste.[17]

Deficiencies are most often associated with malnourishment (in children), malabsorption problems, infantile anemia, premature birth, menkes syndrome, *highly refined diets,* prolonged diarrhea, and excessive intake of zinc, cadmium, or fluoride.[18]

The best food sources for copper are shellfish, dried brewer's yeast, olives, nuts, legumes, cereals, meat, fish, poultry, whole grain bread, and dried fruits.

We should take from 2 to 5 mg of copper daily, or at least make sure that we get the minimum daily requirement. Since our bodies are capable of detoxifying copper and getting rid of it, it is difficult to develop copper poisoning.[19]

Best Food Sources Of Copper

FOOD	Portion	Copper (mg)
Almonds, dried, unblanched, whole	1/4 cup	335
Apricots, dried, sulfured, uncooked	1/4 cup	140
Banana	1 medium	124
Barley, raw	1/4 cup	60
Cashews, dry-roasted	1/4 cup	760
Chicken, dark meat, cooked, without skin	4 oz.	91
Chicken, light meat, cooked, without skin	4 oz.	57
Crab, boiled	3 oz.	4,080
Halibut, steamed	3 oz.	60
Liver, beef, braised	4 oz.	3,161
Mushrooms, raw, pieces	1/2 cup	39
Navy beans, cooked, boiled	1/4 cup	134
Peanuts, boiled	1/4 cup	366
Pecans, dried	1/4 cup	320
Prunes, dried, uncooked	1/4 cup	173
Raisins, seedless, not packed	1/4 cup	112
Sesame seeds, whole dried	1 tbsp.	367
Sunflower seeds, dry-roasted	1/4 cup	586
Walnuts, black, dried	1/4 cup	320
Wheat germ, plain, toasted	1 tbsp.	44
Whole wheat flour	1/2 cup	300

Magnesium

Magnesium is one of the body's major electrolytes, along with potassium, calcium and sodium. Magnesium is involved in many functions of the body, including enzyme and hormonal actions, carbohydrate metabolism, and DNA production. More important is its role in nerve and muscle tissue function and conduction. Magnesium also appears to regulate the balance of calcium and sodium in our cells, particularly in the heart and blood vessels.

Burton M. Altura, Ph.D., of the Down State Medical Center, in Brooklyn, and his wife, Ella Altura, Ph.D., are recognized as the world's experts on magnesium. They believe that mangnesium deficiencies are a factor in many disorders that involve constriction or spasm of the heart and circulatory systems. Their findings indicate that an optimum intake of magnesium can go a long way toward preventing these conditions and alleviating their symptoms.[20]

Other researchers have also associated magnesium deficiencies with heart problems, including arrhythmias and fibrillations, which are types of heartbeat irregularities.[21]

Other deficiency-related problems include weakness, tiredness, vertigo, convulsions, nervousness, muscle cramps and tremors, tongue jerks and tremors, involuntary eye movements, unsteady gait, hyperactivity in children, palpitations, low blood sugar, and painful swallowing.

The therapeutic uses of magnesium are varied. Kenneth Weaver, M.D., of East Tennessee State University, who conducted a study involving 500 women, concluded that migraine headaches are particularly responsive to magnesium therapy.

And Dr. Burton Altura found that high magnesium levels are associated with lower levels of cholesterol. He says:

"Magnesium deficiency is known to be accompanied by an increased tendency of blood to clot. Since magnesium is also known to possess platelet stabilizing action, one must consider the strong possibility that this mineral may either reduce the incidence of, or prevent, thrombosis (blood clotting) in the coronary, pulmonary and cerebral blood vessels which can be life threatening."[22]

Good food sources of magnesium are soy flour, tofu, almonds, soy beans, wheat germ, cashews, brazil nuts, spinach, rye flour, whole wheat flour, peanuts, walnuts, oatmeal, baked potatoes, buckwheat, beef rounds, and peanut butter.

Best Food Sources Of Magnesium

FOODS	Portion	Magnesium (mg)
Almonds, dried, unblanched	1/4 cup	105
Avocado	1/2	40
Banana	1	35
Beef, round, full cut, separable lean only, broiled	3 oz.	24
Beet greens, cooked	1/2 cup	49
Black-eyed peas, dried	1/4 cup	98
Blackstrap molasses	1 tbsp.	52
Brazil nuts, dried, unblanched	1/4 cup	79
Brown rice, cooked	1/2 cup	28
Buckwheat flour, light	1/2 cup	24
Cashews, dry-roasted	1/4 cup	89
Chestnuts, European, roasted	1/2 cup	24
Collards, cooked, chopped	1/2 cup	11
Kidney beans, all types, boiled	1/2 cup	40
Lima beans, baby, boiled	1/2 cup	49
Milk, skim	1 cup	28
Oatmeal, regular, quick	1 cup	56
Peanut butter, smooth	1 tbsp.	25
Peanut butter, defatted	1/4 cup	56
Peanuts, all types, dry-roasted	1/4 cup	64
Pecans, halves, dried	1/4 cup	35
Potato, baked	1 medium	55
Rye flour, light	1/2 cup	74
Salmon, sockeye, canned	4 oz.	33
Shredded wheat, small biscuit	1 cup	55
Soybeans, boiled	1/2 cup	74
Soybeans, dry-roasted	1/4 cup	98
Soy flour, full fat, raw	1/2 cup	180
Spinach, cooked	1/2 cup	79
Spinach, raw, chopped	1/2 cup	22
Swiss, chard, cooked, chopped	1/2 cup	75
Tofu, regular, raw	1/2 cup	127

FOODS	Portion	Magnesium (mg)
Walnuts, black, dried	1/4 cup	63
Wheat germ, toasted	1/4 cup	91
Whole wheat flour	1/2 cup	68

Selenium

This trace mineral is perhaps best known for its association with vitamin E. Selenium and E have been used in the treatment of angina (cardiac-related chest pain), and it was found that the combination led to greater improvement than either nutrient provided by itself. Also, this combination may have an effect on the aging process. Finnish researchers reported that large doses of vitamin E and selenium significantly improved the well-being of nursing home patients. It has also been found that selenium is 50 to 100 times more active in antioxidants than vitamin E.

Selenium may also be a natural anti-cancer agent. Research at the University of North Carolina and the University of Miami revealed that people who have a selenium deficiency, or live in an area with selenium-poor soil, are more prone to cancer.

Gerhard N. Schrauzer, Ph.D., says that selenium stimulates the immune system. "It also alters the metabolism of carcinogenic substances, thus preventing an accumulation of free radicals." Dr. Schrauzer has noted that while selenium is probably one of the least thought-about trace minerals, evidence for its role in preventing a whole list of conditions—especially cancer—keeps accumulating.[23]

Selenium has also been used in the treatment of arthritis, high blood pressure, hair, nail, and skin problems, cataracts, muscular dystrophy, liver disease, and infertility in males.

Selenium deficiency can be caused by diets high in refined and processed foods and eating foods grown in selenium-deficient soil. This condition has also been seen in infants who were fed dry milk rather than breast milk.

Problems associated with selenium deficiency include dental carries in children, hair loss, skin depigmentation, nail problems, and a garlicky breath odor in people who have not eaten garlic.

The two most important points about selenium were probably best summed up by Ara Nahatetian, Ph.D., a researcher at the Massachusetts Institute of Technology.

"Selenium is an essential micronutrient, without it we will die. We also know that taking too much can have harmful effects. What we are trying to find out is how much is absorbed and how much is excreted."[24]

Because large doses of selenium can be toxic, please consult with your physician before taking more than the minimum daily requirement of this (or any other) nutrient.

Manganese

The principle functions of this essential trace element are promotion of growth and the maintenance of a healthy nervous system. It also aids in the synthesis of structural proteins of body cells, is important in the maintenance of healthy bones, and stimulates glycogen storage in the liver. It is a co-factor for vitamins B, C, and E. It is also a co-factor for enzymes, and thus plays a role in the development of healthy joints, nucleic acid synthesis, and the production of female sex hormones and thyroxine.

Manganese has been used in the treatment of schizophrenia, myasthenia gravis, and anemia (it improves the utilization of iron).

Deficiencies are usually related to a diet high in refined and processed foods. While specific deficiency symptoms have not yet been identified, low blood and tissue levels of manganese have been reported in people suffering from diabetes, heart disease, schizophrenia, atherosclerosis, myasthenia gravis, and rheumatoid arthritis.[25]

The best food sources of manganese are cereal, whole wheat breads, nuts, legumes, fruits, green leafy vegetables, liver, root vegetables, meats, and fish. The recommended intake is 2.5 to 5 mg per day.

Minerals are one of the planet's contributions to your well-being. Be sure to take advantage of this mine of vital nutrients.

Don't judge each day by the harvest you reap, but by the seeds you plant.

Robert Lewis Stevenson

18

Supplemental Saviors Begin With the Basics

Proper supplementation may begin with FDA guidelines, but that is not where it ends. Your optimum dosage is determined not only by how vitamins and minerals interact with your body, but by how they interact with each other. I recommend that you do some experimentation under your physician's guidance until you arrive at a formula that is right for you.

As a dieter, you need to be especially aware of the properties of these supplements, for they play an important role in weight loss as well as in health. Some vitamins reduce sugar cravings, others give your metabolism a boost; all are important, so you will benefit yourself by learning as much as you can about them.

The best place to begin is with the vitamin label. I believe that the supplements you buy should offer the minimum basic formula.

SUPPLEMENT	DOSAGE
Vitamin A	25,000 I.U.
Vitamin B	1,000 I.U.
Vitamin B1	100 mg
Vitamin B2	100 mg
Vitamin B6	200 mg
Vitamin E	200 I.U.
Niacin	50 mg
Vitamin C	500 mg

SUPPLEMENT	DOSAGE
Choline	750 mg
Inosito	500 mg
Paba	1,200 mg
Biotin	200 mcg
Vitamin B12	150 mcg
Folic Acid	75 mg
Calcium	1,000 mg
Magnesium	500 mg
Maganese	6.1 mg
Zinc	50 mg
Iron	20 mg
Potassium	25-50 mg
Citrus Bioflavonoid Complex	25 mg
Neutomic Acid	25 mg
Selenium	50 mcg
Chromium	25 mcg
L-glutamine	25 mcg

This basic formula ensures that you will get at least the minimum amount of the vitamins and minerals that you need, without overloading on or neglecting any important nutrient.

You will notice that the recommended formula puts a great deal of emphasis on the water soluble vitamins B and C. It is not uncommon for me to suggest that my patients take extra C, for the healing properties of this vitamin have led to its use in the treatment of conditions ranging from gum disease to cancer.

Like vitamin C, the B-complex vitamins are very important in my diet plan. These nutrients help your body to extract the energy of proteins, fats, and carbohydrates. By taking sufficient amounts of these vitamins, you will be better able to utilize the body's fat mobilizing hormones.

The Magic Formula: Sugar Inhibitors

Dieters will also be happy to know that there are many supplements that can help reduce the craving for sweets and balance the blood sugar. A nonessential amino acid called L-glutamine is one such nutrient. Research has indicated that glutamic acid enhances intelligence, speeds the healing of ulcers, combats fatigue, and helps control alcoholism, schizophrenia, and the craving for sweets.

Nutritionist Roger Williams, Ph.D., was one of the pioneers of L-glutamine research. He and his associates, Drs. L.L. Rogers and R.V. Pelton, at the Clayton Foundation for Research, University of Texas, observed that not only did L-glutamine protect rats against the poisonous effects of alcohol, it stopped their craving for it. (Dr. Rogers also discovered that L-glutamine improved the I.Q. scores of mentally deficient children.)

In his book *Alcoholism: A Nutritional Approach,* Dr. Williams claimed that glutamine reduces the craving for alcohol in humans. The dosage he recommended was 1 to 4 grams a day.

Dr. Williams is far from being the only researcher to report on the link between L-glutamine and reduced alcohol craving. Jerzy Meduski, M.D., Ph.D., a member of the Task Force of Nutrition and Behavior in Los Angeles, also reported on the benefits of this supplement.

"The craving for alcohol seems to be the effect of an imbalance in nutrition. There is no doubt that there is a positive response to nutritional supplementation."[1]

I can personally vouch for the effectiveness of L-glutamine in reducing the desire for sweets. My associate, Dr. Louis Siegal, and I have found that L-glutamine taken in combination with chromium puts a cap on our patients' sweet tooth. The dosage we recommend for most patients is 1,000 mg of L-glutamine and 600 mcg of chromium, taken four times a day (half an hour before each meal and at bedtime).

Chromium has also been found effective in the treatment of high cholesterol levels. An article in *USA Today* stated that, "A natural nutrient available in health-food stores may lower cholesterol and blood sugar as well as act as a safe alternative to anabolic steroids."

The nutrient was tested by chemistry professor Gary W. Evans and his colleagues at Bemidji State University. The investigators gave subjects 1.6 mg of chromium picolinate daily for six weeks and found that:

> ➤ It lowered cholesterol levels an average of 7% in 28 subjects who had high cholesterol.

> ➤ It lowered blood sugar levels an average of 15% in 11 subjects with noninsulin-dependent diabetes.

> ➤ It increased muscle gain in weight lifters.

Because chromium is a natural and effective regulator of insulin, this trace mineral is an integral element in my program. Insulin is required to remove glucose from the blood. When glucose levels are high, as they are shortly after eating, the pancreas secretes insulin, which stimulates the cells to take up the glucose and burn it for energy.

According to one investigator, Richard A. Anderson, Ph.D., of the United States Department of Agriculture and Human Nutrition Research Center, "Chromium makes the insulin more efficient at stimulating the cells. The body needs less to do the job and so blood insulin stays at a healthy lower level."[2]

As we noted earlier, the fat mobilizing hormone is produced only when the body's carbohydrate level is low and the blood sugar level is constant. In a study conducted by Dr. Anderson, chromium supplements or brewer's yeast, which is rich in chromium, was found to normalize glucose metabolism. Volunteers who had slightly elevated blood sugar levels at the beginning of the study showed a drop of about 20 points following chromium supplementation. On the other hand, in subjects with moderately low blood sugar (hypoglycemia), chromium supplementation was associated with an average 10 point increase in blood sugar levels.

As Dr. Anderson explained,

"With chromium you don't have insulin overshooting its target. You don't get too much insulin in the blood or too little. You avoid the seesaws in blood sugar that come as a result of fluctuating insulin levels."[3]

Brewer's yeast has also been used to help regulate blood fats. In one study, subjects who took two tablespoons of chromium-rich brewer's yeast each day for eight weeks showed significant drops in their cholesterol levels. Researcher Clint Elwood, Ph.D., professor of biochemistry at the State University of New York, found that the average decrease in cholesterol was 10%, but that a few of the volunteers had dramatically larger reductions. As Dr. Elwood reported,

"The higher the cholesterol level the better the response was to brewers yeast. But what interested us most was that what we considered to be normal cholesterol levels could also be utilized with brewers yeast. We still don't know the best level of cholesterol for optimal health."

I saw my own cholesterol level drop from 280 to 190 over a period of six months. My program consisted of proper supplementation and a balanced diet, which was moderate in protein, fats and low in sugar and refined carbohydrates.

Our bodies require only 50 to 200 mcg of chromium a day. I may recommend doubling or tripling this amount, depending on a patient's age, weight, and diet. In general, I suggest taking 200 mcg of chromium and 500 mg of L-glutamine three times a day prior to each meal.

As you can see, while all nutrients are vital, some nutrients (to paraphrase Orwell) are more vital than others, depending on your unique requirements. Do be careful, though, not to become so impressed by any one nutrient that you overdo it, as this may defeat your purpose. Think of your supplements as a chain in which every link must be strong. And keep in mind that your supplement needs may be influenced by any number of factors, including your diet. For example, one study indicated that 85% of magnesium, 86% of , and 78% of zinc are lost when the major dietary staple is milk.[4]

Also, let me emphasize that this book is a guide, not a replacement for medical advice. Nor will I claim that I am offering all of the answers: nobody can. Anyone who claims to have the definitive word on health care is sure to eventually wind up in deep water, as the following story by Charles Tremendous Jones illustrates.

"Once a boy was rowing an old-timer across a wide river. The old-timer picked a floating leaf from the water, studied it for a moment and then asked the boy if he knew anything about biology. 'No, I don't,' the boy replied. The old-timer said, 'Son, you've missed twenty-five percent of your life.'

"As they rowed on, the old-timer took a rock from the bottom of the boat. He turned it in his hand studying its coloration and asked the boy, 'Son do you know anything about geology?' The boy sheepishly replied, 'No, I don't sir.' The old-timer said, 'Son, you've missed fifty percent of your life.'

"Twilight was approaching and the old-timer gazed rapidly at the North Star that had begun to twinkle. After a while he asked the boy, 'Son, do you know anything about astronomy?' The boy, head bowed and brow furrowed admitted, 'No, I don't sir.' The old-timer scolded, 'Son, you've missed seventy-five percent of your life!'

"Just then the boy noticed the huge dam upstream beginning to crumble and torrents of water pouring through the break. Quickly he turned to the old-timer and shouted, 'Sir, do you know how to swim?' The old-timer replied, 'No,' to which the boy shouted back, 'Old-timer, *you just lost your life.*'"

You do not have to know everything about nutrition to enjoy good health. You simply need to be willing to learn, before it's too late.

We never stop growing until we stop learning, and people who are learning this simple truth will grow old but never get old.

The excesses of our youth are drafts upon our old age, payable with interest about thirty years after date.

Colton

19

Growth Hormones—Turning Back the Clock

My interest in growth hormones began serendipitously, as a result of my work with athletes and research on steroids. Many of the athletes have asked for guidance on increasing strength and improving muscle tone. They are looking for a natural way to produce the muscle-building effects of steroids and other chemical body builders.

One day I was working with Barbara Bunkowski, winner of the Chrysler Tournament on the LPGA Tour. Barbara, a skilled, disciplined, and dedicated professional athlete, was concerned with building the strength and muscle tone on her left side. Like many other athletes—in fact, like most people, she is interested in inhibiting the aging process. This brought to my mind how wonderful it would be to turn back the clock. And so, began my experimentation with natural amino acids, which stimulate our growth hormones.

"Growth hormone is produced by the pituitary gland in our brain. Experiments sponsored by the National Institute of Aging showed that even in old age there is plenty of growth hormone in the healthy pituitary, but with age it becomes progressively more difficult to release it into your blood stream."[1]

Since the body needs a little help to produce growth hormones as we get older, we can supplement our diets with certain amino acids which are growth hormone releasers. Amino acids, the building blocks of protein, are also the building blocks our our bodies. We need protein to develop muscles, and we need amino acids to make protein. Amino acids are instrumental in regulating our emotions, controlling our cholesterol levels (children rarely have cholesterol problems because their amino acids are working for them), reducing pain, and ridding the body of fat while enhancing muscle tone. In our office, we frequently use amino acids in the treatment of our patients.

A wide range of disorders can be helped by judicious use of amino acids. Phenylalanine, for example, is associated with blood pressure control. Valine, isoleucine, and leucine have been linked with recovery from trauma.[2]

Growth hormones are released while we sleep, triggered by the neurotransmitters serotonin and dopamine. With proper supplementation, you can make sure that your sleep time produces more than dreams.

"Presently, we understand that growth hormone is necessary for proper function of our immune system, the white blood cells, the thymus gland, the spleen, bone marrow. When there is inadequate growth hormone (which we will refer to as GH) the thymus will shrink in size and the white blood cells will not be capable of doing as good a job of locating, killing and eating bacteria, viruses or cancer cells. It is essential to understand that older people release less growth hormone than younger people. It is, however, possible to bring growth hormone (GH) release back up to young adult levels by taking supplements. These supplements are most effective when taken just before bedtime, thus, increase the GH release at a natural pace in a daily cycle. Other factors that stimulate GH release include moderate fasting and exercise. Scientists for many years have studied the decline of GH output with aging."[3]

Essential amino acids are substances which stimulate the release of GH. My two favorites are L-arginine and L-ornithine. Other amino acids include:

L-phenylalanine	L-glutamine	Glycine
L-Leucine	L-methionine	L-isoleucine
L-proline	L-serine	L-tyrosine
L-aspartic acid	L-valine	L-cystine
L-cysteine	L-threonine	L-tryptophan*

(*–As of this writing, L-tryptophan is no longer available, due to its association with eosinophilia-myalgia, a sometimes fatal blood disorder. There is a possibility that the problem can be traced to a particular manufacturer, rather than the supplement itself. Nonetheless, you should absolutely not use this supplement—assuming that you should be able to obtain it—until such time as it is declared safe.)

My own experience is that taking three combined grams of L-arginine and L-ornithine before bedtime not only gave me a more restful night's sleep, but enabled me to build muscle and lose weight at a rapid pace. I found that these supplements help regulate the fat mobilizing hormone. Our metabolism is working while we sleep. Try a simple experiment: weigh yourself before bed, then again in the morning. Don't be surprised if you weigh less. This is why the "fat fighters" (GH) are especially effective when taken before bedtime.

Remember how you could eat as a kid? I've had so many patients say to me, "Doc, when I was young I could eat all I wanted, whenever I wanted. I wish I was young again." I have found that these supplements give the metabolism some of the flexibility of youth, they work like a jump start on our sluggish fat-burning batteries.

Exercise will release growth hormones, although research indicates that this effect ceases by age 30.

I recommend 2 to 3 g. of growth hormone per day, depending on body weight. People under 150 pounds should take 2 g., while those over 150 should take 2 to 3 g. (before bed on an empty stomach). Highly athletic people can also take 1 to 2 g. prior to exercise. It is important that use of GH be conducted under a physician's supervision.

I emphasize that inappropriate use of GH releasers, like improper use of vitamin supplements, can lead to adverse reactions. Children are still producing large amounts of GH, and GH releasers should not be used by anyone who has not completed the full growth cycle. These supplements are recommended only for people 25 or older. Excess GH can cause the skin to grow so rapidly that it can become noticeably thicker and coarser (fortunately, this is reversible upon discontinuation of GH). Consult your nutritionist or physician before using GH.

Food is a good source of GH. Both L-arginine and L-ornithine can be found in relatively high concentrations in chicken, turkey and other fowl. (I don't recommend taking L-arginine or L-ornithine with food, however.

Absorption is maximized when they are taken at bedtime on an empty stomach or prior to exercise.)

I found that L-arginine and L-ornithine have a number of important therapeutic properties. For example, one of my patients developed severe acne throughout his chest and back. After approximately one month on GH releasers, his condition had dramatically improved, and he was able to discontinue the medication he had been taking for it.

And studies, including one conducted by Hans Fisher, Ph.D., professor and chairman of the department of nutrition at Rutgers University, indicate that L-arginine may help the skin heal after major surgery.

"Healing involved formation of scar tissue, and scar tissue is made up of collagen, and collagen, a high percentage of L-arginine and amino acid glycine."[4]

For most people, though, the possibility of weight loss is what makes GH so attractive. I know this is what stimulated my interest in the subject. As a youngster, I was one of those athletes who could consume vast amounts of food without gaining a pound. Shortly after age 30, I found that, although my food consumption had decreased, I was developing a pot belly—a middle-age bulge. Most teenagers can "eat like horses," even if they are not active. But a middle-aged person eating the same food, in the same quantity, during the same hours, and taking the same amount of exercise, will usually gain weight.

But I had sworn not to have excess fat on my body, so I went to work on losing it. I began using growth hormones as part of my own personal fitness program. They were very effective, so I continued to research the subject.

Obese people should not be on "weight loss" diets, they should be on "fat loss" diets.

Most diets do not induce fat loss. Many diets may produce a rapid initial weight loss, but it soon becomes obvious most of what is lost is not fat, but electrolytes (water). The results are therefore temporary.

On my diet, we replace water, so we do not lose water weight. Because this program keeps blood sugar levels balanced through carbohydrate reduction, it promotes release of the fat mobilizing hormone. The stored fat is now a source of energy.

High levels of insulin, which are a natural consequence of carbo-hydrate and fat metabolism, can block the effects of growth hormone.

"Elevated blood sugar causes insulin release. All high glycemic food such as cane sugar, beet sugar, grape sugar, carrots or mashed potato, caused release of insulin which can block the growth hormone receptors and counteract the anti-fat storage effects of growth hormone, and promote the storing of excess calories as body fat."[5]

Conversely, high levels of growth hormone can block the effects of insulin. Therefore, growth hormones promote the conversion of stored fat into energy, which is exactly what my diet is designed to do.

"Growth hormone will alter our body's chemistry so that it will tend to utilize protein to build muscle rather than converting some of the calories and protein to sugar, and then converting that sugar to be stored as body fat. Growth hormone mobilizes stored body fat and makes it available to be burned for energy. Growth hormone discourages your body from converting food that you eat to stored fat."[6]

Growth hormone releasers are also a boom to body builders and weight lifters who are concerned—and rightly so—about the harmful effects of steroids. Steroids are chemical hormone releasers. Athletes who use them are actually injecting animal hormones into their bodies. They are unsafe and illegal.

Because many of my patients are weight lifters and body builders, I am naturally interested in offering them a safe alternative. Several years ago, I had the pleasure of treating Dennis Tinerino, who held the titles of Mr. America, Mr. Universe, and Natural Mr. America. I found him to be bright, articulate, and very interesting. I was impressed because of his commitment to good health, which was at least as important to him as an excellent physique.

The GH releasers I most often recommend for muscle enhancement are L-arginine and L-orinithine. Also, Biotics Research Corporation, of Houston, Texas, offers a product called Amino Sport, which when utilized properly, is an excellent source of amino acids for athletes. My patients have found these supplements to be most effective when taken half an hour before exercise and on an empty stomach.

Once again, the key to proper use of these supplements is balance. The GH releasers can help to revitalize the body's metabolism. However, they do not take the place of proper diet and exercise. There are no shortcuts to health, but there are ways to make it go more smoothly.

Summary

1. Growth hormones should be taken strictly under a physician's guidance; immediately report any side-effects to your doctor.

2. Take them for periods of two weeks at a time.

3. Utilize them to boost your metabolism periodically, whenever metabolism is sluggish.

4. GH should be taken on an empty stomach at bedtime.

5. GH is also effective taken half an hour before exercise.

6. Amino Sport, L-arginine, and L-ornithine are my favorites for weight loss and body toning.

7. GH must be utilized in conjunction with a low-sugar, low-carbohydrate diet for maximum effectiveness.

8. Utilize chromium and L-glutamine to help break sugar, alcohol addiction.

Prejudice is a disease characterized by hardening of the categories.
William Arthur Ward

20

The Dairy News

You won't find the dairy news making the headlines, but perhaps it should. This information has important health ramifications, and if that isn't newsworthy, I don't know what is. If you grew up hearing that, "milk (and by extension other dairy products) is good for you" it may be necessary for you to readjust some of your ideas.

One type of milk is, in fact, very beneficial: mother's milk. Breast feeding is one of the best things a mother can do for her child, for it helps build up an infant's immune system and provides other advantages.

Robert S. Mendelson, M.D., pediatrician and author of *Medical Malpractice, Confessions of a Medical Heretic,* and *How to Raise a Healthy Child in Spite of Your Doctor,* has this to say about the subject:

"Breast feeding lays the foundation for healthy physical and emotional growth. It provides your child and yourself with many additional benefits as well. Mother's milk, time tested for millions of years, is the best nutrient for babies because it is nature's perfect food. It provides your child with all the nutrients he needs for healthy growth for at least the first six months of his life and all responsible nutritional and pediatric authorities acknowledge its superiority over instant infant formulas and cow's milk. Cow's milk is deficient in iron and should not be given to babies for at least six months. Even then it should be introduced with caution, because many babies, perhaps as many as 15%, are allergic to cow's milk. It should be suspected as a potential cause of many illnesses."

Bottle feeding a baby an infant formula is not what nature had in mind. A formula is just that—a chemical concoction that is intended to duplicate an already perfect food. If you breast feed your child, there is no danger that some essential nutrients will be omitted from your milk. This is not true of formula. True, these products are "fortified" with vitamins, which simply indicates that they were not there in the first place. Also, formulas contain added sugar, which paves the way for later sugar addiction. Bottle-fed babies may also be more prone to weight problems.

"Bottle feeding with infant formulas also predisposes infants to lifelong obesity because the products provide the wrong kind of nutrients. Human milk is 1.3% protein. Cow's milk and instant formulas are 3.3% protein or more. That's why one study of 250 full term infants at six weeks of age found that 60% of the bottle fed babies were overweight, compared 19% of those who were breast fed. Excess protein places an unduly heavy load on the kidneys and some children gain weight faster because they retain more fluid. Finally, breast fed babies are permitted to eat until they are satisfied, and you have no ability or need to measure the quantity of milk that your child takes. Formula fed babies are usually placed on a fixed schedule, with a measured amount of milk given at each feeding."[1]

Habits are learned early. A child who is placed on a schedule learns to eat not according to hunger, but according to a timetable.

In addition to the physical benefits of breast feeding, we have the emotional rewards conferred on mother and child.

"One is that a breast fed baby gains from his mother's milk a natural immunity to many allergies and infections that is denied from babies that are bottle fed. Mother's milk contains a unique substance that inhibit the growth of bacteria and viruses, warding your baby critical protection against disease during the most hazardous months of his life. Secondly, the bonding of a mother to a child is regarded as essential to your baby's emotional development and provides emotional rewards for you as well. The nurturing that breast feeding supplies is the ideal way to establish this bond almost from the moment of birth.

"Unless you have received excessive drugs during delivery, which also affected your baby, your desire to begin nursing should be at its peak within 20-30 minutes after birth. From that moment on he should be nursed when he gives evidence of the desire to do so. At the outset this may be as many as 20 times a day."[2]

Dr. Grandly Dick-Read, regarded by many as the father of today's natural childbirth movement, also praises breast feeding: "The newborn baby has only three demands their warmth in the arms of its mother, food from her breast, and security in the knowledge of her presence. Breast feeding satisfies all three."[3]

Given all the evidence in favor of breast feeding, it is amazing that some pediatricians still have reservations about this practice. Pediatricians often recommend taking the child off the breast and putting him or her on formula because the doctor is not satisfied with the weight gain of the breast-fed child. The irony of this was nicely summed up by Dr. Mendelson.

"What their doctor doesn't tell them is that the ritual has no medical significance whatsoever. They aren't told that some formula manufacturer was probably the source of the growth chart that the doctor is using and that he gets them free. At least to an obvious question: why are the formula makers so eager to have your doctor check your baby's weight? Answer. Because the weight gain of breast fed babies may not match the average weight shown on the formula maker's chart. They hope that the pediatrician, instead of reassuring the mother that this is normal and non-threatening will tell her to stop breast feeding and switch to their product, of which he has a reminder in hand. Too often that is exactly what he does and the baby is subsequently denied the immunity and other benefits that breast feeding provides."[4]

Standard growth charts trouble Dr. Mendelson, whose concern is the lack of valid norms for breast-fed versus bottle-fed babies. Somehow, infants thrived for eons before formula manufacturers existed. God did not make a mistake when he created the female breasts. He constructed them so that mothers could provide their children with the essence of life. God did not create En-nulls or Enfamil. It is unfortunate that some pediatricians become so focused on a manufacturer's weight chart that they recommend switching a baby to cow's milk.

Cow's milk is ideal—for calves. That is the animal for whom nature designed this product, and its components are proof of this. For example, all milk products contain a vital substance called casein. But, as I'll explain, there is far more casein in cow's milk than a human can comfortably handle.

Before making a decision, know the facts. Don't be afraid to ask your doctor questions. You can be misled if you only have part of the information you need, as the following story illustrates.

Two men were thrown into the army guardhouse. One prisoner asked his cellmate, "How long are you in for?" The other prisoner replied, "Twenty-four hours." The first prisoner asked what offense he had committed. "I killed the general," he said. Confused, the first prisoner asked, "How come I got 30 days for going AWOL and you only get 24 hours for murdering the general."

He replied, "Because they're hanging me tomorrow."

Humans are the only species that continue to drink milk after they are weaned. If you put a bowl of milk in front of an adult cow, she would probably ignore it and munch on grass. Domesticated animals, such as cats, are different—they will drink milk because humans have tampered with their tastes. The enzymes necessary to break down and digest milk are rennin and lactase. Is it a coincidence that most people no longer produce these enzymes after age three?

This is not to say that you cannot consume dairy products, but it is important to exercise moderation. And dairy products should not be combined with other animal products or with carbohydrates.

Earlier, I referred to white flour, sugar, and salt as the "three whites." Milk is the fourth white. While it is less harmful than the other three, it does present health risks. And it is impossible to consume the four whites in large quantities and remain thin.

Maybe you feel this doesn't apply if you eat the most famous of the dairy "health foods"—yogurt. Perhaps nothing boosted the reputation of this product as much as the famous advertising campaign which featured the Hunza people. The Hunza live in an isolated kingdom in the Himalayas, and the inhabitants are noted for their low (almost non-existent) disease rate and extraordinary longevity; some Hunza people have lived to be 125 years old.

The point of the commercial, of course, is to get people to eat yogurt. I guarantee you, they never heard of Dannon. You can be sure that their yogurt is not processed until all nutritional value has been removed and then loaded with sugar.

In fact, when asked the secret of their longevity, the Mir (king) said that the Hunza people attribute their long lifespan to the naturally hard (heavily mineralized) water that they consume.[5]

So leave the yogurt to the advertisers and drink lots of water.

Yogurt with fruit is also very high in carbohydrates. A single serving contains about 40 g., which puts you close to exceeding your critical carbohydrate level for the day. Even plain milk is rather high in carbohydrates. One glass can contain upwards of 15 grams of carbohydrate. Dairy products are also high in fat. And many people, because they lack the enzymes necessary to break down milk, are lactose-intolerant, meaning dairy products are difficult for them to digest.

In addition, milk has been implicated in many allergies. Many of my patients who suffered from acne, asthma, arthritis and upper respiratory infections found that their problems cleared up once they removed dairy products from their diets.

Before I sustained my knee injury, I believed that I had a healthy diet, even though as a youth I was plagued with acne, and later with upper- respiratory infections. I was warned off chocolate, but other sugar-laden foods and dairy products were never mentioned.

On the contrary, I was told that milk would make me strong. Meat, too, is considered a strengthening food, and many people wash down their meat with milk, not realizing that this combination can cause a digestive overload.

Cow's milk does indeed make cows strong. This drink is intended by nature for a huge, big-boned animal with four stomachs. A calf weighs about 90 pounds at birth and may attain a weight of 2,000 pounds in approximately two years. Humans, on the other hand, enter the world weighing about 5 to 10 pounds, and on the average weight 100 to 200 pounds at maturity. We simply don't need the extra casein that a growing cow requires.

"There is 300 percent more casein in cow's milk than in human's milk. Cows need this for the development of huge bones. Casein coagulates in the stomach and forms large, tough, dense, difficult to digest curds that are adapted to the four stomach digestive apparatus of a cow. Once inside the human system, this thick mass of goo puts a tremendous burden on the body to somehow get rid of it. In other words, a huge amount of energy must be spent dealing with it.

"Unfortunately some of this gooey substance hardens and adheres to the linings of the intestines and prevents the absorption of nutrients into the body. Result, lethargy. Also, the byproducts of milk digestion leave a great deal of toxic mucous in the body. It is very acidic, and some of it is stored in the body until it can be dealt with at a later time. The next time you are going to dust your home, smear some paste all over everything and see how easy it is to dust. Dairy products do the same to the inside of your body. That translates into more weight instead of weight loss. Casein, by the way, is the base of one of the strongest glues used in woodwork." [6]

It is no wonder that people who have a diet high in dairy products are also people whose saliva is highly viscous, and who are prone to hay fever, bronchitis, asthma, sinusitis, ear infections, respiratory infections, and a host of other problems.

We have also been told that we should drink milk for its calcium content, but as I explained in the section on calcium, many other foods, such as fruits, green leafy vegetables, nuts and sesame seeds are better sources of this mineral.

Still, the image of milk as the "perfect beverage" persists. The dairy industry, like the sugar industry, has the money and the power to promote its product.

"In March 1984, the *Los Angeles Times* reported that the Department of Agriculture decided to launch a $140 million advertising campaign to promote milk drinking and help reduce the multi-million dollar surplus."

It's amazing that we would have a surplus given the rate at which dairy products are consumed in this country. We do, though, and you and I are paying for it.

"You can be absolutely certain of one thing, milk is the most political food in America. According to the *Los Angeles Times,* the dairy industry is subsidized (meaning taxpayers foot the bill), to the tune of almost $3 billion a year. That is $342 thousand every hour to buy hundreds of millions of dollars worth of dairy products that would in all likelihood never be eaten. They are sitting in storage and some of them are rotten to the core. The storage bill alone for the surplus that will never be used is $47 million annually."[7]

The nutrients that are contained in milk—and the milk that flows from the udder of a cow does contain vitamins, minerals and other nutrients—often don't survive pasteurization. Harvey and Marilyn Diamond presented an apt analogy of this process.

"What if I were to tell you that there exists a special bomb that, if dropped during war time on a city where fighting was going on, would kill only the enemy and leave our allies unscathed. Would you believe me or think I was lying. What if I were to tell you that I could take a food with some good ingredients and some bad ingredients, adhere to a temperature so hot that it would kill the bad (our enemy) and leave the good (our allies) unscathed? Would you believe that?"[8]

The Diamonds criticism of pasteurized milk is certainly justified by the facts. One of their sources, Dr. William Ellis, noted that "pasteurization destroys the valuable enzymes, making pasteurized milk much worse." The Diamonds also cited a study linking pasteurized milk to heart disease. Yet another example of the nutritional hollowness of pasteurized milk was provided by some puppies and kittens who were fed nothing else. The animals died. But the puppies and kittens fed on raw milk thrived.

Most incredible of all was a study that found that calves fed on pasteurized milk died before maturity in nine out of ten cases. "Calves, the very animal that milk is designed for, can't live if it is pasteurized."[9]

The Diamonds are not alone in their opinion of pasteurized milk.

"Dr. Pottenger conducted a test with three infants. One was breast fed, one was fed raw milk, and one was fed pasteurized milk. The first two infants, those that were breast fed and raw milk were healthy and developed normally. The third infant, the one that was fed pasteurized milk was sickly, small, and developed asthma at the age of eight months."[10]

And pasteurization may be no guarantee that harmful bacteria won't be found in milk.

"The widespread practice of feeding antibiotics to cattle to speed their growth increased potentially deadly bacteria that can affect humans. Seventeen persons became sick and one died because a herd of South Dakota cattle were fed antibiotics."[11]

I'm not recommending that you drink raw milk; I'm suggesting that you moderate your use of dairy products. Milk, like candy and cake, should be an occasional indulgence, not a dietary staple.

Perhaps you are thinking, "Well, if I shouldn't drink milk, and I can't drink soda, and fruit juice isn't recommended, what's left?"

What's left is the core of all these beverages, the most vital part of them—water.

"Ancient man clearly sensed the importance of water and made it a central feature of a great many mythological and religious ceremonies, including that of Genesis. For the Greeks, the Titans Oceanus and Tethys were the parents of creation. Western scientific tradition began in Greece when the Ionian philosopher scientist Thales of Mellitus, who flourished in the 6th and 7th centuries B.C., substituted the natural forces for gods as the courses of natural phenomenon but retained water as the essential principle or element of this cosmology. His successors added only primal elements fire, earth and air and the influence of Aristotle, who taught the doctrine of the four elements."[12]

The body, which is 70% water, is in constant need of this liquid. Yet our values have become so skewed that we would rather drink a beverage whose nucleus is water than to drink water itself. We have polluted not only our oceans, lakes and rivers, but the water reservoir of our own bodies.

One of the reasons we must consume the four whites in moderation is that an overload of these substances will upset our natural water balance. Sodium intake, for example, must be restricted to under 15 mg per day or the body will absorb and store more water than is necessary. Many people who are taking medication for hypertension could control the problem by drinking sufficient water and limiting sodium intake. If we upset the balance of our bodies we take them from a state of ease to a state of "dis-ease," which eventually leads to "disease."

"Water supports all the nutritive processes from digestion absorption to utilization and excretion. From the moment food enters our mouth every process necessary to transform it from our food to blood, bone, muscle and tissue depends on water. Water holds nutrients in a solution and transports all food necessary for life to the various parts of the body."[13]

Water is also the body's chief agent of temperature regulation. If you drain the water from your automobile it will overheat and the engine will burn out. The human machine will suffer a similar fate if deprived of sufficient amounts of water.

While eight, eight-ounce glasses of water per day is the minimum I recommend, you should certainly drink more if you are thirsty.

Water is vital in this weight-loss program. The ketones produced by the breakdown of fat must be transported from the body, and what could do a better job of this than water? I don't recommend carbonated water, which usually contains sodium. In my opinion, the best choices are mountain, spring, and distilled water—which contains nothing but water itself.

Like milk, other dairy products should be consumed in moderation. Cheese is permitted on my diet, but unlimited cheese is certainly not recommended. Many forms of cheese are high in sodium and cholesterol. On the other hand, cheese is a good source of protein and supplies adequate amounts of protein. Cheese makes a good snack for dieters. Many fresh cheeses, such as parmesan, part-skim mozzarella, cottage cheese, pot cheese, farmer cheese, and ricotta, have a moderate fat content. (This is acceptable, as we need a certain amount of fat in our diets.) However, some of the low cholesterol cheeses have a high sodium content, so read the labels carefully.

Low-fat cheese can also be a good choice from the standpoint of your carbohydrate level. While one cup of milk contains 12 grams of carbohydrate, an ounce of Kraft Cracker Barrel Sharp Cheddar Cheese contains only one gram. Use heavy cream rather than milk in your coffee, as a tablespoon of cream contains only a trace amount of carbohydrates.

It is important to keep in mind that sugar will not only push you over your critical carbohydrate level, it will interfere with your ability to break down the fats in dairy products (and other foods, for that matter).

As a youth I was educated to believe that pizza was junk food. It's today's myth that pizza is highly nutritious, but I guarantee that a diet high in pizza is a diet high in cholesterol, high in calories, fat and carbohydrates. It is our purpose to count carbohydrates, not calories. Pizza on occasion is allowable if eaten solely and explicitly on its own. Let me explain.

I owe this discovery to my friend Dr. Jim Gregg, a well-known and respected practitioner in Michigan, and one of the people who has achieved success on my weight loss program. Dr. Gregg and I were attending a conference in Atlanta. One morning, on my way to breakfast I noticed two large pizza boxes outside his room. I said, "You've been doing so well on my diet. How in the world can you sit there at night eating pizza?" His answer was enlightening. "I don't eat the breading of the pizza, I only eat the cheese and the topping." I did a quick calculation, and had to agree that the topping of pizza is perfectly legal on my diet.

One of the first things I did when I was back home was call the Pizza man. After nine months without pizza, I had a great time devouring some pizza topping. And I was delighted when I stepped on the scale the next morning and found that I weighed precisely what I had the day before. This is an excellent example of just how flexible my diet is, and how much you can enjoy your food and lose weight by using a little creativity.

Eggonomics

Eggs can really play havoc with the Dow Jones average of nutritionists. One day they are considered a great source of low-calorie nutrition. The next they are carriers of dreaded cholesterol, and must be avoided at all costs. If eggs were a stock we would grow dizzy watching their rise and fall.

My opinion—and that of many other nutrition experts—is somewhere in the middle of these two extremes. I do feel that eggs are one of the most misunderstood foods on the planet. Eggs, eaten in moderation, are a highly beneficial food.

When people are instructed to steer clear of eggs, their cholesterol content is the reason. I am not saying that your cholesterol level is not important. It is a risk factor in heart attacks, but it's certainly not the only risk factor. Dr. Michael DeBakey, possibly one of the most well-known heart surgeons in the world, has observed that, "About 80% of my sickest patients have the cholesterol levels of normal people."

Furthermore, a certain amount of cholesterol is not only acceptable, but vital.

". . . cholesterol is a complex chemical that is absolutely essential to life. It is the basic molecular building block, from which adrenal hormones, sex hormones, vitamin D, and the bile acids necessary to digestion are formed. Cholesterol forms part of the membranes that surrounds every cell in our body. It is part of the protective covering of nerve fibers; it makes up a large part of the brain, it combines with various proteins to form lipoproteins needed to transport fats used as energy. Recent findings indicate that cholesterol may be essential to normal growth, longevity, and resistance to infection and toxicity."[14]

As always, the key is common sense and balance. While an excess of anything can be dangerous, a lack of certain elements can also be disasterous. According to Dr. Atkins, "Not getting enough fat or cholesterol can cause big problems."[15] He explains that some of his patients on low cholesterol diets have very dry skin. Cholesterol-deficient women may have menstrual problems. He is of the opinion that these people do not have sufficient cholesterol to form the sterol ring, the basic structure of sex hormones. The result can be menstrual irregularities, diminished sex drive, painful intercourse, and/or poor bust development.

It is also interesting to note that not everyone agrees that foods high in cholesterol will elevate your blood cholesterol levels. The dietary cholesterol in shell fish, egg yolks, butter, and other foods provides only about 20 to 30 percent of the cholesterol in the body. Cholesterol is manufactured in the body by the liver and intestines from the metabolism of proteins, fats, and carbohydrates.

"To produce cholesterol the body has a complicated feedback mechanism to operate, which means that the more cholesterol you eat, the less you manufacture. There is a limit to the amount of cholesterol that can be absorbed by your digestive tract, particularly beyond the cholesterol contained in two eggs per day, which is 500 mg. For every 100 mg of cholesterol moved from the daily diet the blood level falls only three points. Eliminating two eggs per day from your diet could only be expected to lower your cholesterol 15 points at most."[16]

Dr. Roslyn Alfin-Slatter of UCLA conducted a study in which 52 young to middle-aged men were fed two extra eggs daily for eight weeks. At the end of this time, there was no significant increase in their cholesterol levels.

"We, like everyone else, have been convinced that when you eat cholesterol, you get cholesterol," Dr. Alfin-Slatter said in an interview, "that we stopped to think that all the studies in the past never tested the normal diet in relation to egg eating. We decided to see what happens. Our findings surprised us as much as anyone else."[17]

Dr. George Mann, professor of medicine at Vanderbilt School of Medicine, had some sharp words about the fear associated with dietary cholesterol,

"The Heart Association committed the nutritional disaster of the century by confusing the association with causation to the endless delight and profit of food companies that employed cholesterol scare tactics in their advertising." [18]

A government report on diet and coronary heart disease in Great Britain pointed an accusing finger at dietary sugar, but not dietary cholesterol.

"There is no certainty that the reduction of cholesterol intake diminishes susceptibility of heart disease. We have found no evidence which relates to a number of eggs to a risk of heart disease." But the panel pointed out that, "The higher the national consumption of sucrose, which would be sugar, the higher the death rate from heart attacks."[19]

On the subject of heart disease and eggs, an interesting extrapolation may be made from findings of noted researcher Dr. Roger J. Williams. He said that the nutrients that are probably most essential in preventing heart disease and arterial disorders are vitamin E, folic acid, vitamin B6, magnesium and vitamin C. Eggs contain every one of these nutrients except vitamin C, and they also supply calcium, iron, phosphorous, vitamin B12, and a trace of vitamin K.

In *Thorson's Complete Guide to Vitamins and Minerals*, it says, "High blood cholesterol levels can be reduced by taking 500 mg vitamin C daily or by taking 3 g nicotinic acid daily."

Our triglyceride levels, like our cholesterol levels, can be important predictors of heart disease. In fact, numerous authorities believe that triglyceride levels are more important than cholesterol levels. Remember, triglycerides are nothing more than stored fat. On Dr. Kaplan's diet, as you break down fat you automatically lower your triglyceride levels. A group of researchers at Harvard used a 26 g. low-carbohydrate diet to treat a group of patients with high triglycerides. In a few weeks, their triglycerides fell from 1,628 to 286, and their cholesterol levels went from 470 to 290.[20]

"Dr. George Bray and his associates demonstrated that triglyceride levels in obese subjects fell over just two weeks on a 60 g. carbohydrate diet. The readings dropped from 184 to 85. The insulin level, another forecaster of heart disease, dropped also."[21]

Research indicates that the average person can safely consume four to six eggs per week. I believe that you are better off eating eggs for breakfast than eating cereal; eggs are high in protein and nutrition (see figures 15, 16, 17), while the popular cereals consist mainly of refined carbohydrates.

What you want to avoid is combining eggs improperly with other foods. Consuming sugar or refined carbohydrates in the same meal with proteins, fats, and starches will immobilize the fat mobilizing hormone. This will force your body to store cholesterol instead of enabling it to use cholesterol where it is needed: in the adrenal hormones, the sex hormones, the bile acids, and the nerve sheaths and transmitters.

I believe my diet is in line with the natural nutrition needs of the human animal. Basically, we are omnivores, not carnivores, vegetarians, or fruitarians. In the infancy of our species, people hunted for food and ate wild berries and other foods from the land. My goal is to help you achieve balance, not to restrict you. So in addition to vegetables, my diet allows you to eat meat, fish, poultry, and, yes, eggs.

Margarine Madness

Today, it is estimated that margarine users outnumber butter users by more than two to one.

This is hardly surprising, for most of us were hearing of the virtues of the former (courtesy of television) before we knew the difference between a polyunsaturated fat and a polysyllable.

We have been led to believe that polyunsaturated fats, especially linoleic acid, can lower body fats and break down saturated fats. So in theory, it seems logical that if we switch to a polyunsaturated oil or margarine, we will be helping to lower the body's serum cholesterol level.

But the facts may not fit this appealing hypothesis. In his book *Super Nutrition*, Richard A. Passwater, Ph.D., explains that,

"The danger of polyunsaturated fats began to be noticed when Dr. Fred A. Kummerow and his colleagues from the University of Illinois at Urbana reported their studies at the 1974 Federation of American Societies for experimental biology meeting of nutritionists and related science. Newspapers carry the story of such titles as 'Margarine Found Health Hazard.' It is a shame that the story didn't make the front sections but that findings showed that fat present in margarine may present a greater health risk than cholesterol rich foods such as beef fat, butter fat, and powdered eggs."

Polyunsaturated fats have also fallen victim to the processed food syndrome, according to Dr. Stuart M. Berger, author of *How To Be Your Own Nutritionist.*[22]

"Polyunsaturated fats can turn chameleon because the sepolyunsaturated margarines contain extra ingredients stabilizers, emulsifiers, and preservatives. (Couldn't this be more dangerous to your health than the saturated fat in butter?) The truth is the real danger of margarine comes not just from such artificial ingredients, but from its heat processing. When vegetable fats are heated to make margarine, they undergo a chemical transformation called hydrogenation, and some of them become what are called trans-fatty acids. Unfortunately, there is good evidence that fatty acids in this form have a significant cancer causing potential."

Dr. Denham Harman, of the University of Nebraska, has concluded, based on animal studies, that the concentrated use of polyunsaturates can shorten a person's life by 15 years.[23]

Recently, a study reported in the Associated Press claimed that men and women who ate the most margarine and certain processed foods had more than twice the heart attack risk. This study, which was presented at the Annual American Heart Association's Epidemiology Meeting, is one of the first to link margarine directly to heart disease. The problem occurs when polyunsaturated oils (which do not pose a heart risk), are modified to make them solid or semi-solid, a process known as hydrogenation. Hydrogenated or partially hydrogenated vegetable oils are used to make margarine, a variety of cookies, potato chips, crackers and other processed foods. (All high in refined carbohydrates.) Dr. Alberto Asherio of the Harvard School of Public Health in Boston analyzed the diets of both heart attack and non-heart attack victims. He found those highest in trans-fatty acids (margarine) had 2.44 times the heart risk of those whose diets were lowest in trans-fatty acids.[24]

I suggest to my patients that they conduct a simple experiment. It involves taking a pat of margarine in one hand and a pat of butter in the other, then rubbing the fingers back and forth. The butter will dissolve, practically liquify, in your hand. The margarine, on the other hand (pun intentional) maintains a thick, coarse texture that is not broken down by the heat given off by the body. If we are not able to break down this viscous, gelatinous substance in our hands, how can the body break it down in the circulatory system?

I'm amazed at the conflicting advice we hear in this society. We are told that dairy products are good for us, and that we should drink milk to build strong bones and eat yogurt to improve our overall health. In the next breath, we are solemnly warned away from butter. Yet butter is nothing more than churned cream.

Butter has been eaten for centuries, while margarine has only been on the market for 30 or 40 years. Butter is a natural food, while margarine is a chemical concoction. The widespread fear of dietary fats makes margarine an advertiser's dream, but it is a consumer's nightmare.

Butter contains *no carbohydrates*, which is why it is allowed on my diet. I'm not suggesting you gorge on it, but by all means use it, as long as it is not combined with a refined carbohydrate. That means no bread and butter, because this mixture can go straight to your waistline.

Fats are essential to the body. They keep your skin and your vital mucous membranes smooth and lubricated.

Most important, they transport the fat-soluble vitamins (A, D, E, K) to the sites where they are needed. Following digestion, fats are absorbed and then oxidized to produce energy, carbon dioxide, and water.

Fats are a reserve of fuel, which is why my dietary principles work. When we cut down on carbohydrates, the fat mobilizing hormone is released, and turns this fat into energy—the purpose for which nature intended it.

Fats are also important in my program because they ward off boredom, which has been the downfall of many a diet. A little butter goes a long way toward adding zest to vegetables. In addition, fats help stabilize blood sugar, and when our blood sugar is under control, our appetite is reduced, so our overall consumption of food—including fat—is reduced naturally.

I find it amazing, day after day, to find that the same people who won't eat eggs for fear of their cholesterol levels will gorge themselves on sweets, starches, and refined carbohydrates. They compound insult to injury by consuming gobs of margarine (they have no fear of margarine's side effects) on their foods. They wash this all down with a glass of milk. The facts are the facts, our country is not the healthiest in the world. It appears to me that chemical nutrition has kept up with medical technology—the result being no major increase in life expectancy over the past 15 to 20 years. Eat wisely, be an educated consumer.

The fellow who says he's too old to learn new tricks probably always was.

21

Cafe Fat Away

Regardless of how well balanced a diet is, or how low in calories (or carbohydrates), it won't work if you don't stay on it. And given the monotony of most weight loss programs, it's hardly surprising that so many dieters see-saw between over-restriction and overindulgence.

I don't expect your kitchen to resemble a chemistry lab—a gourmet restaurant is more like it. The range of foods you are allowed on my diet, along with some imagination, can make eating a pleasure rather than a grim chore.

In this chapter, I'll review the permitted foods and provide some sample menus. Keep in mind, though, that these menus are only suggestions. Provided you remain within the guidelines, you can make your meals as exotic as you desire.

For the first four days, breakfast should consist of one egg, one orange or grapefruit, and a multiple vitamin. Your lunch should consist of a protein in the form of fish or chicken and a green salad with an olive oil and apple cider vinegar dressing. Dinner should consist of the same types of food as lunch. Remember, my diet requires that you have three protein entrees a day, and meals should not be skipped. During this period you may eat as much green salad as you desire. Women should keep protein portions to 6 ounces or less, men to 10 ounces or less.

After the preparatory phase, you will be allowed one or two additional fruits per day. Because this food should be eaten in moderation, watch your portions. A typical portion (i.e., one fruit) might consist of ten small grapes, 1/4 cup of blueberries, 1/4 of a medium size cantaloupe, 1/2 cup of pineapple, or 1/2 cup of strawberries.

Do not eat any fruit after 6:00 p.m.

After week one, you may add a minimum of one and a maximum of two starches a day. I also recommend that you have two tablespoons of miller's bran or an oat bran capsule on a daily basis. These are counted as a free starch, meaning you don't have to count them in your starch allowance. Permitted starches include diet whole wheat bread, which has about 40 calories per slice, but only 6 grams of carbohydrate (check the label). Other allowed starches are unseasoned melba toast (one slice), one Stella Doro bread stick, and/or half of a rice cake.

Your daily diet might look something like this after the four-day preparatory phase:

DAY 1

BREAKFAST
1 egg
1 orange
MID-MORNING SNACK
1 peach
LUNCH
6 oz. cottage cheese
1 cup lettuce
1 cup cucumber
1 slice melba toast
DINNER
9 oz. turkey
1 cup spinach
1 cup squash
DESSERT
diet jello (sugarless, carbohydrate free)

DAY 2

BREAKFAST

herbal tea or coffee (maximum 2 cups of coffee daily,
recommend decaffeinated)

1 orange

LUNCH

6 oz. tuna

caesar salad

SNACK

diet jello

DINNER

6-8 oz. grouper

salad, olive oil/vinegar

1 cup broccoli with melted low-fat cheddar cheese

DESSERT

diet jello

DAY 3

BREAKFAST

2-egg omelet with broccoli and low-fat cheddar cheese

LUNCH

6-10 oz. fish

large green salad

MID-AFTERNOON SNACK

1/2 grapefruit

DINNER

5-7 oz. beef

1/2 cup asparagus

1/2 cup spinach

DAY 4

BREAKFAST
1 grapefruit
cup of coffee
MID-MORNING SNACK
piece of low-fat cheese
LUNCH
shrimp scampi (maximum 10 oz. shrimp)
large salad
SNACK
2 celery sticks with low-fat cream cheese
DINNER
6-8 oz. veal chops
1/2 cup cucumbers
1/2 cup celery
dinner salad
DESSERT
diet jello

DAY 5

BREAKFAST
1 egg
1 orange
LUNCH
caesar salad
9 oz. flounder
1/2 cup celery
1/2 slice diet bread
SNACK
celery stick with 1/2 oz. peanut butter (check label, some
contain sugar)
DINNER
6-8 oz. chicken
1/2 cup green beans
1 cup raw mushrooms

DAY 6

BREAKFAST
1 grapefruit
cup of coffee
   MID-MORNING SNACK
1/2 cup strawberries
   LUNCH
6-8 oz. fresh fish
large salad
   SNACK
4 oz. raw low-fat cheddar cheese
   DINNER
5 oz. beef
1/2 cup cooked broccoli
1/2 cup cooked cauliflower
   DESSERT
diet chocolate pudding

DAY 7

BREAKFAST
1 egg
1 orange
   SNACK
3 oz. low-fat cheese
   LUNCH
8 oz. broiled flounder
green salad
   SNACK
1 apple
   DINNER
8 oz. chicken
green salad
1/2 cup broccoli
1/2 cup cauliflower
   DESSERT
sugarless jello

All meat, fish and poultry portions should range from six to ten ounces for men, and from four to eight ounces for women. If you eat larger portions, the diet will still work provided you eat no refined carbohydrates, but you will reduce at a slower rate. And remember that your eight, eight-ounce glasses of water are important to weight loss.

When you have completed the first phase of this program, you can move to Phase 2. In this phase, you are allowed fats in moderation, as well as condiments and two starches equaling no more than 12 grams of carbohydrates (two pieces of diet bread). If you have a lot of weight to lose, limit yourself to one starch per day.

Your diet in Phase 2 might look something like this:

DAY 1

BREAKFAST
scrambled eggs and turkey bacon
cup of coffee
MID-MORNING SNACK
1 orange
LUNCH
sliced steak
salad
MID-AFTERNOON SNACK
1 small apple
DINNER
caesar salad
chicken cordon bleu
DESSERT
diet jello
diet soda

DAY 2

BREAKFAST
1 orange
cup of coffee
1 slice whole wheat bread
LUNCH
chicken salad with homemade mayonnaise* and celery
1 cup green salad—oil and vinegar

*(Note: The problem with most mayonnaise is that it is made with hydrogenated fats which are associated with clogged arteries and cancer. It is recommended that you make your own mayonnaise using the following recipe.

1 egg white

1/2 tsp. dijon mustard

1 tsp. freshly squeezed lemon juice

1 cup olive oil

Using a food processor, slowly pour olive oil until desired thickness is achieved. You can make larger amounts as well. It will keep in the refrigerator for up to two weeks.)

MID-AFTERNOON SNACK
1 grapefruit
DINNER
assorted grilled seafood with lemon butter sauce
1 cup salad with green peppers, radishes, celery and
scallions
DESSERT
diet jello
chamomile tea

DAY 3

BREAKFAST
low-fat cheese omelet with mushrooms
    LUNCH
shrimp scampi
fresh salad
    SNACK
diet jello
    DINNER
roast Italian chicken marinated in olive oil, garlic, paprika,
onion salt, and parsley
cooked broccoli and cauliflower topped with parmesan
cheese
diet soda
    DESSERT
sugar-free pudding
herbal tea

DAY 4

BREAKFAST
1 orange
1 slice whole wheat bread with butter
cup of coffee
    LUNCH
cheeseburger, no bun
large green salad—olive oil and vinegar

Homemade salad dressing—all natural spices except salt are allowed. You
may include mustard, garlic, scallions, pepper, parsley, oregano or other natural
seasonings. If you must have salt, use a small amount of Morton's Lite Salt.

    SNACK
1 small apple
    DINNER
barbecued steak
any cooked green vegetables
    DESSERT
diet jello

DAY 5
BREAKFAST
soft boiled or poached eggs
1 slice Canadian bacon
LUNCH
shrimp with caesar salad
DINNER
blackened grouper
salad
DESSERT
sugar-free Eskimo Pie (This ice cream bar contains 11 grams of carbohydrate and should be an occasional treat, not a regular dessert.)

DAY 6
BREAKFAST
1 grapefruit
LUNCH
kosher hot dog (no bun) with sauerkraut
DINNER
large salad
fish cooked in olive oil, lemon and garlic
DESSERT
diet jello

DAY 7
BREAKFAST
1 orange
1 slice whole wheat bread
LUNCH
salmon salad
mushroom salad with melted cheese
cooked green peppers topped with parmesan cheese
DINNER
chicken dijon
hearts of lettuce with Italian dressing
DESSERT
diet jello

This diet leaves a lot of room for variation. For example, you may want to have lox as your fish dish. This is fine, as long as you exercise in moderation. Also, I recommend Nova Scotia lox, as it is lower in sodium than other varieties.

Desserts are allowed on this diet, but please don't overdo it simply because they are sugarless. I believe that the best aspects of diet sweeteners is that they will allow our bodies to sample that sweet taste without introducing any changes in our blood sugar levels. I suggest to my patients that they use sugarless products in the form of whole ice cream or ice cream bars (manufactured by Eskimo Pie or Crystal Light Ices), chocolate, candies and soft drinks for the purpose of breaking their addiction to sugar, not perpetuating it. I believe that artificial sweeteners should be used only when the craving for sweets is so strong that the alternative is refined white sugar.

You'll be amazed to see the fat melt from your body as you feast on shrimp scampi, lobster, steak, chicken dijon, caesar salad, fresh fruit, and eggs.

Keep your diet as natural as possible—avoid food with preservatives and canned products. And don't forget to eat plenty of salads. It is important that you eat three square meals a day. If you are inclined to skip meals, you may use my protein drink meal supplement as a substitute.

Eating out on my diet is no problem. At a Chinese restaurant, you may have chicken, shrimp or beef dishes with cooked vegetables. If you are in the mood for Italian food, you may order any unbreaded veal dish that is sautéed or cooked with olive oil. For example, you may have veal marsala, veal piccata, or veal francese. Or you can eat roasted Italian chicken. If you like seafood, your choices are virtually unlimited: shrimp, lobster, or any whole grilled fish. And of course you will have salad and any green vegetable with your meal. The foods that you must avoid in restaurants are bread, potatoes, and of course, desserts.

Because of the flexibility of this diet, my patients enjoy flexibility in their lives. They can eat out, travel, dine at a friend's house and still lose weight. Most important, they can enjoy their meals. If God didn't want us to take pleasure in food, He wouldn't have given us taste buds.

All the phases of this diet, including maintenance (which is where most diets fail), are easy and enjoyable.

Health can lead to happiness, and thinning will lead to winning. Your self-image as well as your outer image will change for the better. You will walk into your next job interview with your head up, your shoulders back, and your stomach flat. You will find that your friends and family will be not only impressed with your appearance, but interested in the secret of your success.

So many Americans are thin people **trapped in fat bodies.** They want to be thin, but nature fights them. The fact is, most of us need to begin watching what we eat by age 30. Our bodies simply don't produce growth hormones and fat mobilizing hormones the way they used to. Recent studies have demonstrated that growth hormones can help restore to our body some of its youthfulness; they help people to lose fat and gain muscle mass. This is why my diet is designed to naturally stimulate these hormones, and return to us some of the youthfulness of the past.

In our culture, looking good is especially important to people. The advertising industry spends billions of dollars creating a certain image, and our society has bought it. I'm not suggesting that you must conform to this stereotype—how many of us can compete with 20-year-old models?—but I am saying that there is no reason not to make the most of yourself.

With this diet, you can lose weight and still experience the joys of eating. You can liberate the slender person who is just waiting to emerge.

*Habit is not to be flung out the window by any man, but coaxed
downstairs a step at a time.*

22

Exercise—
Body Beautiful or
Body Bountiful?

Why in the world are you sitting there reading this book? Take a
walk! Or go for a jog. Ride your bicycle or, if the weather won't permit
that, jump on your exercycle. In order to obtain maximum benefit
from my diet, you must do some form of exercise. It needn't be
strenuous exercise if your physical condition does not permit that, but
it is essential that you get in the habit of moving your body.

If you're not already exercising, you are being left out of a movement that I believe is here to stay. In the '70s, many thought that
exercise was the latest narcissistic fad of the "Me Generation," in the
'80s, it became clear that it was more than the newest yuppie trend;
now, in the early '90s, the sedentary are considered rather eccentric.

"According to the 1978 Pierre study on fitness in American exercise activities—tennis, football, archery, jogging, swimming, bowling, and others draw
almost 300 million devotees in America."[1]

Since there are only 150 million adult Americans, it is obvious that
a lot of them participate in more than one sport.

This enthusiasm is more than understandable in view of recent
findings on the benefits of exercise. For example, a study of Harvard

alumni found that, "Persons with active life styles do live longer than those of us who seek the tranquillity of minimal movement."[2]

People are turning to exercise because they are beginning to acknowledge that a lifestyle that stresses convenience and comfort above all else can produce dire consequences.

"Every year nearly one million Americans die of heart attacks, strokes and related disorders. According to the American Heart Association nearly 40 million Americans have some form of these diseases. Cardiovascular disease is the leading cause of death and chronic disability in the United States. The projected 1983 cost of this problem is $56.9 billion."[3]

I have always believed that exercise strengthens the heart and helps prevent heart attacks. The heart is a muscle, and like any other muscle, it's a case of use it or lose it. It's nice to have my observations confirmed by numerous scientific studies.

"Doctors Ralph Paffenbarger of the Stanford Medical School and Jere Morris of the London School of Hygiene and Tropical Medicine demonstrated that exercise is associated with a lower incidence of heart attacks."[4]

Heart attacks may be one of the most feared conditions in this country, yet a surprising number of people know little about what actually occurs when this disorder strikes.

"The heart is nourished by coronary arteries on its outer surface. When fat is deposited on the inner surfaces of these arteries a plaque forms, which may constrict the flow of blood. If the plaque builds up on an artery to the point where the blood supply is cut off the part of the heart muscle fed by that artery dies. If a large part of the heart muscle dies, the heart can no longer pump blood through the body so the body dies. Heart attack pain ranges from a dull pressure to a sharp, cutting sensation that is like being stuck with a knife. It can occur either at rest or with exertion. It usually arises in the left side of the chest, but can occur anywhere in the chest or upper abdomen. Tests have proven that the pain begins in the left side of the chest and radiates down the left arm, and is brought on by exertion. However, most chest pains people experience are caused by muscle spasms or gas in the intestinal tract and are not always associated with the heart.

"To understand heart disease we must understand how exercise has the ability to offset heart disease. Exercise enlarges all the coronaryarteries which feed the heart. Exercise will increase collateral (auxiliary) circulation so that more than one blood vessel will supply a given area of the heart. If the blood supply becomes blocked in one artery, blood from another will nourish the area and prevent a heart attack. Exercise lowers the concentration of fat in the blood. Fatty plaques obstruct the coronary arteries causing heart attacks. More than 10 years ago John Holloscy, a medical researcher in St. Louis, demonstrated that blood levels of fat, called triglycerides, can be lowered by vigorous activities. Lowering blood fat levels decreased the tendency to form fat plaques that clog the blood vessels. Increased exercise teaches the heart to extract oxygen from the blood more efficiently and increased exercise lowers blood pressure."[5]

Other researchers have also found a correlation between blood fats and exercise.

"The Framingham Study revealed that cholesterol istransported in the blood by high density lipoprotein (HDL) and low density lipoprotein (LDL). LDL is responsible for carrying cholesterol to tissues and depositing it, especially on the walls of the arteries. Conversely, HDL acts like a scavenger—it removes cholesterol from deposits and transports it to the liver where it is disposed. Extensive studies on athletes have shown high levels of HDL and, consequently, low cholesterol levels."[6]

Simply stated, exercise helps remove the bad cholesterol.

I've already explained that dietary changes alone can help to regulate your blood fats. Now imagine the increased benefits when you add exercise to your daily routine.

Exercise has been found to be one of the safest and most effective measures for stimulating the development of new blood vessels, which can bypass diseased arteries. In fact, its hard to think of an organ of the body not helped by exercise. Conditions ranging from diabetes to high blood pressure will respond to this natural therapy. As a chiropractor, I have seen many types of back and neck pain relieved by exercise. And if you suffer from insomnia, a jog (or other form of exercise) during the day may save you from pacing the floors at night.

"Doctors Colin Shapiro of Johannesburg, South Africa and R.B. Zloty of the University of Manitoba, Canada in independent studies demonstrated that the amount of deep sleep you get is proportional to the daytime energy expenditure, the more you exercise the deeper you sleep."[7]

Exercise can also help prevent osteoporosis, a condition characterized by thinning of the bones. Osteoporosis is especially prevalent in post-menopausal women; approximately 6 to 8 million women suffer from this disorder. As a chiropractic physician who takes X-rays of all new patients, I am astounded by the number of women who have osteoporosis and are asymptomatic. "Now there is evidence that regular exercise helps to maintain the density of bones and prevents osteoporosis from developing in the first place."[8]

Of special interest to people on my diet is the fact that exercise helps break down carbohydrates. In fact, the amount of carbohydrates you are allowed to eat on maintenance is correlated with the amount of exercise you take. Refined carbohydrates are still not permissible, of course. But complex carbohydrates in the form of whole grains, whole grain bread and pasta can be incorporated into the diet if the proper exercise and stretching techniques are employed.

As a physician, it is my responsibility to evaluate my patients. I suggest that you perform a self-evaluation. Some of the subjective signs of disease and deterioration include fatigue, jitteriness, unsocial behavior, loss of enthusiasm, loss of appetite, irritability, moodiness, temper tantrums, and high anxiety levels. Physical manifestations of imperfect health include large accumulations of fat around the abdomen (in men), buttocks, and thighs (in women). A loss of muscular strength and endurance (do you get short of breath from climbing the stairs?) are also symptoms of physical deterioration. They are associated with decreased metabolic rate, slowed reaction time, and loss of flexibility.

Albert Schweitzer declared that, "The tragedy of life is what dies inside a man while he lives."[9] In order to fully live our lives, we must constantly challenge ourselves, not only intellectually, but physically as well. I was impressed by a television interview in which former Chicago Bears' coach Mike Ditka discussed a professional athlete who has reached a level so far above his peers that he must prove himself everyday and never rest on his laurels. This kind of attitude can keep us from ever experiencing "declining years," for we will be using each day to grow rather than simply age.

My personal introduction to this philosophy came as something of a shock, even though my "decline" was gradual. I had been an athlete in top condition for many years, so I was unprepared to deal with the fact that I was overweight (200 pounds) and out of shape. But as I thought about it, I realized that my prime years as an athlete were between the ages of 9 and 21. During those 12 years, I participated in athletic events for 3 to 5 hours a day. After I graduated from college, however, my exercise (aerobic and anaerobic) came almost to a standstill. I suppose that I thought that I would always be in good shape. So I smoked, drank, stayed up late at night, and ate large quantities of sugar. I was exercising my mind, but neglecting my body.

One day while I was shaving, I caught a good look at myself in the mirror. I saw that my once flat stomach was now in layers—one overlapping the other. I stared in disbelief at my reflection. You see, a jock never loses that mental image of physical perfection. The picture I saw was worth more than a thousand words—it was worth volumes. At that point I decided that something had to be done.

My first step was an honest evaluation, which is what I recommend for you. Take off your clothes and stand in front of a mirror, and evaluate what you see there. If the image is not to your liking, make an affirmation in which you declare that you look the way you want to look. Then visualize yourself with the body you want. Finally, you must take the action required to produce the results you want.

Aristotle said it best, "The body is the temple of the soul and to reach harmony of body, mind, and spirit it is important to develop physical as well as mental and spiritual qualities."

You have begun thinning, now it is time to take the next step toward winning. Exercise will help you not only to look better but to feel better—it will increase your stamina, raise your energy level, and give you a sense of accomplishment. Exercise will improve not only your physical fitness but your mental alertness. It will provide some protection from degenerative diseases as well as reduce some of the damage caused by fast foods, caffeine, alcohol and cigarettes.

Physical fitness is the first step toward freedom—freedom from the bonds of disease and the shackles of a poor self-image.

The excuses people have for not exercising simply amaze me. I have had patients tell me that they don't want to begin exercising because when they get bored and quit, the muscles they develop will turn to fat. The answer to that, of course, is—don't quit! Physical fitness is not drudgery, it is one of life's pleasures. As Dr. Maxwell Maltz, author of

Psychocybernetics, points out, "It's fun to be fit, to eat right and to discipline yourself to do these things. Do them for 30 days, and they become a habit that's harder not to do on the 31st day than it is to do."

If you begin your program slowly, with a 30 day plan, you'll find that "inch by inch, it's a cinch."

I have also had patients tell me that they fear exercise will bring on a heart attack. This is one myth I would really like to dispel.

"According to Dr. R. Roy J. Shepard, a professor of preventive medicine at the University of Toronto, the chance that heart attack will occur in a normal man during one half hour of heavy exercise is 1 in 5 million. In a normal woman the chance is 1 in 17 million."[10]

This is not to say that I dismiss my patients' concerns. Whenever I am discussing an exercise program with middle-aged patients, I make sure to ask them whether they have a history of chest pain, diabetes, high blood pressure or heart disease. Many have told me that, yes, they have experienced chest pains, but that a resting electrocardiogram performed by their medical physician did not detect any abnormalities. It is my experience that a resting electrocardiogram often fails to detect blocked coronary arteries. The most reliable test for predicting susceptibility to heart attacks is the stress electrocardiograph, which is conducted while the patient exercises.

"Dr. Myrvin Ellestad of Long Beach, California, found that 40% of his patients who showed abnormalities during the stress electrocardiogram had a heart attack within five years. However, other studies indicate that a poor result on a stress electrocardiogram can be improved after the patient undergoes a medically supervised exercise program."[11]

I recommend that before embarking on an exercise program, you undergo a complete physical examination conducted by a cardiologist. This is especially important if you have been inactive and consider yourself out of shape. Explain to the doctor that you plan to begin exercising, and follow his or her advice on the matter.

Chances are, your doctor will support you in your program. These days, exercise is not only recommended as a preventative for heart disease, but is utilized by doctors around the world in the rehabilitation of heart attack patients. Dr. Terence Cavanaugh of Toronto, Canada, took eight post-heart attack patients to compete in the Boston Marathon. Seven of them finished and none suffered any adverse effects. Dr. Jack Scaff, a Hawaii-based cardiologist, encourages his heart patients to run in a Honolulu Marathon. Doctors Noel Nequin of Illinois, Joe Rodgers of Michigan, Pat Gorman of Washington, D.C., and Herman Hellerstein of Ohio are among the many cardiologists who use jogging as therapy for heart patients.[12]

Naturally, these patients are medically supervised, as you should be if any abnormalities are detected.

You have available to you a smorgasbord of fitness techniques. In Florida, where I live, you can't step out the door without seeing people involved in virtually every form of exercise. They walk, golf, play tennis and racquetball, jog, ride bicycles, swim, and surf. They're clearly enjoying themselves as they raise their resistance to disease, increase their self-confidence, and trim their bodies. It sure beats a pill.

I often say to my patients, "Try not to re-create the round wheel." Our ancestors didn't suffer from the problems that come with a sedentary lifestyle. They remained strong and healthy through vigorous outdoor work, such as chopping, digging, planting, hunting, and building. They had to do this to survive. And so do we, although for different reasons.

The industrial revolution brought us many conveniences. Thanks to washing machines, we don't have to go down to the creek to launder our clothing. We can jump on a power mower to keep our lawns trim. We don't walk or ride our bicycles because now we have cars. We don't climb stairs if an elevator is available. Modern amenities can be wonderful, but they can also deprive us of the vitally needed exercise that was all in a day's work for our forebears. Without daily exercise, we store our unreleased energy as fat. We lose touch with our physical well-being. We lose touch with the life energy that surges within us.

There are no shortcuts to good health, and if we do not accept this truism, we will find ourselves in the position of the young contractor in a story told by Tremendous Jones.

It seems this young contractor was married to a contractor's daughter. The father-in-law wanted to give the young man a boost in his career.

"Son," he said, "I don't want you to start at the bottom where I did. So I want you to go out and build the most tremendous house this town has ever seen, put the best of everything in it, make it a palace, and turn it over to me."

Well, this was an opportunity to make a killing. He hurried out to slap together a building that would survive two fairly stiff gales.

In short order he was back to dear old dad. "Well, Dad, it's finished."

"Is it a palace like I asked?"

"Yes-siree, Dad."

"Is it really the finest house ever built, Son?"

"Yes-siree, Dad."

"All right, where is the bill? Is there a good profit in it for you?"

"Yes-siree, Dad."

"Very good. Here is your check, and where is the deed?"

As he looked at the deed, the father said, "I didn't tell you why I wanted that house to be the best house ever built. I wanted to do something special for you and my daughter to show you how much I love you. . . . Here, take the deed, go live in the house—you built it for yourself."

The young gold-bricker crept out a shattered, frustrated man. He thought he was making a fortune at his father-in-law's expense by saving money on inferior material and short-cuts, but he cheated only himself.

Exercise, like diet, takes time and discipline—gimmicks won't hasten the process. You are building a new, better life, so don't skimp on the materials. Now let's discuss the specifics of your foundation for good health.

Stretching

Stretching is essential for making a stress-free transition from a sendentary condition to an active condition and for reversing the process. It helps to keep our muscles supple and flexible and prepares them for the activities ahead.

Stretching is a must for participants in strenuous sports such as basketball, football, tennis, and even golf, a game which affects the biomechanics of the lumbar spine.

In my years of practice, I've treated many top amateur and professional golfers, including Billy Caspar, Nathaniel Crosby, Steve Hart, Sue Fogelman, Mike Weeks, Randy Erskine, Jim Carr, Kim Bauer, and Barbara Bunkowski, to name just a few. The one common fault I find in both the amateurs and the pros lies in their pre- and post-exercise routine—or rather, the lack of one. A runner will stretch for one hour prior to a hundred yard dash that will take under 10 seconds to complete. A golfer will prepare for a four-hour game by hitting golf balls. The exhausted player will then head for the 19th hole (the lounge).

Golfers, like all other athletes, must do proper warm-up and cool-down exercises, the most important of which is stretching. Stretching will help prevent common injuries such as pulled muscles, shin splints, tendentious, and bursitis.

If you have been a non-exerciser, then you really need to maintain a warm-up and cool-down routine. Warming up is the process that gets your blood flowing. It enables you to test the effects of a specific movement before you do it more strenuously. It increases your body's flexibility, and gives it fair warning that you are about to undertake some new and unusual activities. During the warm-up period, your heart rate will begin to climb slowly rather than abruptly. Therefore, oxygen will be distributed through working tissues at a more even and comfortable pace. Each exercise has a specific warm-up program, all of which begin with stretching.

Some experts believe that cooling down is even more important than warming up. It is during the cooling-down period that your heart gradually adjusts to a lighter load, and eventually returns back to its normal resting pulse. The cool-down period also is when the body begins the removal of metabolic waste, and prevents blood from pooling in the legs. It is easy to cool down; simply continue your exercise at a reduced pace. If you were jogging, for example, switch to a walk. Continue your cool down until the heart returns to normal or to a beat below 100 per minute.

As a chiropractor, I specialize in the biomechanics of the human body. It is my job to help people make the most of their physical potential, especially in a practice that includes so many athletes. I have worked with members of the Minnesota Twins, Cincinnati Reds, Toronto Blue Jays, California Angels, Montreal Expos, Miami Heat, New York Knickerbockers, Boston Celtics, the United States Basketball League, the PGA and the LPGA. My clients include world class tennis players, weight lifters, and dancers. Some of these extremely gifted people do not include stretching in their pre-workout routines. When I have questioned this, I've been told that stretching is a form of exercise associated strictly with pre-season training.

But once I persuade them to make it part of every workout, they are delighted with the results. I have had patients tell me that stretching helps them to avoid not only injuries, but aches, pains and strains as well. Furthermore, it often improves performance.

"Muhammad Ali, one of the greatest boxing champions the world has ever known stretched for 45 minutes prior to each workout."[13]

Stretching, like all forms of exercise, should be adjusted to your individual needs and condition, particularly muscle structure, flexibility, and varying tension levels. Done correctly, stretching feels good. It is important not to overdo it—this is not a contest to see how far you can push yourself. Respect your limitations. If you haven't touched your toes in 20 years, don't make this your goal the first time you stretch.

The key to stretching is regularity. It should be done slowly, methodically, and daily. Stretching not only loosens and invigorates us, it enables us to get in touch with our muscles, an important element in safe exercising.

Virtually anyone can learn to stretch, regardless of age or flexibility. And whether you are sedentary or extremely active, the stretching techniques are the same.

I recommend that you go through your stretching routine three times a day: first thing in the morning (if you have a dog or cat, you've notice that these little animals instinctively know enough to stretch upon arising), prior to any form of exercise, and before bedtime. Since this activity can be performed just about anywhere, you may also stretch to release nervous tension caused by sitting or standing for too long a period, or simply to relieve stiffness.

You will find that regular stretching will reduce muscle tension, improve coordination, increase range of motion, and develop your body awareness and flexibility.

It will help ease your body into an exercise routine. Remember, you have to walk before you can run. And speaking of walking. . . .

Walking

"The prescription without medicine; weight control without diet; the cosmetic that is sold in no drug store; the tranquilizer without a pill; (psycho) therapy without a psychoanalyst; the fountain of youth that is no legend; a true magic, a psycho physical alchemy which transforms the body and mind."

This lyrical description from *The Magic of Walking*, by Aaron Sussmand and Ruth Goode, sums up the value of this exercise.

Walking is easy, invigorating, healthy, fun, and inexpensive. You don't have to buy a new wardrobe or join a spa. Just open your door, pick a direction and start walking. Take your spouse, child, grandchild or pet with you. You'll find that walking is a great way to spend "quality time" with them.

And walking can easily be fit into your daily routine. Walk up the stairs instead of taking an elevator; stroll to the store instead of using your car; stride across the golf course instead of riding in a cart

Anyone who is not disabled can walk regardless of age or muscle condition. This is why when patients who have been advised to exercise say, "Dr. Kaplan, I don't know where to start," I suggest they begin with a good brisk walk. Sometimes the simplest answer is the right one.

People instinctively understood the value of walking long before we had hard scientific evidence to prove it.

Hippocrates, patron saint of medicine, mentioned walking 40 times in one chapter on digestive diseases, and prescribed brief walks, short walks, long walks, after dinner walks, and night walks.

"The late Harry Truman, President of the United States of America, when asked why he took his famous early morning stroll said, 'I believe it will make me live longer.' Mr. Truman was 88 years old when he died."[14]

Walking can increase cardiovascular endurance, which is certainly a condition worth working toward.

"Cardiovascular endurance is the ability of the heart to perform more work than is usual, more economically, for a prolonged period and the heart's ability to recover quickly upon cessation of the activity. An efficient cardiovascular system is capable of adjusting the flow of blood in order to supply oxygen to the necessary tissue and to remove chemical byproducts produced in muscular contraction."[15]

People who are unaccustomed to regular exercise should begin with short excursions. For a more precise indication of just how far you should extend yourself, I recommend the walking fitness test developed by Dr. James Rippe and his colleagues at the University of Massachusetts. Dr. Rippe recommends this test for people between the ages of 30 and 69 unless:

> ➤ They have known health problems.
> ➤ They are greatly overweight.
> ➤ They are extremely inactive.

People who fit into any of these categories are advised to see their doctors for an assessment.

The Walking Test

Put on comfortable clothes and shoes and find a flat smooth course of one mile in length. Use a school facility if you can, or measure off one mile at any other safe place such as a large shopping center parking lot. Walk the mile as fast as you can comfortably. Don't stroll unless that's your true best effort, but push yourself a little. Time your walk.

How to know when you are pushing yourself too hard

You could obviously check your pulse. As we said, it should never go above your maximal rate. But there is an easier way to gauge your effort and you should learn it right now. It's called the Borg Scale of Perceived Exertion and in most cases it will give you a safe understanding of your exertion level, the scale looks like this:

Rating Of Perceived Exertion

6
7—very very light
8
9—very light
10
11—fairly light
12
13—somewhat hard (moderately hard)
14
15—hard
16
17—very hard
18

19—very very hard maximal

(G.V. Borg, *Medicine and Science in Sports and Exercise*)

Regardless of your fitness level, consider 6 an easy stroll. Regardless of your fitness level consider 19 an effort that feels as if it will kill you. For the purpose of your fitness test, you want to feel that your effort is about 12 to 13 somewhat hard but a level at which you can still speak without gasping for breath. Your one mile walk will tell you right now it's not important how long it takes you to cover the distance. Some of you might need to take a little camping gear along. Some of you might rightfully decide to stop walking after a few hundred feet. Definitely stop if you begin to feel uncomfortable. Watch out for mud puddles. But if you make it, here is how your time stacks up against the rest of the world.

Fitness Level	Male Time	Female Time
Excellent	10 min. 12 sec.	11 min. 40 sec.
Good	10:13 – 11:42	11:41 – 13:08
High Average	11:43 – 13:13	13:09 – 14:36
Low Average	13:14 – 14:44	14:37 – 16:04
Fair	14:45 – 16:23	16:05 – 17:32
Poor	16:24 or above	17:33 or above

"If you don't have any physical handicaps and you really did try anything over 13 minutes for men or 14 minutes for women means you really do need to take a very serious interest in your health and don't think your age is an excuse here either. Being older doesn't necessarily mean that you are automatically weaker in cardiovascular sense. But don't be discouraged."[16]

Walking needn't be competitive, nor do you have to continually test yourself. It is my recommendation that you begin your program by walking approximately 10 minutes per day for the first week, and that you increase the time by 5 to 10 minutes per week. Within a 6 to 10 week period, you will be walking approximately one hour per day. As you build up your stamina, you can further increase the distance you cover. After about four months, you will be walking approximately three to four miles in an hour.

It is recommended that you record your results in a notebook, which you can use as a guide in clocking aerobic activity.

If you're not walking, you're losing out. Not only are you neglecting an important health benefit, you are missing many of the experiences this planet has to offer. The world simply doesn't look the same from behind a windshield.

Aerobic and Anaerobic Exercises

Our bodies derive energy from fuel in one of two ways: through the aerobic metabolism and through the anaerobic metabolism.

Aerobic metabolism refers to the production of energy requiring oxygen. Much like a fire, aerobic metabolism needs oxygen in order to burn. Anaerobic metabolism, on the other hand, is a process that releases energy to the body without the presence of oxygen.

Aerobic exercises include walking, running, jogging, rowing, swimming, skiing, biking, basketball, football, tennis, or any other movement that requires the use of large muscle groups for sustained periods of time.

Anaerobic exercise will help increase muscle strength and keep the body toned. Weight lifting is the primary form of anaerobic exercise.

Many of my female patients are involved in aerobic dancing, and the question I most commonly hear is, "Is this exercise safe, or will I injure myself?" This is a query for which there is no clear-cut answer, but in general I feel that aerobic dancing can be safe provided it is done properly: Check out the qualifications of your instructor. There are no formal standards to establish credentials in this field, so you'll have to go by word-of-mouth and your own impressions.

Choose your aerobics center carefully. Unless you are a professional dancer, you should find a place that teaches low-impact aerobics, which are designed to provide the same cardiovascular benefits as high-impact aerobics while minimizing physical trauma. One of the primary techniques in low-impact aerobics involves keeping one foot on the ground at all times. By doing this, you will reduce the impact of jumping but will still gain the benefit of increased heart rate through exaggerated movement such as high steps, lunges, and vigorous arm motions. Many people eventually move from low-impact to high-impact aerobics. Remember, though, impact is impact—injury can occur unless you exercise with care.

Be patient. Too many people want to get into shape immediately, after years of sedentary habits. Don't push your body too hard too soon. If you do, the resulting aches, pains, and injuries will quickly dampen your enthusiasm for exercise. While you can expect some soreness, stretching exercises will help relieve these new-found twinges.

Some people like to combine aerobic and anaerobic exercises. If you choose to follow such a course, it is helpful to understand that these two types of activities produce quite different reactions in the body.

"Aerobic metabolism is a slow reacting process. It does not react instantly to an immediate increase in energy requirements such as a sudden sprint in the rain from the car to the store when your individual cells gasp for breath. At that point, sugar in the cells begins to breakdown and form lactic acid, releasing energy—anaerobic metabolism.

"Lactic acid is a by-product of metabolism. During intense activity, the acid builds up in our cells. When lactic acid production is greater than the body's ability to remove it, your blood and muscles become acidic. Your muscles don't work as well in this acidic state and you fatigue quickly."[17]

Sugar and dairy products increase the acidity in the body. Remove these products from your diet for a more active, beneficial, rewarding exercise routine.

Anaerobic exercise is hard exercise. It shortens muscles and makes them more vulnerable to pulls and strains. Therefore, this form of exercise is not for everyone, and should be conducted under the guidance of a professional instructor. And proper stretching is an absolute must for people who choose an anaerobic routine.

Jogging

This form of aerobic exercise consists of alternating brisk walking and running at a slow to moderate pace. Jogging is particularly valuable as a graduated program of exercise that may be adapted for people of all ages. I enjoy this activity a great deal, and presently jog 9 to 10 miles a week.

"News coverage of the late President John F. Kennedy jogging along the beach brought the nation's attention to this form of exercise. But in the late 1960s it was called the latest health craze when *Time* magazine reported 5 million people in America were jogging. In 1982 the estimated number was between 35-40 million."[18]

President Bill Clinton and ex-president George Bush both kept up their jogging regimens even during their presidential campaigns. As a physician, I feel a lot more confident in the leadership abilities of a man who has the stamina, endurance, and discipline to take control of his own life on a daily basis.

The popularity of jogging is largely due to the accumulated data of physicians, cardiologists, and physiologists. They have produced an impressive body of evidence attesting to the beneficial effects of jogging on the heart and lungs. Jogging increases endurance and confidence, improves appearance, reduces weight, and enhances overall health.

Like walking, jogging is a noncompetitive exercise that requires no specialized skill or equipment (although you should invest in high-quality, comfortable footwear). Jogging is also a natural transition for the person who no longer finds walking challenging enough, but is not ready to embark on an extremely strenuous exercise program.

"Jogging combines the desirable qualities of walking and, in addition, offers higher caloric expenditure in a slightly shorter period of time. Jogging is the natural addition to the exercise program of the individual who has increased his rate of walking to four miles per hour."

If jogging seems too hard on your body, you can always revert back to brisk walking, which offers the same cardiovascular effects without the risk of trauma. However, I believe that, for many people, repeated jogging will improve the mechanical efficiency of the body. I also feel that by setting distance goals and increasing stamina, the jogger will enjoy increased mental alertness and an improved sense of overall well-being.

Cycling

"Today in America there are over 80 million cyclists. A recent Department of Interior study revealed that bicycling has grown faster than any other summertime activity with an unusual growth rate of over 10%. Over 60 cities in more than 20 states now have bike ways provided for the increased ease, safety and enjoyment of cyclists."[19]

No wonder cycling is so popular. It combines fun, fitness and transportation. It confers many of the same health benefits as walking, jogging, and running. Cycling can be enjoyed as a solo exercise, or with companions. These days, solitude is a scarce commodity. It is often difficult for a successful man or woman to find some private moments.

Cycling enables you spend some time with yourself as you exercise.

Or, you can spend some time with your family. Cycling is one activity in which children and adults can participate on a nearly equal level. It can be enjoyed by people of almost any age, regardless of sex, body build and fitness level.

Because we move our location as well as our bodies during cycling, we are less likely to experience the boredom that sometimes occurs when we exercise at home or in a spa. Cycling increases our aerobic capacity and involves nearly all of the muscle groups of the body.

The pedal action strengthens the legs, arms, back and abdomen. It also induces good breathing, stimulates the circulation and does wonders in shaping the body. It develops endurance—the real basis for lifelong physical activity.

If you haven't been on a bicycle since childhood, give it a try—you never lose this skill.

Swimming

Swimming differs from other cardiovascular endurance activities in two important respects. First, the water provides the exerciser with buoyancy. Second, it allows free active movements with far less effort, so that even weaker body parts may be exercised. Swimming does not present the hazards associated with many other activities.

Swimming is a non-traumatic form of exercise which minimizes the occurrence of numerous joint injuries such as bursitis, tendentious, muscle strains and sprains are therefore minimized.

Hydrotherapy is extensively utilized in the rehabilitation of athletes to speed the healing of those who have been injured or are recovering from surgery.

The handicapped can also benefit from swimming. Amputees and people with joint impairments, who are otherwise healthy, can participate in activities in the water. These people might otherwise be denied the benefits of cardiovascular endurance type exercises.

The ability to swim is also important for safety reasons—your own life or someone else's could depend on it. In Florida, children are trained in water safety at an early age. My oldest son, Michael, was able to swim at age two and swam the length of the pool by age four. Jason, my younger son, was able to swim at age three.

Swimming, like cycling and walking, is a very versatile sport. It can be practiced by people of all ages and both sexes, and by people of varying fitness levels. It provides the body with a high degree of strength and flexibility. And it is a sport that is pleasurable, induces relaxation, and can be enjoyed by the entire family.

Skipping Rope

Jump rope is an activity that has always been associated—incongruously enough—with school girls and boxers. But those of us who fall somewhere between these two extremes can also benefit from skipping rope.

Speaking of boxers, I recently had the opportunity to watch Sugar Ray Leonard work out. I was amazed by what that man can do with a rope—the speed, stamina and hand-eye coordination he exhibited had me entranced.

Non-athletes can also benefit from this inexpensive endurance-building activity. Rope skipping helps us to develop balance, rhythm, agility, and hand-eye-foot coordination. It can produce the same cardiovascular fitness effects as jogging, swimming, walking, and cycling.

Jump rope can be utilized safely by people of all ages—and occupations. An executive would find it heavy going to take weights along on a business trip, but it's no problem at all to pack a rope in your suitcase. And even the smallest motel room offers enough space to accommodate this activity.

Jump rope can also be combined with other activities.

Skipping at a pace of 70-80 skips per minute using a work rest ratio of 3 to 1 for a total of 30 minutes will provide the minimal daily requirement for exercise. A more beneficial program, however, would be a 15 minute skip period combined with 15 minutes more of some other form of vigorous exercise.

These are just a few of the many activities you can employ to increase your cardiovascular capacity, lower your blood pressure, and increase your productivity. Once again, it is important to undergo a complete physical examination prior to beginning an exercise program, and I suggest that your exam include a stress test and a blood pressure check.

The stress test does more than indicate the presence of heart disease. It can indicate your physical work capacity. In other words, a stress test lets you know how much exercise you can safely tolerate at a given time. When you have your next annual physical, the stress test is one way to calibrate your improvement.

Another way of keeping tabs on your improvement is through regular blood pressure testing. Many patients have asked me, "Doc, what does all this blood pressure stuff mean?" It's a good question, given the importance of the system, so I think it's worth an explanation here.

Your blood system is a closed system. Therefore, the blood exerts pressure on the vessels at all times. Your blood pressure is determined by measuring in millimeters of mercury the pressure applied to all of the interior walls of your arteries. The results are recorded as an inverted fraction, e.g., 120/80.

The top number indicates your systolic reading, which represents the pressure that is on the vessels while the heart pumps. The bottom number, the diastolic reading, indicates the pressure between heart beats.

When either the systolic of diastolic pressure moves out of the statistically normal range, the reading may indicate that the patient has high blood pressure, or hypertension. "Normal" blood pressure varies somewhat from person to person, so your physician needs to evaluate your condition. If there is a problem, be sure to have your pressure checked periodically.

Hypertension has been called "the silent killer," because it may produce no symptoms in the victim. It will, however, create a great deal of damage. When blood pressure is within normal ranges, the pressure itself does no damage to the arteries. Conversely, pressure that remains high over a period of time can damage and weaken the artery walls, reducing their elasticity. High blood pressure places a strain on the heart and forces it to work harder, eventually leading to congestive heart failure.

High blood pressure can often be reduced by the removal of salt and salt products from the diet, weight loss (assuming you are overweight), and exercise.

Through the course of this chapter we have determined that exercise will increase the ability and capacity of the heart. We must understand that the heart is a muscle and, like every other muscle, it will atrophy if it is not exercised.

As you can see, you can get a lot of mileage from exercise. It can trim you down, tone you up, increase cardiovascular fitness, improve lung function, increase bone density, lower blood pressure and improve the elasticity of your blood vessels.

Is exercise a magic bullet? No, and neither is anything else. But exercise is a powerful weapon against obesity, heart disease, poor muscle tone and many other undesirable conditions.

Your exercise program, like your diet, begins in your mind. Make it your goal to achieve optimum fitness. Use your affirmations—at least three times a day affirm that your are the person you want to be. You don't have to emulate Arnold Schwarzenegger or Jane Fonda—your goal is to be the best that *you* can be. You need not compete against anyone but yourself.

Give yourself a chance to adapt—to your new eating habits, your new exercise program, and your new attitude. In time, you will find yourself exuding the confidence that comes from having a healthy outlook and a healthy body.

Think of your exercise program as a metaphor for your life. The key words are "progress" and "improvement." It is important not to stress the body, but it is also important to stretch its capabilities. We must walk up one more step, jog for five extra minutes, swim two more laps. Your warm-up and cool-down exercises, and your stretching, should never be neglected.

In the early stages of the program, slow and steady work is preferable to rapid, intense work. As the body adapts and our physiological mechanisms adjust to the workload, speed and endurance can be increased. Baseball spring training provides a perfect analogy for the pace I recommend. Pitchers don't throw at their maximum velocity on the first day of practice. Nor do they pitch nine full innings on their first outing. They increase their pitching velocity and endurance slowly. This enables them to maintain peak performance for longer periods and, because the body has a chance to adapt, numerous injuries are prevented.

"In order to obtain the optimum cardiovascular response to heart rate during exercise, the pulse (heart rate) should reach a peak rate of 60-90% of the maximum heart rate reserved or 50-85% of the maximum oxygen uptake (VO2/MAX)."[20]

I recommend that you exercise a minimum of three to five days per week. In time, you'll develop a healthy "addiction" to your activities. Ask a jogger not to jog for a couple of weeks, and listen to what he or she says. (The answer may not be polite.) Any physician can tell you that the primary worry of injured athletes is that they will be unable to exercise. I have no problem with people who are addicted to looking and feeling good. Individuals who lose weight and exercise regularly are on a natural high. They are confident, tranquil and suffer less from anxiety and tension. They run their lives rather than get run over by them. These are the people who concentrate better, perform better, and live happier, more productive lives. Dr. Maltz said it takes only 30 consecutive days of doing something to develop a habit, so set a 30-day goal.

Don't get discouraged if your initial attempts don't match your aspirations. Any improvement is significant, so don't downplay even your modest achievements. If you miss a day, a week, even a month of exercise, don't give up.

Given the nature of this book, it would be impractical for me to cover all of the exercises available in greater detail. Many experts have written fine books on the subject, and I highly recommend that you consult these works. My goal is to plant seeds; you will harvest the crop. The purpose of this book is to guide you down the proper path, to lead you to greater physical, emotional and social well-being.

I promise that if you follow these guidelines, you will lose weight. You will increase your energy levels, reduce your blood sugar, and notice an improvement in your attitude. And I guarantee that if you stick with the principles outlined here, you will maintain your gains—and your (weight) losses. Many diets enable you to lose weight, but in the form of muscle and water. My diet will enable you to lose fat, and lose it once and for all.

If you treat your body like a valued friend, it will return the compliment.

The common curse of mankind, folly and ignorance.
William Shakespeare

23

Fiber Phobia

Considering the great American obsession with fiber, it is surprising that so few people are in possession of the facts about this substance. Fiber is one of the best things that has happened to the cereal industry; to hear their commercials, you would think they invented it. However, cereal is not the only—or even the best—source of fiber. And fiber is not just a breakfast food.

Fiber is the structural and stabilizing part of the plant cell that cannot be digested by enzymes or other digestive secretions. The chief benefit of fiber is derived from its ability to move the feces through the digestive system at a rapid pace. Fiber expands and soaks up liquid like a sponge, thus adding bulk to our diet and aiding in the elimination of waste.

Fiber is associated with the prevention of colon/rectal cancer, diverticulosis, hemorrhoids, appendicitis, hiatus hernia, and a number of other conditions. And fiber is especially important to dieters, because it reduces the appetite by producing a feeling of fullness.

Thanks to certain technological "improvements," fiber may be lacking in your diet. According to Dr. Pritikin, author of *The Pritikin Program for Diet and Exercise,* "Anyone on the so called 'normal American Diet' doesn't get enough fiber." As he explains it:

"Over a century ago, some genius made it possible to mill a new low fiber flour and bake pretty new white breads and pastries. While these new products may have looked more elegant, they have less fiber. With less fiber came an assortment of pathologies, such as a virtual epidemic of diverticular disease, appendicitis and hiatus hernia." (The same milling process that eliminates fiber also removes many of the micro nutrients (vitamins, minerals) essential to our health.)

Changing eating patterns have also contributed to the problem.

"Since people eat about 1/10th as much bread today as they did 100 years ago they have lost even most of the fiber that is found in white bread. We do eat more fruit and vegetables, but not enough to compensate for the loss of grain fiber."

Fiber can be broken down into a form of complex carbohydrate. And while carbohydrate-containing foods provide us with fiber, it is important to keep in mind that not all carbohydrates were created equal. Let us categorize carbohydrates into four basic subgroups. We will grade them by their nutritional quality.

Category A-1—Complex Unrefined

This category consists of all vegetables, whole grains, whole cereals, nuts, seeds, legumes, and greens.

Category B-2—Simple Unrefined

All fruit, milk, yogurt, buttermilk, raw honey, sugar cane and molasses are in this category.

Category C-3—Refined

Here we have flour, cornstarch, white rice, potato starch, bread, crackers, and pasta.

Category D-4—Refined

This category includes sugar, honey, corn syrup, dextrose, fructose, lactose (powdered skim milk), glucose, maltose (barley malt), maple sugar, and sorbitol.

As this list explains, carbohydrates are divided not only into re-fined/unrefined groups, but further subdivided as simple—sugars, which must be avoided at all costs—and complex, the category into which starches fit.

The carbohydrates in Category 4 are the least desirable. They will provide the greatest stimulus for insulin release and reduce the potency of the fat mobilizing hormone. Conversely, those in Category A-1 are the best, as they provide the least stimulus.

The carbohydrates in Category 1 are allowed in moderation until you reach maintenance. I often begin my day with a 100% natural (no sugar added) bran muffin, spread with natural peanut butter. Since I love peanut butter (the kind with no sugar added), I have hit on an enjoyable way to get both protein and fiber in one meal.

In the Preparatory Phase of the diet, though, carbohydrate intake must be restricted; even cooked vegetables are not allowed. The more weight you have to lose, the more carbohydrate and fat-restrictive your diet must be.

But you needn't worry about not getting sufficient fiber in this phase, since you are permitted to have plenty of green salads, an excellent source of fiber. Leafy vegetables provide unabsorbable carbohydrates and some of the bulk necessary for normal bowel function. Because they are unabsorbable, these complex carbohydrates push through the digestive system and add virtually no convertible (countable) carbohydrate to the diet. Salad is also rich in vitamins, and since I don't ask you to eliminate dressing, it is also very tasty.

Many of my patients supplement their diets with a raw fiber capsule. I personally take an oat bran supplement which contains 533 mg of fiber. (Oat bran has also achieved fame for its cholesterol-reducing properties.) I recommend two fiber capsules two times a day, taken with an 8 ounce glass of water. I have found that this practice helps to keep my patients regular and has not caused any weight problems. These capsules also work quickly to suppress the appetite.

A change in diet can make someone prone to constipation. Usually this happens when the dieter fails to consume sufficient salad and raw vegetables, but some people simply have sluggish bowels. This is why fiber capsules can be so useful. I have also had occasion to recommend a preparation called herbplus. This is a combination of herbs, including fig concentrate, aloes, senna leaves, licorice, basil flowers and leaves, anise, black currant, uva hesi, dandelion, marjoram leaves and senna pods. These ingredients stimulate the bowel naturally. I want to emphasize the "naturally," because pharmaceutical laxatives work by irritating the bowel. The herbplus preparation contains ingredients that have been used for centuries. Cleopatra, noted for her velvety, unblemished complexion, knew the value of such herbs. "Cleopatra's 'beauty secret' was her regular cleansing of the system with the mildly laxative leaves of senna to prevent constipation and keep her intestinal tract clear."[1]

Of course, sufficient dietary fiber will also keep your intestinal tract clear, but don't look for it in a commercial cereal box. If you read the labels on these products, you'll see that the emphasis is on sugar and carbohydrates rather than fiber.

Since many children begin their day with a bowl of cereal, they are consuming a large allotment of carbohydrates at this one meal. Take a certain cereal, Raisen Bran, which is advertised as being rich in fiber—for example. A serving of this cereal contains 31 g. of carbohydrate. Add half a cup of skim milk, and this breakfast is now a 37 g. carbohydrate meal. Granted, Raisin Bran contains wheat and wheat bran, as well as raisins. But it also offers sugar, corn syrup, malt, and other assorted flavorings, in addition to a whopping 290 mg serving of sodium. Naturally, the child will be given a glass of processed, pasteurized orange juice with breakfast. This adds another 20 g. of carbohydrate, so breakfast is now up to 57 g. (An orange, which contains roughage, would be a better choice.) If we must go below 40 g. of carbohydrate to lose weight, and keep to 40 to 60 g. to maintain weight, then this meal is dangerously close to going over the limit.

Children, because of their activity levels, can handle larger amounts of carbohydrates. Refined and processed carbohydrates will act upon their bodies like sugar. A steady diet high in refined carbohydrates will make it hard for the child to sit in school and concentrate. His body innately wants him to be active to burn up the carbohydrates.

It is no wonder that our schools are crowded with obese and hyperactive children.

My recommendation for children is a wholesome breakfast like fresh fruit, oatmeal, and natural bran muffins. More and more children today are overweight, hyperactive and have learning disabilities. Many children take an assortment of suppressive medications during their growth years. Let us not just treat the symptoms, but let us find the cause.

Raisin Bran is far from being the only cereal that makes us pay heavily for our fiber. I was raised on cereal which was considered nutritious. Yet it contains 20 g. of carbohydrates (26 with milk) and 290 mg of sodium. It also contains wheat oat flour, wheat starch, *sugar,* calcium carbonate and assorted other ingredients. Then there is nutri-grain cereal which does not have sugar added. It does, however, have a carbohydrate count of 32 g. (38 g. with milk), and 230 mg of sodium. Don't assume that a product purchased at a health food store will automatically be healthy for you. One brand-name cereal has 22 g. of carbohydrate an ounce, and 28 g. when you add half a cup of skim milk. Another provides 26 g. of carbohydrate (32 g. with skim milk) and 300 mg of sodium.

The cereal industry has educated us about the benefits of their products, but the education is somewhat slanted. Cereal is easy to prepare, and convenient to eat, but it is not 100% nutritious. And, yes, cereal is vitamin enriched. Have you ever wondered why?

"In the process of milling and refining, over twenty-six essential elements are either damaged or removed from the flour. The 'enrichment' process puts back a tiny, unusable percentage of these."[2]

Unlike the human animal, other animals are not susceptible to hype from the cereal industry.

"Dr. Edward Taub at a west coast university put a box of Fruitloops in a cage with rats. The rats ate the box and left the Fruitloops."[3]

It is also important to keep in mind that cereal is mixed with milk. You already know my feelings about this dairy product, and the combination of milk and cereal is a digestive disaster. Whenever a liquid is consumed, water is the first thing to leave the stomach during digestion. We are thus left with a coagulation of thick dense curds, which require tremendous digestive energy to break down.

The curd is a concentrated protein, the cereal is a starch. These are totally incompatible food groups that will spoil and rot in your stomach. It is no wonder that our children are whiny, hyperactive and sluggish, and that so many of them suffer from poor attention spans.

I'm not trying to give you a fiber phobia, I just want you to get your fiber from the best sources. Look for stone ground cereal and bread. They are more natural and higher in fiber. These products are allowed on maintenance. After Phase 1, you may occasionally have wheatless bread such as millet and oat bread.

It is best to begin the day with fruit or protein. The latter is especially important for children. "Children need one and a half to two times more protein per pound of body weight than adults and babies need three times more."[4]

What I have learned from working with my patients is that most people can tolerate the complex, unrefined carbohydrates that are found in category A of my chart. I do, however, caution them about the second group of carbohydrates. Even though I believe that fruit is a vital part of a well-balanced diet, it does contain sugar (fructose), which when eaten recklessly can elicit a greater insulin response than starches. It is for this reason that fruit is allowed only in moderation, and only during the day, which is when our bodies have the ability to utilize and burn natural sugars.

In the evening hours, the body will not burn them off, but will store them. Thus, the carbohydrates allowed on my diet must always come from category 1, which offers better blood sugar control.

Once you are on maintenance, you can easily afford to eat up to four fruits per day. Fruits are healthy, tasty, and a good source of fiber.

One of the primary worries of people on any diet is that they will not get sufficient fiber. On certain programs, such as the liquid protein diet (LPD), this may indeed present a problem. While the basic principle of the LPD is sound, the wrong mechanics are implemented. The LPD supplies necessary nutrients, but it lacks fiber. As a result, the digestive system may become sluggish, and when food is reintroduced, it may create a digestive overload. Weight may therefore be regained.

You don't have to be concerned about that on my diet, for you are allowed an unlimited amount of selected high-fiber foods in the form of salads and raw vegetables, which are the most natural and nutritious sources of fiber. One of my goals in writing this chapter was to let you know that you can get the fiber you need without the refined carbohydrates you don't need.

I realize that it's easy to be seduced by the claims of the rich and powerful cereal industry. Your supermarket undoubtedly has an entire aisle devoted to this much-advertised product. The solution to this dilemma is as easy as avoiding that particular section—and heading for the produce department instead.

Nothing gives one person so much advantage over another as to remain always cool and unruffled under all circumstances.
                                                                Thomas Jefferson

24

Stress To Kill

The time and place in which we live offers us more opportunity than has been enjoyed by any culture in history. But one of the by-products of modern living is stress. As a chiropractor, one of my functions is to help people to reduce the effects of stress, for it can cause significant health problems. We can't completely avoid stress, but we can minimize it—in fact, we must minimize it.

There are two types of stress: internal and external. Within these two categories there are various degrees of mental, emotional, and physical stress. More important than the stress itself, is the ability of the body to adapt to it. The body can react favorably to stress, in which case no harm is done. Conversely, an adverse reaction will produce adverse consequences. The degree to which a person reacts to stress is subjective, and some people have a higher tolerance than others.

While some people thrive on stress, my opinion as a physician is that these sturdy souls are in the minority. I have found that most people suffer from numerous ailments when their stress tolerance is exceeded. I am one of them. Stress may lead to diseases such as hypertension, atherosclerosis, and heart disease. It can cause irritability, insomnia, anxiety, anger, frustration, and a variety of other unpleasant emotions. Stress can decrease the quality of life, cause premature aging, and even hasten death.

Obesity is an especially dangerous form of physical stress. When we overeat, the digestive system is burdened by the need to break down the excess food we consume. Obesity also leads to numerous diseases as the immune system of the body becomes fatigued and sluggish.

If you asked 100 people what their greatest source of stress was, chances are that 99 of them would say, "My job." This is especially true of the super-achievers whose jobs involve a great deal of responsibility and require top performance at all times. Because they are expected to set an example for everyone else, they may be unable to let themselves go and relax. The result is a more or less constant state of performance stress.

These are the people who can often benefit most from my program. Proper diet, exercise, and nutritional supplements are important, because stress will take its toll on the body as well as the emotions. Two other items that can help reduce stress are the herbs valerian root and kava kava. As I said before, a body not at ease is in a state of "dis-ease," which can eventually lead to disease. One of my goals is to teach you to listen to your body, and to use your emotional reactions as a stress barometer.

One of the greatest natural stress reducers is exercise. The mood elevating effects of exercise have been widely documented. Various theories have been proposed to explain this effect. Some experts believe exercise increases the level of certain hormones in the brain, thus producing a feeling of well-being. Others claim that the beneficial effects of exercise are due to increased blood supply, which in turn increases the oxygen level throughout the circulatory system and brain. Whatever the reason, the message is clear: you can exercise a good deal of your stress away. The over prescription of valium and other drugs might stop if more people used the natural and beneficial tranquilizer they have available to them.

"Herbert De Vries, Professor of Physical Education at the University of Southern California, tested muscle tension in a group of subjects after half had exercised and half had taken tranquilizers. His studies showed that even the minimal exercise that you would get in a fifteen minute walk is more relaxing than a tranquilizer."[1]

Stress can also be relieved by chiropractic, massage and all forms of rest, relaxation and sleep. Relaxation is a neuromuscular skill that is innate to some people, but must be learned by others. Massage, which is relaxing and invigorating at the same time, is an excellent route to neuromuscular relaxation.

Relaxation is becoming a lost art in our culture. It is important that we learn some techniques that will enable us to take advantage of this restorative.

Nothing is more relaxing than a good night's sleep. Unfortunately, insomnia is rampant in this country. Sleeplessness can be caused by anxiety or depression, as well as by physical problems. It can also be the bane of creative people, whose minds are always on the go; by the end of the day they have built up such mental momentum that they can't stop it.

Bad habits—intake of sugar, refined carbohydrates, salt, caffeine, nicotine and alcohol—can also interfere with our ability to sleep. Many of the stressed-out people I see in my office not only have severe structural problems which I associate with their nervous systems, but are dependent on one of these substances.

Try replacing these bad habits with a good one—exercise. As I noted in Chapter 22, exercise can help promote deep, restful sleep. And in the morning, nothing will invigorate you more than ten minutes on a stationary bicycle or some flexibility calisthenics. Nothing will have a more positive impact on your self-esteem than seeing your new-found physique in the mirror. Exercise will remove stress from your life, and that's a fact.

Stress and Diet

The interaction of improper diet and stress contributes to the plight of many ulcer patients. It is commonly believed that ulcers are caused solely by emotional conditions. I disagree. An ulcer, which Webster's defines as, "A necrotic or eroded sore that often discharges pus. Something that festers and corrupts like an open sore," is frequently caused by dietary stress. And the two substances most often responsible are sugar and dairy products.

My mother provided a perfect example of this problem. When she was diagnosed as suffering from ulcers, the prescribed treatment included extensive intake of dairy products. But mother's diet was high in dairy products prior to her condition; with greater intake of them, her condition worsened.

Another relative of mine was also found to have ulcers, and he too was put on a bland diet that included an abundance of dairy products. The irony is that he had consumed a pint of ice cream a day for at least 20 years. To add insult to injury, he was also taking one aspirin a day (which can worsen stomach problems) for prevention of heart disease. Although he is a handsome, bright, successful man, like most of us, he believes what he is told, even when there is evidence to contradict it. I reviewed his diet, which did not prohibit sugar and encouraged dairy products.

I explained to him the benefits of a program without sugar and dairy products, but since his true addiction (and probably the cause of his problem) was the ice cream, he was thrilled with his new diet. Before his bout with the ulcers, he had had his gall bladder removed—once again, he was suffering from an organ which had been irritated by dairy products and fat. His body screamed for help, but rather than put out the fire he continued to feed it.

As I explained earlier, sugar creates excess stomach acid and dairy products are hard to digest; both of them will act as an irritant. Yet dairy products—which include sugar-laden ice cream—are regularly prescribed to help heal ulcers.

"For years ulcer sufferers were advised to consume milk to ease the pain. Natural hygienists voiced their disbelief of such absurd advice from the beginning, knowing that acid-forming foods are the worst thing for an ulcer sufferer, and all dairy products, except butter, are acid forming. The natural hygienists were first scoffed at by the elite credentialed health experts. But check with medical professional or dietitians today and they will now agree with the very hygienists they used to attack. Dairy products aggravate ulcers.

"Ulcerative colitis is another extremely painful and uncomfortable ailment. Frequently it is a precursor to colon cancer. Dairy products not only contribute to colitis, but removal of dairy products results in a dramatic improvement of colitis."[2]

All too often, we worsen dietary stress by the "remedies" we use to relieve it. We get upset about something, (which causes our blood sugar levels to jump) and eat the wrong foods (sugar) to console ourselves. Our stomachs, in response to this external and internal stress, produce excess acid. So we run to the medicine cabinet, and then it's "plop, plop, fizz, fizz, oh what a relief it is."

The facts and the commercial jingle don't quite match, however. Three leading gastroenterologists told a senate subcommittee that aspirin and patent medicines containing aspirin can aggravate the stomach disorders they are supposed to relieve.[3]

Dr. J. Donald Ostrow, an associate professor of medicine at the University of Pennsylvania, had patients whose gastrointestinal hemorrhages were engendered by aspirin preparations. In 5 of the 18 patients (greater than 25%), the preparation was Alka-Seltzer.

"People take it to relieve stomach distress, temporarily it seems to work. As the antacid effects subside, the pain returns, more severe than before. This leads to another dose of Alka-Seltzer and so on, with more pain, more Alka-Seltzer, until the patient ends up bleeding in the hospital. Dr. Ostrow estimated that every four months in this country some 600,000 individuals use Alka-Seltzer to excess, ending up worse than before."[4]

How then, do we avoid dietary stress in the first place? In his book, *Sweet and Dangerous,* John Yudkin, eminent British physician, biochemist and Emeritus professor of nutrition at London University, discusses his own bout with ulcers. He was given the standard advice—take it easy, avoid spicy foods, eat small meals, delay surgery.

He took antacid for stomach distress. Nonetheless, his stomach problems persisted. Dr. Yudkin began to gain weight, so he went on a diet, cutting down on sugar and refined carbohydrates. In a few months his stomach symptoms disappeared. This led him to some experimentation.

The results of his two year study with 41 patients who were placed on low carbohydrate diets was impressive, to say the least. While two patients claimed to be worse off, and 11 said they noted no appreciable change, 28 (almost two-thirds) reported that they were much better off. As Dr. Yudkin noted, "sugar irritates the lining of the upper alimentary canal, the esophagus, stomach, duodenum."[5]

Internal or external, stress is stress. So watch what you eat, and become an educated consumer. Don't take a medicine unless you are aware of its side-effects. If it is a prescribed drug, ask your doctor for information about it.

Cigarette Smoking

Ever since the 1960s, federal law has required that tobacco companies place warnings from the Surgeon General on all cigarette packs. The studies done on cigarette smoking over the years have produced astonishing findings. Smoking has been associated with lung cancer, emphysema, bronchitis, cardiovascular disease, arteriosclerosis, vascular disease, gastrointestinal distress, urinary tract disease, nerve-related disease, and many other maladies. Yet people continue to smoke.

With the advent of low tar and nicotine cigarettes, many people began to rationalize the habit. But these cigarettes are also hazardous.

As an ex-smoker, the questions I most always ask smokers are, "Why do you smoke?" and "Do you enjoy smoking?" These questions are always the most difficult to answer.

It is important to understand that smoking effects the quality as well as the quantity of your life. This book, with its emphasis on good health, might never have been written without my mother. I believe that she was a victim of her smoking habit. The damage she suffered did not cause her to quit—she felt that it was too late. It is never too late.

If you need a reason to quit, consider this list compiled by the American Cancer Society:

Why You Should Quit Smoking

Risks of Smoking	Benefits of Quitting
Shortened life expectancy	
Risk proportional to amount smoked. A 25-year-old who smokes two packs a day can expect to live 8.3 years less than non-smoking contemporary.	After 10 to 15 years, an ex-smoker's risk approaches that of those who never smoked.
Lung cancer	
Cigarettes are major cause in both men and women. Overall, smokers' risk is 10 times higher than non-smokers.	After 10 to 15 years, an ex-smoker's risk approaches that of those who never smoked.
Larynx cancer	
Smoking increases risk by 2.9 to 17.7 fold that of non-smokers.	General reduction in risk, reaching normal after 10 years.
Mouth cancer	
Smokers have three to ten times as many oral cancers as non-smokers. Alcohol may act as a synergist, enhancing effect of smoking.	Reducing or eliminating smoking/drinking lowers risk in first few years. Risk drops to level of non-smokers in 10 to 15 years.

Risks of Smoking	**Benefits of Quitting**
Cancer of esophagus	
Smoking increases risk of fatal cancer two to nine times. Alcohol acts as synergist.	Since risk is proportional to dose, reducing or eliminating smoking/drinking should lower risk.
Cancer of the bladder	
Smokers have 7 to 10 times greater risk. Synergistic with certain occupational exposures.	Risk decreases gradually to that of non-smokers over 7 years.
Cancer of pancreas	
Risk of fatal cancer is 2 to 5 times higher than for non-smokers.	Since risk seems related to dose, stopping smoking should reduce it.
Coronary heart disease	
Smoking a major factor, causing 120,000 excess heart deaths each year.	Risk decreases sharply after one year. After ten years, risk is same as for those who never smoked.
Bronchitis and emphysema	
Smokers face 4 to 25 times greater risk of death, lung damage even in young smokers.	Cough and oputum disappear within a few weeks. Lung function may improve; deterioration slowed.
Stillbirth and low birth weight	
Smoking mothers have more stillbirths and babies both at below normal weight, with greater vulnerability to disease and death.	If mother stopped smoking before the fourth month of pregnancy, risk to fetus is eliminated.
Peptic ulcer	
Smokers get more ulcers and are more likely to die from them; cure more difficult in smokers.	Ex-smokers get ulcers, too, but they heal faster and more completely than in smokers.
Drug and test effects	
Smoking changes pharmacological effects of many medicines; changes results of diagnostic tests and increases risk of blood clots from oral contraceptives.	Most blood factors raised by smoking return to normal after quitting. Non-smokers on birth control pill have much lower risks of hazardous clots and heart attacks.

Alcohol

Alcohol, the great social lubricant, is often used to combat stress; it relaxes muscles and decreases anxiety. But alcohol used to excess can be a source of stress. And it is one of the major drug problems in the United States.

"According to the National Council on Alcoholism there are 3.3 million alcoholics and problem drinkers age 14-17, 10 million aged 18-65 and 1.6 million over 65, a total of nearly 5 million alcoholics. Approximately 5 million Americans have alcohol related health problems. As a central nervous system depressant alcohol does not increase either physical or mental ability, nor does it dilate the cornea vessels as some believe. Studies show that even in low or moderate amounts, alcohol actually increases the workload of the heart. Moderate amounts significantly impair visual and motor coordination in the ability to estimate speed and distance of objects and judgements of passage of time. Sexual function is diminished by even a moderate amount of alcohol. Addiction to alcohol is characterized by tolerance and physical dependence. Illnesses associated with alcohol abuse include cirrhosis, gastritis, pancreatitis, nutritional disorders, organic brain disease, coronary artery disease and hypertension. Over 50% of all highway fatalities are directly related to alcohol abuse."[6]

Alcohol and nicotine are drugs—that is, products that have the capacity to alter the natural chemistry of the body. *Newsweek* recently reported that drug abuse has become America's number one problem in business. Drugs in today's society have moved into the corporate board rooms, courtrooms, airline hangars, nuclear plants, factories, construction sites and even our schools. Drugs and alcohol are by-products of stress. People utilize these substances to alleviate their problems, not realizing that they are actually feeding them. Stress can be reduced by proper diet, proper exercise, and proper health habits. Any dependency is an addiction, any addiction is a problem, and problems are a major source of stress.

Alcohol creates biochemical stress within the body. When it enters the blood it stimulates an increased production of our stress hormone no-repinephrine. This hormone mobilizes all our resources to fight stress. The fact that alcohol stimulates norepinephrine production suggests that regular drinking takes its toll on the body's capacity to cope with stressful life situations.

Caffeine

Most of my patients are more reluctant to give up caffeine than any other drug. In fact, most of them do not realize that it *is* a drug.

"The Department of Health, Education and Welfare lists caffeine as addictive along with nicotine and heroin and admits that if caffeine were a new drug the manufacturer would have a great difficulty in getting a license to sell it and would no doubt be available only by prescription.[7]

"Caffeine, which is introduced into our bodies via coffee, tea or soda, is a socially acceptable addiction. For many people, it would be unAmerican to start the day without that morning 'pick-me-up.' But, ultimately, this substance lets you down. Coffee drinkers experience the three distinct signs of addiction: tolerance to the drug, withdrawal symptoms when it is removed, and craving upon deprivation.

"Coffee has also been associated with a number of diseases, and elimination of caffeine may bring relief from certain disorders.

"Coffee has been linked with several types of cancer, including leukemia and pancreatic cancer. For men coffee has been associated with cancer of the prostate and intestines, and for women to the lung, larynx, the breast and ovarian cancer.

"In an Ohio State University study of women who completely eliminated caffeine from their diet found that within six months 65% of them no longer had breast cysts.[8]

"Caffeine has also been linked to high blood pressure, ulcers, diabetes, psychosis and birth defects. And a little caffeine can go a long way

"Caffeine is an addiction that can bring upon symptoms of anxiety, restlessness, agitation, muscle tremors, headaches, sensory disturbances, cardiovascular symptoms and gastrointestinal complaints. Caffeine can result from an intake of 500–600 mg of caffeine a day which is approximately only 2–4 cups of coffee or 7–9 cups of tea."[9]

An estimated 90 million Americans drink 6 to 7 cups of coffee a day. And this doesn't take into account the consumption of caffeine through soft drinks. (I always recommend that my patients drink caffeine-free soft drinks.) The average American—and this includes children—consumes approximately 200 mg of caffeine per day, which is double what it takes to affect the body significantly. And 20% to 30% of us consume more than 500 mg of caffeine daily, an amount double what doctors consider a large drug dose.

Caffeine acts as a stimulant, a fact that U.S. students who need to study all night and Middle East Muslims who wish to pray all night have long recognized. Caffeine encourages the body to produce insulin, which depletes the body of normal energy and lowers the blood sugar, thus decreasing the production of the fat mobilizing hormone. Caffeine also encourages the release of the hormones epinephrine and norepinephrine, and with the release of these anti-stress hormones the heart beats faster, blood pressure rises, the stomach jumps, the bowels react, and blood vessels constrict.

The primary appeal of caffeine is the sudden, sharp surge of energy it provides. But this boost is deceptive. True, the mind feels more alert and the body more stimulated at first, but when the effects wear off, rebound sets in.

"One mug of coffee contains enough caffeine to raise the metabolism 10%–25%, which is the equivalent of 10 mg of amphetamine. The body goes into overdrive but when the effects of the coffee wear off in 2 1/2 to 3 or 4 hours the body feels the effects of having drawn on its energy reserves it goes into a slump and feels more fatigued than ever."[10]

These are the very same symptoms that are associated with hypoglycemia. Because caffeine is an insulin releaser it can cause irritability, performance irregularity, and obesity.

Use caffeine only on occasion and in moderation, and never drink more than two cups of coffee per day.

Children

It is important that we help our children to avoid soft drinks with caffeine, as they will create the same biochemical stress that they do in adults. And stress is not only an adult disorder—it can and does adversely affect children. Studies have shown that stress can increase a child's risk of infection and reduce the body's resistance to disease. So parents, keep your children away from products with caffeine.

Although the substances discussed here are often used in reaction to stress, they obviously only worsen the condition. The substances that can be used to combat stress are vitamins, especially the antioxidants. And because vitamins can help us to cope with stress, they can also better enable us to overcome our addictions to harmful substances.

The Dow Jones of life is bound to have its ups and downs. But the shortcuts to stress relief—drugs, alcohol, nicotine, caffeine, sugar—will lead only to dead ends.

When we remove these bad habits we are on our way to mastering stress, for our self-control helps to develop our inner strength. With this strength, we can build a happy and healthy lifestyle, one in which we can manage circumstances rather than be victimized by them. An enhanced self-image will enable us to plan our lives and live our plans. We will be less susceptible to obesity and diseases. (It has always been my belief that obesity and disease are synonymous—remove one and you eliminate the other.)

Many addictions (sugar, alcohol, caffeine, tobacco) are often behavioral in nature. These may also trigger anxiety disorders by altering your blood chemistry. St. John's Wort, a herb, may assist you in addictive behavioral disorders. Adults should take approximately 1,000 mg per day. Children should take 300 mg per 50 lbs of body weight. For example, a 100 pound child should take 600 mg. Always cousult your physician before beginning any type of regimen though.

I believe that with some guidance, a certain amount of discipline, and a lot of dedication, we can achieve a happier, healthier existence. Stress, like disease, will be always with us, but we can reduce it and learn not to let it run us. Befriend yourself, learn from your failures, and acknowledge your successes. Accept that plans do not always work out and that worrying will not improve matters. Most of all, be willing to accept that the life you deserve is available to you. With the right habits, you can live a longer, more fulfilled life.

The first wealth is health.

Ralph Waldo Emerson

25

Chiropractic— Myth or Miracle?

Chiropractic is now taking its rightful place in the mainstream of the healing arts. Today, this profession is accepted by the public, insurance companies, and even many medical doctors.

Chiropractors have come a long way in a relatively short time, for not so very long ago it was quite acceptable to dismiss this profession as a form of quackery. The American Medical Association (AMA) was especially hard on chiropractic. This powerful organization represents the interests of approximately 225,000 medical doctors; it is the most powerful medical organization in the world and has the second strongest lobby (after the Aerospace industry) in the United States. But we've had our day in court—and we won.

"On August 27, 1987, a United States Federal Court in Chicago found that the American Medical Association and various affiliated organizations, such as the American College of Radiology, had between 1966 and 1980 pursued an illegal conspiracy designed to contain and destroy the chiropractic profession. The conspiracy was planned from 1963 because the AMA's dismay at the degree to which individual medical doctors were choosing to practice in association with chiropractors, undermining the medical monopoly on private and hospital health care services. American Medical Association activities were not always in the best interest of chiropractic. They always tried to leave a less-than-favorable impression of chiropractic. Yet today chiropractic stands alone as the largest natural health care profession in the world.

"Chiropractic is now the third largest primary health care profession in the Western world after medicine and dentistry. There are approximately 36,000 chiropractors in the United States, 3,000 in Canada, 2,000 in Australia, 1,000 in Japan, 300 in France and 1 in 300 each of Belgium, Denmark, Great Britain, Italy, Norway, Sweden, Switzerland, New Zealand and South Africa. The profession is established, though in small numbers, in other European countries, Asia, Africa, the Middle East and South America.[1]

"Chiropractic and chiropractors are like the spine itself; often misunderstood and overlooked. A profession that claims to be the world's largest natural healing art, however, shouldn't be taken lightly."[2]

According to some estimates, more than 10 million people a year visit chiropractors, and one fourth of the U.S. population has been to a chiropractor at one time or another.[3]

These figures are especially impressive in view of the fact that chiropractic is still a young profession. Chiropractic (from the Greek, meaning "treatment by hand") was conceived by Daniel David ("D.D.") Palmer, who was able to eliminate the deafness of a custodian named Harvey Lillard. D.D. Palmer began his career as a teacher. He was a religious man, known for his fervor for reading and study. His interests were science and the development of humanity, a combination reflected in today's chiropractic profession. He eventually founded the Palmer School of Chiropractic in Davenport, Iowa.

But it was Palmer's son, Bartlett J. ("B.J.") Palmer, who was responsible for the phenomenal growth of the profession. B.J. Palmer wrote and published 40 books, and owned the first radio station west of the Mississippi (one of his employees, Ronald Reagan, went on to a career with which we are all familiar). Under this flamboyant and controversial man, the school grew from 24 students in 1906 to 3,100 in 1923. And the growth of the student body was accompanied by a growth in credibility and respectability.

True, the medical profession was still wary, but the public was accepting chiropractic treatment for a wide range of ills. Chiropractors used an important technique in building their practices—*results*. Results are what brought chiropractic to its place as the third largest primary health care profession in the western world, and results led to the victory over the AMA.

Chiropractors are far from being glorified masseurs. The number of hours devoted to science in chiropractic school actually surpasses the medical school requirements.

Chiropractic Class Hours (minimum)	Subject	Medical Class Hours (minimum)
520	Anatomy	508
420	Physiology	326
271	Pathology	335
300	Chemistry	325
114	Bacteriology	130
370	Diagnosis	374
320	Neurology	112
217	X-ray	148
65	Psychiatry	144
65	Obstetrics & Gynecology	198
225	Orthopedics	156
2,887	Total Hours	2,756

Each health care profession concentrates on a specific avenue of approach. In dentistry, it is the drill, while in medicine it is drugs. But for the doctor of chiropractic, the avenue of approach is through the spine. Spinal manipulation dates back to Hippocrates, the father of medicine, and Galen, the prince of physicians. As Hippocrates told us, "Look well to the spine for the cause of disease."

The brain and the spinal cord are the first organs to develop in human beings. They are the only organs of the body wholly encased in bone. (The brain is encased in the skull or cranium, while the spinal cord is encased in the spinal, or vertebral, column.) The brain communicates with the body through the spinal cord, which by spinal nerves branches out through openings in between bones (called foramen) of the spinal column to every organ, tissue, and cell in the body. Together, the brain and spinal cord form the central nervous system, which is the master communication system for the entire body.

The vertebrae of the spinal column consist of 24 moveable segments, separated by little pads called disks. The vertebrae are stacked like building blocks, one on top of another. The engineering of this structure enables us to bend, twist, and turn. When the brain is sending the appropriate signals, messages travel down the spinal cord out from and in between the vertebrae to every organ and muscle group in the body. If all is well and there is no interference, the body functions as it was designed to. However, periodically, through strenuous physical activity, trauma, or toxicity, one or more of these segments can be knocked out of alignment, a condition known as subluxation. A subluxation acts in much the same way as the pinching of a fuel line. The gas will not effectively pass through the pinched line to the engine, and thus we have an engine malfunction. Because nerves exit the spinal cord through openings, a subluxation causes interference with the normal activities of the nerves. This interference can disturb function throughout the body and cause many diseases.

Modern doctors of chiropractic work directly with the nerves because they understand that the nerves control and coordinate the functions, organs and systems of the entire body. The system is vast and complex; it has been estimated that there are approximately 20 billion neurons throughout the nervous system, and 10 billion in the brain alone. Nerve impulses not only give us the ability to experience sensation, they make it possible for the individual to carry out movement. It is the nervous system, which transmits all sensations to the brain, that makes it possible for us to see, smell, taste, touch and hear. And our nerves maintain the perfect balance of the body.

In Florida, temperatures often go above 100 degrees. But our internal thermostat will keep our body temperature at a constant 98.6 degrees. In Chicago, where temperatures often plummet to 20 degrees or less, our body will likewise maintain a body temperature of 98.6. The intelligence we refer to as innate intelligence keeps this thermostat accurate. But it is our nervous system that allows this mechanism to work as it should.

It is the nervous system that makes it possible for us to swallow and move our bowels. The nervous system controls the liver, lungs, spleen, pancreas, gall bladder, and kidneys. Perfect health, natural health, is possible only when you have a complete, perfect, normally functioning nervous system.

Conversely, when there is interference with the nerve energy signals, a problem of some type will develop. An estimated 90% of all interference with nerves originates in the spinal area. Vertebrae slip out of position and pinch the nerves, thus diminishing or perhaps cutting off the vital life force of the body. A misaligned bone will not necessarily cause pain at the time, but it will eventually give rise to symptoms. The symptoms will proliferate unless the bone is put into its proper place so that the nerve can be freed. And this is where chiropractic comes in.

Nature's Way

My introduction to chiropractic came in childhood, when my uncle Al Brenner used to treat my father and brother for hay fever. Once a week, they would visit him for a spinal adjustment. The obvious question, of course, is how can a spinal adjustment affect a respiratory ailment?

Chiropractors have received bad publicity because of mistaken notions of what the profession claimed to do. Many people have stated that chiropractors believe that they can cure cancer and other debilitating diseases. I want to make it clear that this is absolutely untrue. Chiropractors cannot "cure" anything—what they do is enable the body to cure itself. (Drugs also do not cure, they assist the body by aiding it's internal defense mechanisms.) When a chiropractor performs a spinal adjustment, the nerve impingement is relieved, thus allowing the body's healing powers to take over. Chiropractors know that the power that created the body has the power to heal the body.

The medicine of the future is not the administration of more complicated, more potent, and potentially more hazardous drugs, it is natural healing. Simply stated, the job of chiropractors is to utilize their extensive training to understand and release the body's inherent recuperative powers. This process may begin literally at birth, for newborns are prone to subluxation, which blocks the natural healing mechanism.

"Dr. Abraham Towbin, M.D., is a medical neuropathologist of Harvard Medical School. He is one of the many world authorities investigating the relationship between the birth process and spinal damage. He found in one of his many studies that nearly 1 out of every 3 still-born infants examined appeared to have actually died of cervical injuries during childbirth. Other studies have also linked spinal injury as a result of the birth process to a host of other conditions such as mental retardation, epilepsy, amyotonia cerebral palsy, hyperactivity and various paralytic neuropathies or diseases of the nervous system. In one of many published articles Dr. Towbin states, 'During the last part of delivery, during the final extraction of the fetus, mechanical stress imposed by obstetrical manipulation, even the application of standard orthodox procedures can be intolerable to the fetus.'"[4]

Chiropractors have long advocated the examination of children. We believe that this examination should take place as early as birth. The adage, "As the twig is bent, thus is the tree inclined," is especially true in our profession.

In the medical profession, the focus is on the treatment of symptoms. If a person has a headache, she will be given something to mask the pain; if someone has high blood pressure, he will take a medication to bring it down. But chiropractic takes the view that the cause, not just the symptoms, must be understood and treated in order for health to be restored and maintained. Once the cause is treated, the symptoms will disappear. A chiropractor is inclined to ask, "Why in a class of 30 children did 3 develop chicken pox while the other 27 did not? Why did one worker come down with a headache while the other did not?" We know that spinal misalignments (subluxations) disturb nerve function and thus alter the function of the organs, the tissues, and the cells of the body. Chiropractors work with the nervous system because we recognize that therein resides the innate intelligence of the body.

The only difference between a live person and a dead body is the energy that flows through a living human being. We call this the life force. As a chiropractic student working on my first cadaver, I was awed by the profound difference between life and death. That corpse had every nerve, organ and tissue I had. The only difference—and it was a huge one—was the energy flowing in my body. The true meaning of this was brought home to me the night of my mother's death. I went to the hospital and saw my mother lying there. Only three hours before, she was so full of life. Although she looked at peace, I could not help thinking of her as she was such a short time ago, when the life force—a force that humans cannot duplicate—was animating her.

When the life force is flowing as it should, the human body is perfect—a marvelous system working in complete harmony. Perhaps no organ demonstrates this so well as the heart.

"The human heart beats about 100,000 times every 24 hours. Consider the fact that the heart and its pumping system, which scientists have attempted to duplicate without success, pumps six quarts of blood through over 96,000 miles of blood vessels. This is in equivalent of 6,300 gallons being pumped per day, this is almost 115 million gallons in only 15 years. The six quarts of blood are made up of over 24 trillion cells that make three to five thousand trips throughout the body every day. Seven million new blood cells are produced every second. This pumping system has the capability of working non-stop for decades without ever missing a beat."[5]

The human body harbors an intelligence that is unmatched in power, capacity, and adaptability. A mother instinctively recognizes this; she has a personal understanding of the infinite wisdom of the miracle of the sperm and the egg, which will combine to form a fully-functioning human being. She understands this without any special training or education. And she therefore has a special faith in her own body and the body of her child.

As a physician, one of my tasks is to recognize this perfection. It is the function of the chiropractor to help the body maintain its perfect balance, because if this balance is off even a fraction, the body will no longer be at ease.

Recently, my father underwent quadruple bypass surgery. His very talented surgeon cut open his chest, spread apart his ribs, removed the diseased vessels and replaced them with new ones. My biggest concern, obviously, was my father's prognosis. "How's my father, Doc, will he be alright?" Dr. Richard Faro, to whom I will be forever indebted, replied, "Your father is doing very well. I've done my job, it's now up to your father." It was now up to my father. This surgeon, who had the ability to reconstruct the damaged vessels of the heart, understood that the body must heal itself. The body must close the wounds created by the surgeon's scalpel. The body must mend the bones broken by the surgeon's tools.

To a chiropractor, symptoms are not nuisances—they are warnings. If for example, a person's blood pressure is too high, and the problem is dietary rather than structural, medication will not correct the problem. In all likelihood, dietary changes, such as reduced salt consumption, will relieve the condition. (Once again, I must emphasize that you should never adjust your medication without a physician's approval.)

Chiropractors know that it takes time to become ill, and we let our patients know that it also takes time to become well. Pain is always the first thing to come and the last to leave. Smothering the symptoms is not the answer. All licensed medical doctors take the Hippocratic Oath, which provides guidelines for ethical practice. Yet how many doctors follow the philosophy of that oath, which advocates working in harmony with the body, not controlling it?

Hippocrates knew that it wasn't the doctor who cured the disease. Rather, an inborn force within the body was responsible for restoring health. Hippocrates believed that the doctor had an obligation to work with this force and support the healing properties of nature. The philosophy of Hippocrates and the philosophy of the chiropractic are one and the same.

The premise and philosophy of chiropractic are really not hard to understand. Quite simply, chiropractic teaches that within the body there are well-established survival mechanisms designed to maintain a state of good health. That the innate intelligence that is working in our bodies at all times, whether or not we are aware of it, has the ability to relay signals to and from the brain and spinal cord to all tissues in the body. We do not have to tell our bodies when to digest our food. We do not have to tell our lungs to breathe. We do not have to tell our hearts how many times to beat. The body in its infinite wisdom goes on and continues to do its job automatically, never asking for a day off. Have you ever sat and realized that your body, brain, and nervous system, along with every muscle, tissue and organ in the body has never for one day, for one hour, for one minute taken time off? It continues to duplicate itself, replicate itself, regenerate itself, so that our lives can continue in harmony with nature.

Throughout history, people have searched for the elusive fountain of youth. They have been on an endless quest for eternal health, youth, and well-being. We have spent billions of dollars on drugs, potions, elixirs, fad diets, health spas, cosmetic surgery—but only in recent years have we begun to study health, and not just disease.

Over the past year, my clinics have had over 40,000 patient visits. And the greatest benefit I can offer them is an education on this thing called health, a term Webster's dictionary defines as, "A condition of wholeness in which all of the organs are functioning 100% all the time."

We as physicians understand that disease is a degenerative state, and that halting this degeneration is the first step toward regeneration. It is my informed opinion that through chiropractic care, the body's healing powers and internal awareness are increased.

Medical Doctors Recognize Chiropractic Benefits

The medical profession is beginning to share this view. Many medical doctors have conducted honest, open-minded investigations of chiropractic, and the response has been favorable.

"Chiropractic's position and status today with the American College of Surgeons is as follows: The American College of Surgeons says, 'There are no ethical or collective restraints to full professional cooperation between doctors of chiropractic and medical physicians. Such cooperation should include referrals, group practice, participation of all health care delivery systems, treatment and services in and through hospitals, participation in student exchange, programs between chiropractic and medical colleges in cooperation and research in continuing programs.' The American College of Radiology says, 'There are and should be no ethical or collective impediments to inter professional association in cooperation between doctors of chiropractic and medical radiologists in any setting where such association may occur, such as in a hospital, private practice, research, education, care of a patient, or other legal arrangement.' The American Hospital Association says, 'The AHA has no objection to a hospital granting privileges to doctors of chiropractic for the purposes of administering chiropractic treatment furthering the clinical education and training of doctors of chiropractic or having X-rays, clinical laboratory tests and reports there are made for doctors of chiropractic and their patients and/or previously taken X-rays, clinical laboratory tests and reports made available to them upon patient authorization.'"[6]

Individual physicians have also praised the results possible through chiropractic.

Ills Traced to Vertebrae

"It may never occur to them (his/her medical colleagues) that the headaches, stomach trouble, neuritis, or nervous irritability they are attempting to cure may be due to nothing more serious than a displaced vertebrae which any competent chiropractor can restore in ten seconds."[7] Rubin Herman, M.D.

Chiropractic Adjustment Works (referring to severe headaches during and after specific movements of the head)

" . . . a chiropractic adjustment will work on the cervical region. We find in the case of hypertension a drop from 25 to 30 mm Hg right after the adjustment is given."[8] K. Gutzeit, M.D.

Performs Miraculous Cures

"From personal experience alone, I am of the opinion that many patients suffer from some type of dislocation on the vertebral structures. There is no doubt that the consciousness of the orthopedic surgeon was aroused originally by the success of bone-setters, the early manipulators, and more recently the chiropractors. The latter group has undoubtedly performed their miraculous cures in individuals who have been misdiagnosed and mistreated by the practitioner of internist."[9] Harold T. Hyman, *American Journal of Medical Science.*

Patients Find Relief

"It is quite easy to replace the vertebrae with a moderate amount of manipulation, and . . . many patients find relief in the hands of chiropractors."[10] James Brailsford, M.D.

Chiropractic First . . . Surgery Last

"It is better that the chiropractor treat these patients than to have them treated by a physician who thinks only in terms of surgery."[11] H.B. Gotten, M.D.

Chiropractic Succeeds Where Medicine Fails

"Few medical practitioners could recommend manipulation because they were barred against it by their oath; however, it is indisputable that the exponents of chiropractic had brought relief to many patients in the past, after orthodox treatment had been tried and failed."[12] John Mennell, M.D.

Results for Medically "Incurable"

"There was a time when I looked at chiropractic through a pair of bifocal lenses, the upper plus prejudice, the lower plus lack of investigation. But because medicine, with all its adjuncts, had failed to reach the complicated ailments of my invalid wife, I, like a drowning man, grasped for anything in sight.

"I learned of chiropractic through a friend of mine. I went at once to a school of chiropractic, and to my surprise, they were actually getting results on cases that were hopelessly incurable from the standpoint of medicine. I soon saw that the theory they were working on was plausible and met the approval of common sense. All of this opened up a new field of thought to me which had never been presented through the study of medicine. The sooner the medical profession recognized the work of the chiropractor, the better! S/he is doing a work that medicine cannot do. S/he belongs exclusively to the specialists and should be recognized."[13] M.E. King, M.D.

Misaligned Spine Affects Organs

"It is possible that a slight irregularity in the disposition of the vertebrae by 'strangling' certain spinal nerves at their exit from the spine can have considerable organic effects, as the chiropractic school maintains."[14] R.F. Allendy, M.D.

Medical Doctors Treated by Chiropractors

"Most physicians are opposed to vertebral manipulations, yet they do not hesitate to correct other bony or articular displacements. This attitude causes them to have themselves taken care of by . . . chiropractors."[15] James Cyria, M.D.

Often Only Cure

"The 600 cases that we have observed over a period of four years have taught us super abundantly that vertebrotherapy . . . often . . . constitutes the only means of curing, and that in a manner which is at times spectacular . . . the manipulations extolled by chiropractors are multiple and varied, and do not concern back pain only."[16] Charles Rocher, M.D.

Gaining Favor Among Doctors

"An explanatory introduction to chiropractic is no longer necessary. The manipulation of the spine, or at least a strong interest in it, is gaining favor in a wide circle of doctors. Among patients it has almost become the fashion to let oneself be treated by chiropractic, be it by the few in Germany who have been trained professionally in the United States or by physicians who have familiarized themselves with this method of treatment."[17] G. Zillinger, M.D.

Chiropractic Enriches Medical Disciplines

"The great possibilities of chiropractic lie in the exactly purposeful removal of a blocking of the spinal dynamics. Chiropractic does not belong, therefore, in the realm of a medical specialty; rather does it cut across all medical disciplines, not superseding them, restraining them, but broadening, uniting, and enriching them."[18] Albert Cramer, M.D.

Chiropractors Make People Better

"We must now realize that the world is not full of cripples produced by chiropractors. Chiropractors do not make people worse, they make an awful lot of them better."[19] W.J.S. Melvin, M.D.

Value Not Appreciated

"Subluxations of vertebrae occur in all parts of the spine and in all degrees. When the dislocation is so slight as not to affect the spinal cord, it will still produce disturbances in the spinal nerves, passing off through the spinal foramina (Channels). The value of (chiropractic) has not been fully appreciated."[20] James P. Warbassee, M.D.

Athletes and Other Celebrities

It is my good fortune to have a practice that includes many dynamic, successful and interesting patients. In the course of my career, I have treated numerous professional athletes.

Athletes have historically been more open to chiropractic than the population at large, because they are more in tune with their bodies. They especially appreciate our noninvasive, nonsurgical, nondrug treatment approach. They understand that good posture, good nutrition and appropriate exercise, combined with spinal adjustments, produce a strong, well-balanced body that is more resistant to disease and injury. Because of the results we have achieved with these high-profile patients, chiropractic is becoming increasingly important in the field of sports medicine.

Chiropractic is now represented in the U.S. Olympics. The 1976 Winter Games at Lake Placid, New York, marked the first time that a chiropractic doctor was accepted as an Olympic team physician. Participating athletes insisted that a chiropractor be included. The practice of having a chiropractor on staff was continued in the 1984, 1988 and 1992 Olympics.

Athletes made it all but impossible to ignore the benefits of chiropractic. Kareem Abdul Jabar of the Los Angeles Lakers has visited chiropractors for headaches. Famed runner Mary Decker of the U.S. Olympics consulted a chiropractor following a fall during the 1984 games. With the aid of Sid Williams, Life Foundation and Life Chiropractic College (of which Williams is president) represented the 1986 U.S.A. Goodwill Games in Moscow. Twenty chiropractors were involved in caring for athletes from all over the world.

Chiropractic is perhaps best known as a safe and effective treatment for back pain, an ailment no athlete can afford. Jeffery Saal, M.D., of the San Francisco Spine Institute, achieved fame by prescribing surgery for football star Joe Montana. Nonetheless, in an interview with *USA Today* he said that, "Surgeons generally use the wrong criteria in deciding to operate. At least twice as many operations as necessary are performed for ruptured discs in the lower back." He and his brother Dr. Joel Saal conducted a three year study and reported the following conclusions:

"More than 20 percent of patients with (lower back) disc problems have surgery but less than 10 percent may really need it if there are no other problems, such as stenosis, or narrowing of the spine."

In other words, 50% of lower-back disc surgery is unnecessary, according to a top orthopedic specialist. I believe that surgery is sometimes indicated, but only when all else fails. Chiropractic should be the first option, surgery the last.

Joe Montana of the world champion San Francisco 49ers has had back surgery, and today he is an outspoken advocate of chiropractic. A special on his experience with chiropractic was aired on national television prior to the 1990 Super Bowl.

As a chiropractor, I not only treat injuries, I make it my business to research the origin of the problem. My purpose is to understand the underlying causes of malfunctions in the human body, and to restore communication between the different areas of the body. The spine and nervous system—the master communication system—are my primary areas of expertise.

Athletes are especially prone to injury because of the rigorous training programs in which they are involved, so a good deal of my practice is oriented toward sports medicine. Many of my patients have also become my friends. I am especially gratified by the friendship of Jeff Reardon, one of baseballs premier relief pitchers, and one of the nicest gentlemen I have ever met. Jeff first came to my office for treatment of neck and shoulder problems. The diagnostic workup, which included X-rays, indicated a severe subluxation of the lower cervical segments. This resulted not only in neck and shoulder pain, but in a condition known as *brachial radiculitis*, an inflammation of the nerves that travel down the arm. In addition, Jeff had a history of elbow problems.

In the review analysis, I explained to Jeff how removing this interference would eliminate the inflammation and thus enhance his performance. I utilized chiropractic adjustments to relieve the nerve interference, and worked with Jeff kinesiologically, educating him on techniques to strengthen the weakened muscle tissue. This treatment and self-help makes it possible to maintain the body at 100%.

It is a rare pleasure to work with someone of Jeff's caliber. He recently became the first pitcher in the history of the major leagues to get 40 saves in both the American and the National Leagues. In addition to his other accomplishments, Jeff has won the Rolaid's Relief Award, Reliever of the Decade. He has dedicated his life to baseball, and the fact that he is as devoted to his profession as I am to mine is an added bond between us. I found Jeff easy to work with. He maintains a conditioning program 365 days a year in order that he will always be capable of delivering a peak performance. He also has an excellent understanding of the biomechanics of the body. This combination has me convinced that he will one day be a member of the Hall of Fame.

One of my peak experiences as an athletic spectator and a physician was attending the 1987 World Series at Jeff's invitation. He continued the success that started in the playoffs with the Detroit Tigers by pitching the final outs in both the league and world championship series.

An article by Tom D'Angelo in *Today's Chiropractic* had this to say about Jeff:

"At 32, Reardon has enjoyed eight successful seasons in the big leagues. With 193 saves—including a career high 41 in 1985 (he surpassed that number with 42 in 1988), the year he won the Rolaid's Relief Award. Last year he finished regular season with 31 saves, and added three more in the post season. Reardon was on the mound when the Twins clinched the American League West title, the American League Pennant, and the World Series. Just as important he pitched the entire season pain-free. Although he worked with the Twins training staff during the season (Reardon never consulted a chiropractor during the season) he gives most of the credit to Dr. Kaplan. 'My arm didn't hurt me the whole year,' Reardon said. 'He's helped me a lot.'"

I do not claim credit for the success of Jeff Reardon or any of the other athletes and celebrities I have treated. Chiropractic techniques and the cooperation of the patient deserve the praise.

Tennis players are another group that seeks chiropractic care. An article in *Tennis Magazine*[21] revealed that Billy Jean King, Tracy Austin and Wendy Turnbough utilize chiropractic to help relieve aches and pains and keep them in top condition on the court. Other pros who visit chiropractors include Elliot Telscher, Stan Smith, Ivan Lendel, John McEnroe, Jimmy Connors, and Kevin Curren.

"'Word gets out,' said King in the article. 'If I'm happy, or if Lendel is happy, then the others say, 'Well if you're going to do it, then I'm going to do it.' She noted that, 'A lot more players and athletes are going to chiropractors now. Even up to 10 years ago, any time you went to an M.D. he would tell you not to go (to a chiropractor). I used to get this kind of information and finally I just went, and quite frankly, there is no comparison. If my neck went out on me, I used to wait about 21 days—I could just about time it—before I could do anything again. I'd just go to the chiropractor and get manipulation, and I could play every day.'"[22]

I feel thankful and blessed to be a chiropractor. The reason this book is so important to me is that it is one of the first of its kind to be written by a chiropractor, someone who is trained to work with the natural healing energy of the human body.

Chiropractic has arrived because the public is no longer willing to settle for less than optimal health. And they are beginning to realize that good health cannot be procured from a pill, a potion or a lotion. They have been deceived once too often by the media and the advertising industry. The chiropractic approach, one that combines proper nutrition, water, rest, exercise, and a properly functioning nervous system, is being eagerly accepted by a public that is sick and tired of being sick and tired.

As has been true of many important movements, celebrities have led the way in this one.

> Doc Severinsen—"Whenever I travel I seek the benefits of this great profession of chiropractic."

> Marlo Thomas—"Chiropractic solved my neck and shoulder pains; it put me back on my feet. I think chiropractic is great!"

> James Arness—"Chiropractic care is the only real, long-lasting relief that I have found for my neck pain due to an old injury."

> George Kennedy—"A chiropractor accomplished in three weeks what the army doctors haven't been able to do in two years."

> Peter Fonda—"Regular chiropractic adjustments go hand-in-hand with good health."

> Liza Minelli—"I rely on regular chiropractic care to keep in shape for my strenuous type of acting and singing."

> Chuck Connors—"I depended on chiropractic care when I was an athlete. I depend on it now as a busy film and TV actor."

> Jane Russell—"I credit chiropractic care for maintaining my health to keep up the pace of my career."

> Robert Goulet—"I wouldn't be without my regular schedule of chiropractic adjustments because of my very strenuous schedule."

> Jeane Dixon—"I am walking today because of chiropractic care I received years ago. I predict a great future for the science of chiropractic."

> Melvin Belli—"I had headaches for over 30 years until I tried chiropractic. They have completely disappeared."

> Bob Cummings—"I have been a great devotee of chiropractic all my life. My father was a medical doctor who kept well using chiropractic."

> Ken Berry—"My success as an entertainer would not be possible if it weren't for chiropractic."

> Carol Lawrence—"Chiropractic keeps me in shape for my life as a TV, stage and screen star, wife and mother."

> Jack LaLanne—"The spine is the lifeline. A lot of people should go to a chiropractor but they don't know it."

> Clint Walker—"Without chiropractic care, I couldn't have existed with my work as a TV and film actor."

And the list goes on and on. Other celebrities who use chiropractic include Marla Maples Trump and family, Jim Kelly, Billy Casper, Gary Carter, Bruce Jenner, Robert Parish, Dave Cowens, Bruce Willis, Demi Moore, Arnold Schwarzenegger, Princess Diana, Burt Reynolds, Mickey Rooney, Jane Fonda, Muhammad Ali, Tim Witherspoon, Jack Nicklaus, Arnold Palmer, Cybil Shepard (married a chiropractor), Mitzi Gaynor, Eva Gabor, Glen Ford, George McCarthy, Doug McClure, and Evander Holyfield.

Mark Eaton of the Utah Jazz says of chiropractic, "I've gotten addicted to feeling good."[23]

You needn't be rich and famous to feel like a million dollars. Chiropractic is not for the select few, but for everyone who wants to enjoy optimum well-being. Nor is chiropractic acclaimed only in the U.S.; people throughout the world are discovering the benefits of this healing art.

Germany

"Chiropractic is scientifically well founded, is one of the most effective neurotherapeutic measures known, and belongs in the very center of medicine."[24]

England

"Seventeen percent of my patients require manipulation and it is a tragic fact that the average physician learns of manipulation after his patient has been helped by someone outside the medical profession."[25] Albert Cramer, M.D.

Switzerland

"The attitude of clinical medicine toward chiropractic has radically changed. . . . In the mid-1930s, it was denounced. . . . Today, however, many medical doctors are in favor of chiropractic and consider it to be an excellent therapeutic measure from certain diseases having their origin in changes within the spinal column."[26] H. DeBrunner, M.D.

Australia

"There can be no disease which does not disturb the nerve cells concerned. If the cause of the disturbance of these conducting nerves can be ascertained or removed, the patient will be cured. If not, treatment merely diverts from the truth."[27] R.J. Berry, M.D.

Canada

"The addition of chiropractic maneuvers to general management permits treatment of the cause rather than effect."[28] R.A. Leeman, M.D.

Scotland

"Spinal manipulation is a method of treatment which has been long neglected by the medical profession. In spite of the efforts of men . . . to demonstrate its value, there is still much prejudice against it and ignorance regarding the rational understanding of the treatment and methods for carrying it out."[29] T. Millar, The Clinical Journal

Russia

"(In) many pathological processes . . . the nervous component remains from beginning to end the factor that determines their general state."[30] A.D. Speransky.

Great Britain

"It is regrettable that patients suffering from slight congestive spinal lesion should be advised to seek relief in a popular pain killer. No wonder that the manipulator who can, in a short time, often relieve intolerable backache receives warm appreciation."[31] *British Journal of Physical Medicine*

Denmark

"Manipulative treatment, which previously in this country was given exclusively by chiropractors, has in latter years been taken up by some physicians, among others, the writer, who has found that this therapy is of significant value. . . . It must be emphasized that it requires great clinical experience and great technical skill to perform these manipulations. . . . If the physiotherapists want to use manipulative treatment, they ought to get an education just as thorough as that of chiropractors."[32] Dr. Boje, Senior physician at Rigs Hospital, Copenhagen

France

"The 600 cases that we have observed over a period of four years have taught us super-abundantly that vertebro-therapy . . . often . . . constitutes the only means of curing, and that in a manner which is at times spectacular . . . the manipulations extolled by the chiropractors are multiple and varied, and do not concern back pains only."[33] Charles M. Rocher, M.D.

Argentina

"Chiropractic is a useful therapeutic method worthy of being introduced into the patrimony of medicine. We regard it as very fitting . . . to create a school of chiropractors, with the object of making known to physicians the existence of this therapeutic method and its accomplishments. . . and with the highly social objective of bringing the benefits of chirotherapy to even the humblest classes."[34] Ministry of Public Health and Welfare

Germany

"Since the introduction of chiropractic methods in our polyclinic . . . it must undoubtedly be recognized that the percentage of success is great. . . . No physical or psychic damage was done to the patients not successfully treated. Those not handled successfully were almost exclusively those who did not come regularly for treatment. This method is worth being brought to the attention of the widest possible medical circles."[35] A.A. Hochfield

A Cost-Effective Treatment

The spiraling cost of health care has convinced many individuals and organizations to look favorably upon chiropractic. In the past 20 years, numerous studies have documented the cost-effectiveness of chiropractic care. In a paper entitled, "Health Economics and Chiropractic", prominent Australian economist John Dillon says that,

"Undoubtedly in terms of economic appraisal of the current health scene . . . chiropractic is in a very strong position. Compared to medical services, it is an extremely cheap avenue of health care for those who seek it. Unlike primary medical practice, it does not spiral costs into the system through ancillary and specialist services, hospitalization and pharmaceutics. On average, a dollar spent on a chiropractor's causes no further costs."

In Australia and Sweden, chiropractic has been found so cost-effective that increased government funding for chiropractic services has been recommended.

The cost-effectiveness of chiropractic is explained not only by its lower price, but by the improvement it can produce in people with certain chronic problems. Back pain, for example, is a widespread problem that is costly not only in terms of dollars spent, but in productivity lost.

"Surveys of chiropractic practice in a number of countries confirm that approximately 90% of chiropractic patients have headache, neck pain and back pain. In the western world 80% of the population will experience disabling low-back pain during their lives. At any given time 6.8% of the adult U.S. population is experiencing a bout of back pain that has been continuing for more than two weeks. Thirty percent of WCB claims by injured workers are for back pain (more than twice the percentage of any other complaint) and, because of the acknowledged poor medical management of this complaint and the huge cost of chronic cases, these 30% of claims generate 60% of total WCB compensation costs. In 1985 U.S. workers compensation boards disbursed $6 billion for low-back pain. The estimated total annual cost of back pain in the U.K. in 1982 was . . . millions of pounds."

Research indicates that spinal manipulation for the treatment of acute back pain has a success rate greater than 90%.

Back pain is becoming a major headache for the insurance industry. Back problems composed the second most common medical diagnosis related group (DRG) for all hospital discharges in 1987. Among surgical DRG's, back and neck problems ranked third behind cesarean section and tubal ligation. Liberty Mutual found their average cost per case of compensable low back pain to be $6,800 in 1986.

These are scary statistics considering back pain is the most costly ailment of working age adults. Dr. Arthur White, M.D., a world-renowned orthopedic surgeon, states that over 90% of back surgeries performed in the United States in 1991 were unnecessary. *Spine*, a respected orthopedic magazine reports 40% of patients undergoing low back surgery continue to have pain with 10% of those being worse after surgery.

"Mr. Larry Edwards, Manager of Medical Services Texas Employers' Insurance Association, Dallas. No one knows the true cost and, as the manager of a large

U.S. insurance association has confessed, 'the insurance industry should be and is being criticized for an obvious lack of statistical data on the costs of back related injuries. What we have, however, is scary.'"

It's especially scary in view of the fact that conventional medical treatment has had limited success with this problem.

The high cost of medical management of low-back pain is a major subject in scientific literature in recent years, which reveals:

A. Surgery and chemonucleolysis have been subject to high failure rates and unacceptable costs, and are now used rarely, with under 1% of patients.

B. Bedrest, which promotes 'illness behavior' and huge compensation costs has now been proven ineffective. It has been a general medical first response to back pain. It is being outspokenly rejected by leaders in medicine—most notably in recent months by Gordon Waddell, in work which won the 1987 Volvo Prize for spinal clinical research.

C. The basic approach to treatment now recommended is on a chiropractic model—early active treatment to restore spinal function and prevent onset of illness behavior.

One of the studies I am most pleased with was conducted by Dr. Steve Silverman, an excellent chiropractor and a personal friend.

"In a trial study Silverman, a Florida chiropractor, was sent a consecutive series of 100 patients with persistent low back or neck pain by AV-MED, a large South Florida health maintenance organization (HMO). Faced with fixed funding per patient, and prohibitive rates and costs of surgery, Dr. Herbert Davis, M.D., AV-MED's medical director, agreed to a study wherein the next 100 patients requiring hospital evaluation with a view to surgery would first be sent for chiropractic evaluation and, if appropriate, care. Comments are:

A.   Patients had already been seen by 1.6 M.D.s on average.

B.   2% had already been hospitalized.

C.   12% had been confirmed medically as requiring surgery.

D.   Chiropractic care consisted of spinal adjustment supplemented with physical therapy modalities, remedial exercise programs and advice.

E.   Average number of visits per patient was 12.1, average cost per patient $326.76.

F.   This was total cost—there were no referred costs for outside diagnostic investigations, other health care practitioners, or hospitalization.

G.   No patient, including the 12 medically diagnosed as needing surgery, required surgery.

H.   At six month follow-up 86% had used no further chiropractic or medical services.

I.   AV-MED advised an average cost of neck/back surgery at the time as $20,000. Accordingly AV-MED considers it savedapproximately $225,000 (medical and sur gical costs, less cost of chiropractic care) on the 12 confirmed surgical cases alone.

Following the trial AV-MED established a corporate policy requiring all patients to receive chiropractic assessment before referral to hospital for back and neck pain."[36]

Yet another Florida study compared chiropractic to other forms of treatment.

"The Foundation of Chiropractic Education and Research (FCER), with the cooperation of the Florida Dept. of Labor and Employment Security, Division of Workers' Compensation, recently completed a comprehensive analysis of Florida's workers' compensation claims for back-related injuries. The analysis compares the cost of treatment for patients of chiropractic, medical, and osteopathic doctors, and includes the costs of both hospital and non-hospital services for back-related injuries. Conclusions of the study excluded the costs for surgical procedures.

"Data for this analysis were compiled from all cases reported to the State of Florida during its 1985-86 fiscal year. The analysis covered the costs of all major diagnostic and treatment procedures and hospital services by type of physician."

Conclusions:

> Chiropractic patients had the lowest rate of incurring compensable injuries when compared to medical doctors.

> Of the patients who incurred compensable injuries, chiropractic patients were less likely to be hospitalized for treatment.

> When the average cost and number of services were compared, chiropractic care evidenced a relatively cost-effective approach to the management of work-related injuries.

> The estimated average cost of care, compared across all the major categories of treatments, was substantially higher for medical patients.

> The average cost of chiropractic services and prescribed procedures was significantly less than the corresponding costs of medical doctors.

The Rand Study concluded:

Spinal manipulation is the most commonly used conservative treatment for low back pain in the United States. It is the treatment supported by the most research in its effectiveness in terms of early results and long term benefits.[37]

Chiropractic has always been the people's doctor. Most of the chiropractors I know are willing to work with any patient regardless of ability to pay. It is good to know that third-party payers are also beginning to recognize the value of this treatment. Without the principles of chiropractic this book would not exist, for I believe that chiropractic is as important to good health as proper diet, exercise, and rest.

Study after study from the Rand Corporation to the *British Medical Journal* recognize the benefits of chiropractic care. Chiropractic is the safe choice, the cost effective choice, and the smart choice. It's not different to go to a chiropractic anymore, it's just smart.

If you have a health problem, it is highly probable that you also have a chiropractic problem. If your weight is a concern, it is possible that some form of nerve interference is making it impossible for your body to properly digest and utilize food.

In Ephesians 4:16, the Apostle Paul says, *All the body, by being harmoniously joined together were being made to cooperate through every joint that gives what is needed, according to each respective member in due measure, makes for the growth of the body for building up itself."* The human body has not changed since Biblical times, and Paul's statement is as true now as it ever was.

Chiropractic is not a myth, it is a reality, and within the scope of chiropractic, miracles are taking place with every adjustment. Chiropractic has arrived, and it is here to stay.

Nothing in this world is so powerful as an idea whose time has come.

Victor Hugo

26

Kaplan's Diet Commandments

The Diet in Review

1. Drink eight, eight ounce glasses of water a day. No substitutes.

2. Eat only permitted foods, but eat as often as you wish (minimum, three meals a day).

3. Initially (forever, if possible) avoid all foods containing the three whites: sugar, white flour, salt. It is our objective to avoid all sugar and refined carbohydrates.

4. We count carbohydrates, not calories. Follow these guidelines:
   Carbohydrates
   PHASE 1 — 10 g. or less

   PHASE 2 — 20 g. or less

   PHASE 3 — under 40 g.

   PHASE 4 (maintenance) — 40 to 60 g.
   (Note: Week 1 equals Phase 1; week 2 equals Phase 2, etc.)
   *Keep fat intake between 40 and 60 g. per day. Under 40 g. will allow quicker weight loss. In excess of 60 g. will lead to weight gain. These numbers are estimates; you must determine your own critical carbohydrate level through experimentation or use of ketostix. By staying at or below your personal critical carbohydrate level, you will stay within your desired weight.

5. Take a multivitamin three times a day. Review Chapter 18 for dosages.

6. **PHASE 1**

    BREAKFAST

    1 egg and 1 orange, or 1 whole grapefruit

    LUNCH

    1 protein (chicken, fish, veal, or beef) prepared any way except breaded. A green salad with oil and vinegar (preferably olive oil and apple cider vinegar).

    DINNER

    Follow same regimen as lunch.

    SNACKS

    Any protein, salad, or raw vegetable

    DESSERT

    Diet (no carbohydrate) jello

Permitted foods:

Meat:

Steak (trim fat), corned beef, veal, lean hamburger. No organ meat with fillers (e.g., hot dogs, meat balls, corned beef hash, many sausages). Do not eat red meat more than once a day or four times per week.

Fish:

Any fresh or saltwater fish. Lobster (butter allowed after Phase 1), shrimp, crab (no more than twice a week). Do not use breading in preparation. Oysters, clams, scallops and pickled fish are allowed in limited quantities later in the program.

Condiments:

Morton's light salt, in moderation. All natural spices. Mustard in moderation. No catsup, nothing with sugar or M.S.G. Horseradish, apple cider vinegar and vanilla are allowed.

Fats:

Butter (no margarine), cold pressed oils (preferably olive, sesame, sunflower, safflower). Four teaspoons of cream. Homemade mayonnaise.

Beverages:

Only one cup of regular coffee. Unlimited herbal tea. After Phase 1 you are allowed two caffeine-free diet sodas (no more than 2 g. of carbohydrate) per day.

Alcohol:

Not permitted until maintenance. (If you need to lose as little as 10 pounds, this may occur as early as week 3.) After Phase 3, you may drink any alcohol without juice or sugar mixers (e.g., scotch and club soda, vodka on the rocks, rum and diet coke, gin and tonic). Keep in mind that on this diet, one ounce of alcohol equals 15 g. of carbohydrate. If you have more than three drinks you will exceed your critical carbohydrate level. (I recommend red wine.)

Vegetables allowed on Phase 1:

Asparagus	Okra
Avocado	Olives (green or black)
Bamboo shoots	Onions
Bean sprouts	Peppers
Beans (string or waxed)	Pumpkin
Beet greens	Rhubarb
Broccoli	Sauerkraut
Cabbage	Snow pea pods
Cauliflower	Spinach

No-No Foods:

Banana	Cornstarch	Pancakes
Beans	Crackers	Potatoes
Bread (white)	Dates	Raisins
Cake	Figs	Rice spaghetti
Candy	Flour	Sugar
Cashews	Honey	Sweet pickles
Catsup	Ice cream	Sweet relish
Cookies	Jam or jelly	Sweetened anything
Corn	Macaroni	

7. After Phase 1, you are allowed: 1 cup of any cooked green vegetable with dinner; breakfast meat (e.g., turkey bacon, ham, turkey sausage) in moderation; omelets; two fruits daily (but never after 6:00 p.m.). If you are on an intense exercise program, you may add one extra fruit; sugarless jello.

8. **PHASE 2**

   A. If you have not lost weight on Phase 1, repeat it, and remove your one fruit.

   B. If you have lost 3 to 7 pounds and are exercising, you may add a second fruit (I recommend an apple, orange or grapefruit). No fruit juice!

   C. You may add 1/2 cup of cooked vegetables, or one cup if you are athletic. (No more than one cup, total.)

   D. Cheese (4 ounces) is allowed, cheese spreads are not; you may add cottage cheese.

   E. You may add a moderate amount of onion to your salads, but scallions are preferable.

   F. You may have kosher frankfurters and scallops once a week.

   G. You may have one slice of melba toast per day.

9. You must keep a diary of everything you eat and drink.

10. If you experience pain or any other symptoms *see your physician immediately.*

11. You are not allowed starches (e.g., pasta, potatoes). They will react like a sugar on your metabolism.

12. You may exercise as much as you wish after the first four days. It is during this time that your body will begin to break down fat for fuel.

13. **PHASE 3**

   If you've lost 3 to 7 pounds you may proceed to Phase 3. If you have not lost, continue on Phase 2. If you have gained, return to Phase 1.
   Continue on Phase 3 for two weeks after reaching your desired weight.

   A. You may add another 1 1/2 cups of allowed cooked vegetables (total, 2 cups daily if you are athletic).

   B. You may have sugarless, low carbohydrate chocolate pudding. You may use heavy cream to make a whipped cream topping.

   C. You may add one more fruit, or have an extra fruit in place of bread.

   D. You may have 4 ounces of unsalted peanuts.

Group 1*	Group 2**	Group 3***
Pecans	Peanuts	Chestnuts
Walnuts	Almonds	Cashews
Brazil nuts	Pistachios	Macadamia nuts
	Pignolia nuts	

*—Best choice; **—Allowed; ***—Not allowed

E. Oysters, clams, mussels, and pickled fish are allowed in moderation, once a week.

F. You are allowed one more piece of bread (I recommend diet bread) per day. A man on an active schedule is allowed two pieces of bread, containing no more than 6 g. of carbohydrate per slice.

14. If you experience weakness, add more salt and increase your vitamin and mineral intake.

15. Drugs, including amphetamines, diuretics and estrogen, are contraindicated. Do not, however, discontinue prescribed medication without your physician's approval. (Note: this diet will have a diuretic effect.)

16. If you are constipated, take three oat bran capsules with water before each meal. (I recommend 100% natural oat fiber with herbs, containing 533 mg of fiber.) If constipation persists, I recommend a mild natural laxative (senna).

17. **PHASE 4—Maintenance**

    Review Chapter 28, "The Magic of Maintenance." You may continue to add 5 to 10 g. of carbohydrate per week until you gain weight (three pounds is significant), then use the following formula to lose any excess weight:

    Phase 1—3 days; Phase 2—3 days; Phase 3—3 days

    This should put you at the same weight (or less) as when you first commenced on Phase 4. By utilizing this simple formula you will control your metabolism and never be fat again. On maintenance, you will get a more clear idea of your critical carbohydrate level. For example, if you gain weight on Phase 4, this means you should never again exceed 15 to 30 g. of additional carbohydrates (keeping in mind that when you started Phase 4 you were allowed to add 5 to 10 g. Of carbohy drate per week). Assuming you do not gain weight, Phase 4 would look like this:

Week 1—5 to 10 g. of additional carbohydrate
Week 2—10 to 20 g. of additional carbohydrate
Week 3—15 to 30 g. of additional carbohydrate

18. Never move into the next phase of this diet until you are on a "losing streak."

19. This is an effective diet whose principles you can follow for the rest of your life. The average person will lose 5 to 7 pounds the first week of my diet, then an average of 3 pounds per week (the key word here is "average" if you lose one pound one week, and 5 pounds the next, this averages out to 3 pounds per week).

This system and formula will afford you freedom from the fear of ever being fat and fatigued again. By utilizing the super formulas in this book and by following my basic principles of maintenance you will be able to achieve a lifetime of success through weight control. The important thing is not how fast you lose weight on my diet, but how easy it is to stay on it. Even people who cheat don't get discouraged on my diet. They simply return to Phase 1, which is still very liberal. Where else could you find a diet that will allow you turkey bacon and eggs for breakfast, hamburger (no bun) for lunch, steak and scampi with green salad for dinner, and sugarless jello for dessert? All for under 10 g. of carbohydrate. This diet is not only easy, it's effective. Bon appetit, everyone!

The greatest discovery of any generation is that human beings can alter their lives by altering their attitude of mind.
                                                        Albert Schweitzer

27

Dietary Detours

Mountain climbers know that before they reach the peak, they will land on many plateaus. In dieting, there are also plateaus—called unwanted stabilization. This condition causes the body to become stuck at a certain weight, even when the dieter is faithfully following the program. This chapter offers techniques to help you break free from the plateaus and get back on your journey to the top.

The following graph shows a typical weight-loss pattern on my program.

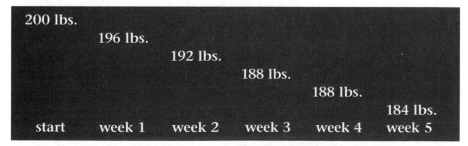

As you can see, the typical dieter loses approximately 3–4 pounds per week, with a total loss of 9–12 pounds after three weeks. But the following week, even though the diet was followed, the body stalled.

This is when you must remind yourself that this is a fat loss diet; you are not losing water and muscle. No proper diet will produce constant weight loss. Although unwanted, stabilization is a normal phase, so don't panic if a day or even a week passes without a change in the reading on your scale.

On the other hand, sometimes stabilization is inadvertently induced and therefore unwarranted. When this occurs, you can take advantage of the weight jolters described here. They will "shock" your metabolism, thus enabling your body to break down fat and remove weight at an accelerated pace.

Do not, however, expect to lose weight at an extremely rapid rate. Rapid weight loss is unhealthy and can make you vulnerable to future problems. It can also be unwise as a long-term strategy, for you may fool yourself into thinking that weight loss is easy, and thus slip back into your old habits—and regain the weight you shed so quickly.

During any diet, the body will go through three stages:

1. Reduction

2. Stabilization

3. Weight gain

All three stages are normal, but patients often become frustrated during the last two. I recommend that you monitor your results, utilizing the "Dow Jones" principle of my program. Watch your weight as you would a stock in which you have invested your life savings. In a way you have, for health is undeniably a more valuable commodity than money, and sometimes harder to come by. After all, you can inherit wealth, but you can only earn health. Another principle I want you to keep in mind is Newton's Law of Gravity: What goes up must come down. This applies to weight as much as it does to apples falling from trees.

Every morning upon awakening, you should step naked onto the scale. More often than not, this will encourage you. But there will come a day when the reading will not budge. If approximately two weeks go by without weight loss, you can then bombard your body with what I call the "Protein-Fruit Blitz." This is one of three ways to stimulate your metabolism. It is generally effective, but if it doesn't work for you, then you can also try:

> ➤ Modified Stillman's zero carbohydrate diet.

> ➤ Increased growth hormone intake in conjunction with Phase 1.

With all of these methods, it is essential that you continue to drink eight glasses of water a day, and keep taking your vitamin supplements. None of these three techniques should be implemented for more than three consecutive days or more often than twice a month. After three days on any of these regimens, return to Phase 1 of the program.

It is also essential that you consult regularly with your physician, and immediately report any adverse side-effects.

The Protein-Fruit Blitz will hyperstimulate your metabolism. It must be followed exactly as it is described here in order to produce results.

Protein-Fruit Blitz
(Apple-Egg-Orange Break)

BREAKFAST
> One medium apple
> One medium orange
> One egg

LUNCH
> One medium apple
> One medium orange
> One egg

DINNER
> One medium apple
> One medium orange
> One egg

If you are unsatisfied with the results of this method, you may try one of the other two techniques:

Modified Stillman Diet

BREAKFAST
> One egg

LUNCH
> 6-8 oz. protein (preferably chicken or fish)

DINNER
> 6-8 oz. protein raw green salad

(Another variation on this theme is the Protein Sparing Modified Fast, described in *Super Energy Diet*. The developer of this program, Dr. George Brackburn of the Massachusetts Institute of Technology, notes that while fasting—no food at all—is a very effective weight-loss method, a prolonged fast can lead to the loss of protein and essential body tissue. By adding 400 to 600 calories of lean protein, the nitrogen balance of the body is maintained, and there is no net loss of protein. Dr. Brackburn's diet consists of beverages and 6 to 8 ounces of lean meat, fish, or fowl a day, and virtually nothing else. I personally feel that the Modified Stillman Diet is safer and more effective.)

GROWTH HORMONES/PHASE 1

Follow Phase 1 of the diet or the Modified Stillman Diet and increase your growth hormones (arginine, ornithine) to 2 g. every four (waking) hours. (An increase in growth hormones alone may give your body the boost it needs; try doubling the dosage; instead of taking 1,000 mg of arginine/ornithine, take 2,000 mg.)

In rare instances, none of these techniques work for the patient. This may indicate that the person is suffering from a metabolic problem. I want to emphasize that this is the exception and not the rule. But if after giving these methods an honest try you are still unable to lose weight, consult a physician; it is possible that you have a thyroid problem. Please don't despair if this is the case; it's only a roadblock, not the end of the road.

"Dr. Irving Perlstein in Louisville, found that approximately 15% of the seriously overweight produced antibodies to their own thyroid hormone. When he gave them large doses of synthetic thyroid, the antibodies were neutralized so the patients could achieve a normal weight loss when placed on a high protein, low carbohydrate, low fat, frequent small feeding diet."[1]

If you've gotten this far on the diet, I know that you are now a believer, a member of the "I Feel Great Club." Don't allow what appears to be a setback set you back. Weight loss takes time, patience and perseverance. And even when it seems that "nothing is happening," you may be sure that important changes are taking place. This principle is beautifully illustrated in an anecdote by Joel Weldon featured in Dave Dean's book, *Now Is Your Time To Win.*

"The Chinese Bamboo Tree is a remarkable tree. The Chinese plant the seed for the tree, water it, fertilize it, but the first year nothing happens. Then the second year they continue watering and fertilizing it, but still nothing. The third year nothing. The fourth year they continue to water and fertilize it, with no evident results. Then during the fifth year, in six weeks the Chinese Bamboo

Tree grows 90 feet. But it grows 90 feet in just those six weeks. If during any of those six years they hadn't watered or fertilized the seed daily, there would have been no Chinese Bamboo Tree."

Don't be deceived by appearances—something *is* happening as long as you stay on the diet. Just continue to follow the principles, and remember—Now Is Your Time To Be Thin.

One of the common denominators in people with bad health habits—whether it is lack of exercise, smoking, drinking, or overeating—is that they are always looking for a detour and/or escape route from a new, healthy lifestyle. They hunt for reasons to return to their old ways, and in some cases manage to find them. Discouragement is a major pitfall in any diet, as the following story by A.L. Williams indicates:

It seems that one day the devil was going out of business, and he decided to sell all his tools to whomever would pay the price. On the night of the sale they were all attractively displayed. Malice, Hate, Envy, Jealousy, Greed, Sensuality and Deceit were among them. To the side, though, lay a harmless wedge shaped tool, which had been used more than the rest.

Someone asked the devil, "What's that? It's priced so high."

The devil answered, "That's Discouragement."

"But why is it priced so much higher than the rest?" The onlooker persisted.

"Because," replied the devil, "with that tool I can pry open and get inside a person's consciousness when I couldn't get near with any of the others. Once discouragement gets inside, I can let all the other tools do their work."

We probably confront some form of discouragement every day. How we handle this emotion determines whether we succeed or fail in reaching our goals. Discouragement is only a pit stop—it's not the pits unless you allow it to be.

Fatigue is sometimes a factor in weight-loss programs, and like stabilization, it can lure the dieter back to old habits. Before you go running for a candy bar to "boost" your energy, consider some possible causes of this problem.

Low intake of sodium or potassium can leave you feeling tired, so you might add some salt and consume at least one extra orange per day.

You must also be vigilant about hidden sources of sugar and refined carbohydrates—they tend to lurk where you least expect them. For example, many vitamins have sugar coating or a sugar filler. I learned this the hard way when I purchased chewable vitamin C tablets for our children from a company that supposedly dealt only in natural products.

Our children loved these vitamins; it was like dessert time when when we took out the bottle. They loved the vitamins so much that I put on my Sherlock Holmes hat and investigated the bottle. Sure enough, sugar was utilized as a filler. Even I, a physician and educated consumer, assumed that my vitamin company was selling me a 100% natural product.

Sugar can also be hidden in cough syrup, lozenges, chewing gum, mints, salad dressings, cole slaw, sweet pickle relish, tuna fish, tartar sauce, and a number of other foods you would be unlikely to suspect. So be sure to read labels carefully.

Like sugar, carbohydrates can cause you to feel tired. I have found that a decrease in carbohydrate intake will enable you to obtain more fuel from free fatty acids and ketone bodies, thus increasing your energy level.

If your energy level is low, I recommend that you return to Phase 1, consuming only protein and raw green salads.

Another substance that can cause fatigue is caffeine. As I noted earlier, caffeine is a highly addictive substance, and abrupt withdrawal can cause symptoms such as nervousness, insomnia, and headaches. This is why I recommend that you remove caffeine from your diet gradually.

Increasing your vitamin intake may help you to combat fatigue. Normally, you would be taking two or three multivitamins per day, but if you feel fatigued it might be advisable to double your intake. I have found folic acid to be a highly effective energy restorative.

"Doctors at the Fitsimmons Army Hospital discovered that there are patients who are hypoglycemic but who do worse on a low carbohydrate diet because of the specific enzyme called fructose 1, 6 diphosphatase, is deficient. They discovered that could be treated effectively with the vitamin folic acid in doses of 15 mg daily."[2]

It is amazing how people will rationalize cheating on a diet. They convince themselves that a little of this or a little of that won't hurt. The fact is though, that as little as 10 g. of carbohydrate can inhibit ketosis, fat mobilization, and weight loss. While this small amount of carbohydrate may not cause you to gain weight, it can keep you from losing. On this program, carbohydrates will be reintroduced into your diet at the right time—i.e., when you have lost the appropriate amount of weight.

While most people are aware that too much food will halt weight loss, few realize that too little can have the same effect. Don't skip meals in an attempt to hasten the process. If you do not provide your body with adequate proteins or fats, it will not be able to work to its potential. The metabolism becomes sluggish, and the result is stabilization. If you want to keep a fire hot, you must feed it. The same is true of your metabolism; we want to heat it up so it can melt down fat. Skipping a meal can also lead to overindulgence at the next meal, which leads to digestive overload—a major cause of sluggish metabolism.

I recommend that you eat six small meals or snacks per day. This provides a constant source of energy and prevents insulin rebound. Laboratory experiments have shown that animals fed large meals rather than frequent snacks gain more weight and have an increased production of blood lipids.

The same is true for humans.

"Dr. Paul Fabry of the Institute for Clinical and Experimental Medicine, in Prague, found in both children and adults that far apart meals, especially huge dinners, led to weight gain, raised cholesterol levels, decreased glucose tolerance, and even increased the rate of heart disease."[3]

My rule of thumb for dieters who are stuck in any way is: *Return to Phase 1.*

This is the metabolic switch, which we turn on simply by eliminating carbohydrates from our diet. But, because each person is unique, it may take some experimentation to determine your critical carbohydrate level. Your best guides are ketostix and common sense.

For example, during week 1, if you find yourself overly fatigued, you might first try introducing more salt into your diet. If this doesn't work, you can increase your fruit intake to three per day and increase your vitamin intake. Add 15 mg of folic acid two times a day. If after three days your energy level is up and your weight is down, you may introduce 1/2 cup of cooked green vegetables into your diet. Cooked vegetables are a form of complex carbohydrates that do not generally interfere with weight loss. However, any increase in fruits or vegetables may lead to stabilization. So once your energy is restored, and if stabilization occurs, try gradually reducing your fruits and/or cooked vegetables.

You must watch what you drink as well as what you eat. If your diet or exercise program depletes certain nutrients, such as salt and potassium, sugary beverages are not the answer. I am dismayed by the number of athletes who consume Gatorade. This beverage contains nothing but water, sucrose (refined sugar), glucose (more refined sugar), salt, sodium citrate (more salt), and yellow dyes 5 and 6. The label states—in small print, to be sure—"Contains no fruit juice." Extra salt and a potassium supplement are the answer, not this imitation fruit drink.

And speaking of exercise, one of the best ways to get past unwanted stabilization is to increase your activity level. Exercise wakes up sluggish hormones and stabilizes your blood sugar. It also puts an extra demand for fuel on the body, and stored fat, as we know, can be converted into energy.

You may be surprised to learn that cigarette smoking has been linked to slower rates of weight loss. In many cases, smoking interferes with the correction of hypoglycemia. Naturally, I'm not in favor of smoking in any case. However, it can be especially harmful for dieters since it plays havoc with their blood sugar and metabolism. Quitting smoking will help balance the blood sugar, thus you will not continually crave food. If you can quit, by all means do so. If you cannot, at least cut down on your cigarettes.

Modern medicine offers numerous methods to quit smoking, from group therapy to the FDA-approved nicotine gum and patch, which is available by prescription and helps eliminate the nicotine craving under a physician's guidance.

The sole purpose of this book is to plant seeds that you will one day harvest as crops of improved health and well-being. I want to help you understand that certain indiscretions can affect and/or cause weight stabilization.

Alcohol can cause weight stabilization by stimulating insulin production. As I mentioned, although alcohol contains only a trace of carbohydrate, to your body each ounce of liquor represents 15 g. of carbohydrate. (Other high-carbohydrate beverages, even if they are "diet" drinks, will also stimulate insulin production.) This is why no alcohol is permitted during the early phases of this diet. If you slip up and have a few drinks and discover a few extra pounds, return to Phase 1. It's like a game of Monopoly—if you're "bad" you go to jail. But in Phase 1 you can eat steak and scampi, which is hardly prison cuisine.

Drugs and Dieting

Drugs are a major factor in weight stabilization. Many medications can induce hypoglycemia, and thus interfere with weight loss. If you are taking prescription medication, it is imperative that you review this diet with your physician. Hormones, amphetamines, diuretics, antihistamines, anti-inflammatory drugs, antidepressants, analgesics, anticoagulants, antibiotics, and tranquilizers are but a few of the drugs that may lead to stabilization.

Watch out for over-the-counter drugs, too. Even good old aspirin can interfere with weight loss. And, if possible, cut out drugs containing caffeine, which stimulates insulin production. Excedrin, a very popular form of aspirin, is one non-prescription drug that is high in caffeine.

Many people who carry extra pounds do so in the form of what we call water weight. I know that many of my female patients take diuretics during their menstrual cycle to reduce the puffiness or edema that occurs at this time. In addition, many people take diuretics to reduce high blood pressure.

Because of the large amounts of water we drink on this diet, diuretics are one form of medication that should never be taken on this diet. Keep in mind that this diet, especially during the first few weeks, is a potent diuretic on its own. The combination of a diuretic and the diet will cause too much water loss at too rapid a pace, and deplete your body of potassium, sodium, and calcium. This can result in such symptoms as exhaustion, cramps, and muscular weakness.

Should you experience these symptoms, discontinue the diet and contact your physician. (I am confident, however, that if you follow the guidelines, you won't develop any problems.)

I usually recommend to my patients that they discontinue the use of diuretics for a minimum of one week before even beginning the diet. *Do not discontinue any medication without the approval of your physician.* While I am not an advocate of drug therapy, I am aware that certain conditions do require medication. If you are not comfortable with the type of treatment offered by your doctor, and wish to explore more natural avenues of health care, then I suggest that you consult a chiropractor, osteopath, or medical doctor/nutritionist.

You must also avoid diet pills while on this program. The purpose of these drugs is appetite suppression, and you will find that carbohydrate restriction alone will take care of this. While diet pills will enable you to reduce your intake of calories, and thus lose weight, they can boomerang very badly. When you discontinue the drugs, your body will attempt to readjust. In the process, hunger will increase, and a series of biological changes will occur. This can lead to weight gain despite dieting. Diet pills are a crutch. My goal is to help you lose weight and keep it off without reliance on artificial support.

Another drug that you must watch carefully is estrogen. This hormone, which is taken by many women to reduce the symptoms of menopause and is an ingredient in many birth control pills, has been linked with numerous disorders.

Not only is it associated with breast and other cancers, it can greatly magnify insulin problems. Estrogen increases insulin production, causing the patient to become more sugar intolerant. As a result, the dieter may experience weight stabilization.

There are numerous types of oral contraceptives which do not contain estrogen. I am not in favor of birth control pills—I believe any medication that causes hormonal interruption or confusion can lead to an assortment of health problems down the road. As for menopause symptoms, my experience with patients undergoing this change is that high doses of vitamins C and E make an excellent substitute for estrogen.

Anti-depressants and tranquilizers will often produce hyperinsulism. I have found that patients who use lithium or Prozac are prone to weight gain.

One drug that is especially hazardous is valium. I recommend anyone taking this popular tranquilizer read Barbara Gordon's best-selling book, *I'm Dancing As Fast As I Can.* Since the publication of this story of addiction, valium sales have dropped 40%. I find it especially ironic that people take this drug to "feel better."

"Valium was the number one all time best selling drug which carries as its indications tension, anxiety, fatigue, depressive symptoms, acute agitation, trauma, hallucinosis, skeletal muscle spasm specicity. Its side effects include fatigue, depression, confusion, trauma, hyperexcited states, anxiety, hallucinations and increased muscle specicity."[4]

There doesn't seem to be much difference between the problems and the solution.

It is my recommendation that you discuss all medications you are taking with your physician, and explain your desire to lose weight. I have never found a drug that could cure a problem. Drugs can only mask and/or alter symptoms.

The United States probably spends more money on health care than any other country; if health could be bottled we would be the healthiest nation in the world. But will all the advances in modern medicine, life expectancy has not significantly increased over the last 40 years. Most medical problems can be helped without medical intervention. We turn to modern medicine to keep us healthy, but the facts indicate we may be looking in the wrong direction.

"In recent years much has been made over doctor strikes, doctors who have striked throughout the country because of the increased prices of malpractice insurance. But one of the things that has been found throughout the world is that when doctors strike, the mortality rates drop. The first strike was in Saskatchewan, Canada, in the late '60s. The second was in Los Angeles where, according to Professor Milton Roemer of UCLA Schools of Public Health, 'the mortality rate during the strike dropped by 17%. The third strike was in Colombia, South America, where the mortality rate dropped by 37%. The fourth was in Israel. During an 85-day strike the mortality dropped by 50%."

These statistics came to the attention of morticians. "So the morticians did a study of their own and they discovered the last time the mortality rate dropped that low was 20 years previously at the time of the last doctor's strike."[5]

I am not implying that I am opposed to doctors or hospitals. But the fact is, today's doctors are becoming more like business people and today's hospitals are big business. What we need is more education and less economics.

For example, many of my patients have high blood pressure, yet continue to consume large amounts of salt and sodium. We have found that by removing these dietary irritants, blood pressure can often be controlled naturally.

Another instance of natural health care is provided by the Pritikin Program, which has proven especially beneficial for heart disease patients. The Pritikin Program is an excellent regimen, consisting of proper diet, exercise, and health education. The Pritikin diet emphasizes extensive intake of complex carbohydrates and limited protein and fats. You may wonder how I can advocate a diet that seems almost the opposite of the one I have designed. The answer is that complex carbohydrates, such as those found in fruits, vegetables, and whole grains, are not the cause of obesity in America. The villains are refined carbohydrates and sugars. While I maintain that it is not a good idea to combine proteins and carbohydrates, the Pritikin Program is nonetheless a beneficial one. Because it is a bland diet, it is difficult to live your entire life by its rules, but it is an excellent rehabilitative program for people who have abused their bodies.

My diet will also increase the body's resistance to disease. A perfect example is provided by my patient John K., an executive who came to me with a cholesterol level of 240. After following my program, his cholesterol dropped to 196.

There was a two-week period in which John's weight stabilized. He became frustrated and began to cheat. Then his weight was no longer stable—his "Dow Jones" was going up. However, John was able to turn his stabilization phase into a growth phase. We worked on his attitude, put him back on Phase 1 and he began to lose weight again. Eventually, stabilization set in once more, but this time he was ready for it. He kept to the diet and, over the next four weeks, lost 12 more pounds. John was happy, and feeling healthier than ever.

John was not deprived at any point on the diet. My program is designed to allow you to maintain a normal and healthy lifestyle while you lose. It has been over four years since I lost my weight, and I continue to dine well at the finest restaurants. We recently went on a cruise with two of our closest friends, Billy and Denise M. These two people are extremely stimulating and intelligent, and Billy especially expects any statement to be backed up by evidence. Yet these extremely bright people were most bewildered by the way I ate during the seven day Caribbean cruise. Or rather, bewildered by the fact that I would routinely eat two entrees per meal yet gained no weight. The secret, of course, was that I consumed no desserts, bread, or other refined carbohydrates, but ate protein, fruits, and vegetables instead.

Perhaps the most important aspect of my diet is that it allows you to control your metabolism and not vice versa. When you use the Dow Jones principle of weight control, you are president of the corporation known as your body. Try to look at stabilization as one of the inevitable fluctuations of the market, but one which you can control. (Later, we will discuss maintenance, which is in effect a desirable form of stabilization—stabilization at your ideal weight.) By monitoring the changes in your body, you can learn to determine when it's time to unload some stock, i.e., make some changes in your routine.

As you become more familiar with your body, you will learn to recognize the conditions that lead to weight stabilization. Some of them may surprise you. For example, did you realize that stress can affect your weight? Stressful situations can create an imbalance in the body. Not only can hypoglycemia cause stress, stress can cause hypoglycemia, and we've learned that this condition can interfere with weight loss. On the next page are listed some potential stress triggers, along with some useful antidotes.

Stress Triggers	**Stress Inhibitors**
1. Caffeine	1. Chiropractic Care
2. Sugar	2. Proper Diet
3. Tobacco	3. Exercise
4. Refined Carbohydrates	4. Positive Mental Attitude

Stress Triggers	Stress Inhibitors
5. Salt	5. Meditation
6. Overeating	6. Massage
7. Alcohol	7. Breathing
8. Medication	8. Sleep
(Tranquilizers)	9. Aromatherapy
	10. Kava Kava/Valerian Root

There's no doubt that stress can sabotage a diet and health program. If you wander from the path and cheat, don't get down on yourself! Just start all over again with Phase 1. The removal of carbohydrates will provide you with the metabolic regulation and blood sugar control you need during this stressful period.

I should note that depression is a form of stress, and that it can often lead to fatigue. If your emotional problems seem overwhelming, don't hesitate to seek professional help.

Fortunately, we take a more enlightened view of psychotherapy these days. Professional counseling can help you take charge of your health, your body, and your life. A line from a Dave Mason song tells us that, "The world is at your fingertips, no one can make it better than you." It is essential for you to understand that you control your destiny.

A perfect example is Gary Carter who endured numerous surgeries on his knees. Instead of giving up, he got up, and worked harder. No wonder Gary was an 11-time, all-star catcher. A remarkable statistic for one of sports most physically demanding positions. The principle of success comes not from looking back, but ahead.

Vince Lombardi and Mike Ditka, two of the greatest motivators of all time, understood this success principle well. Their philosophy was that an all-pro athlete is someone who understands that it is necessary to prove oneself every day. Their definition of an old-pro: an all-pro who rests on his laurels rather than continue to prove himself.

This is true not only in sports, but in life. A man spends many years of his life courting a woman to be his wife and then upon his marriage he forgets the principles that made this woman fall in love, and vice versa. We must not only court our spouses, but "court" our health if we are to maintain it. Look back on your life and honestly consider the dreams, aspirations, and ideals you left behind. Try to recapture the youthful motivation and spirit that is necessary to follow this program, for it is more than a diet, it is a way of life.

Diets are by their nature temporary. Consider talk show hostess Oprah Winfrey, who lost so much weight on a liquid protein diet. But what happened when she was suddenly confronted with real food? She provided the answer when she publicly attributed her weight gain to the liquid diet which she used to shed pounds. She explained that when she began eating solid food again, her body was not capable of properly breaking down and digesting it. An article in *USA Today* discussed this dilemma.

"John Madden, famous sportscaster says he trimmed 55 pounds on a two-month, doctor-supervised liquid protein diet. And word is NBC 'Today Show' host Bryant Gumbel and New York Mayor Ed Koch shed extra pounds on similar diets. Experts say the advantage to such a program is dieters can lose a lot of weight quickly. But keeping weight off is uncertain."[6]

Protein drinks are utilized by my patients as an occasional supplement, not as a total diet program. Although my powder is supplemented with vitamins, fiber, and protein, I don't expect it to be used indefinitely as a food substitute. I find that in general, it is far more satisfying to eat your meals than to drink them.

Good health is not to be taken lightly, but laughter can improve your physical as well as emotional state. "Good humor is an integral part of wellness and health," says Vera Robinson, a professor of Nursing at California State University, "This is being taught more and more at universities."[7]

Dr. William Fry, a psychiatrist at Stanford Medical School, says that laughing 100 to 200 times a day is good exercise—equivalent to about ten minutes of rowing. As he explains it, "And here's what happens when you're breaking up over Letterman's stupid pet tricks: heart, lungs, torso and back get a short workout."

When you laugh, catecholamines—hormones that speed blood flow and accelerate healing—are released. If you laugh very forcefully, the muscles in your legs and arms are also stimulated. After you've finished chuckling, your heart rate, blood pressure, and muscular tension will subside, leaving you feeling relaxed. As Dr. Fry says,

"Having a humorous attitude is beneficial in its negative stress producing emotions such as anger, fear, and depression. These are linked to a variety of illnesses which also make illnesses last longer, and laughter . . . may also help reduce heart disease risk and high blood pressure."

Dr. Martin Seligman, at the University of Pennsylvania, found that pessimistic thinking impairs health and job performance. A study of 1,100 Metropolitan Life Insurance salesmen revealed that optimists outsold pessimists by 20%. Dr. Seligman says, "If you begin removing negative thoughts, it should ease the depression, raise achievement in the work place and increase physical health."

When you reach that plateau called stabilization, laugh at it—laugh at it hard. Give your body the benefit of those healthy natural stimulants. Your improved attitude will help you bypass the detour of stabilization and put you back on the road to reduction.

*You, the individual, can do more for your own health and well being
than any doctor, any hospital, any drug, any exotic medical service.*
Joseph Califano,
Former U.S. Secretary of Health,
Education and Welfare

28

The Magic of Maintenance

Congratulations! If you have reached this phase in the program I
am certain that you look and feel better than you ever did before. In
fact, you may be doing so well that a nagging voice is telling you it
can't last. Don't listen to it. One of the ways in which my program
differs from others is that weight loss and other benefits can be
permanent.

The term maintenance is self-explanatory. You will maintain your
new look and your new lifestyle. Evaluation is an essential element in
this process. Continue to keep a food diary. Watch the scale faithfully,
because constant monitoring will prevent those extra pounds from
sneaking up on you. And listen to what your body tells you. Your body
communicates with you via symptoms. If you experience fatigue,
depression, or a ferocious appetite, beware! You are probably over your
carbohydrate limit.

During maintenance, you can begin to add many of the foods that
have been restricted while you were in the weight loss phases. This must
be done slowly and cautiously, however. I recommend that you take it
one week at a time, taking care not to overload your metabolism. The
two pounds that you gain will be four pounds before you know it, and
eight pounds more quickly than you suspect.

Once more, the Dow Jones principle applies. You must monitor and graph your weight, and modify your diet accordingly. If your weight goes up, you are no longer maintaining, you are gaining. At this point, you should return to Phase 1 until you are back to your desired weight.

It is possible to gain two to three pounds simply from excess salt consumption, which can lead to water retention. This is not a signal to cut back on water consumption; you must continue to drink eight, eight ounce glasses of water during maintenance. It has been proven that one of the best ways to overcome the problem of water retention is to give your body what it needs, which is more water. Your body will not continue to store water if you provide it in abundance. By drinking large quantities of water, you will enable your body to release the water it has stored.

Salt, on the other hand, can only be tolerated in small quantities. The more salt you eat, the more water your system retains. If you must use salt, buy "Morton's Light Salt." And don't forget that salt, usually called sodium, is hidden in many foods, including packaged meats, ham, bacon, diet sodas and even some drinking water. You can sometimes get back to your ideal weight simply by reducing your intake of salt. Other factors that can lead to fluid retention are alcohol consumption and sunburn.

Excess carbohydrate consumption is a primary cause of weight gain. I hope that by now you realize that you are probably allergic and addicted to carbohydrates—most overweight people are. Some people find it difficult to understand this concept, because carbohydrates are "natural." Well, tobacco and opium are also "natural" and both are also highly addictive. While reducing, 40 g. or less is the average recommended carbohydrate allotment. During maintenance, 40 to 60 g. of carbohydrate is usually acceptable. But this will vary from person to person. And carbohydrates, like salt, can be hidden. Even those convenient pink packets of artificial sweetener may contain up to 10 g. of carbohydrates, so read labels carefully.

If you decide to continue using alcohol and caffeine, do so only in moderation, and don't expect your results to be as significant. As I have explained, one ounce of alcohol equals 15 g. of carbohydrate on this diet. Also, excess alcohol can induce a vitamin deficiency, and like sugar—which is how it reacts in your body—alcohol can aggravate hypoglycemia.

Attitude is also extremely important in maintenance. Weight Watchers uses the expression "Kissing the mirror" to describe the self-admiration of newly thin people. While I certainly appreciate the advantages of self-esteem, it is important not to give way to complacency. You can't afford to get careless once you have reached your goal. Maintenance is like cruise control—even though the rate of speed is on automatic, you can't take your hands from the wheel or your eyes from the road.

This is why you must proceed with care when reintroducing certain foods into your diet. You will be allowed more fresh fruit and grains, and even certain starches, such as potatoes. Maintenance is the phase of the diet in which you can begin to add whole grains back into your diet. Add nutritious foods such as buckwheat, oatmeal, lentils, wild and brown rice, and maize (in moderation).

I suggest, however, that you continue to avoid beans and white rice. You are allowed bread; I recommend the natural grain light variety. I am not concerned with calories, since a slice of bread contains only about 40 of these units. Carbohydrate content is what you must consider, and most light wheat breads contain only 6 g. per slice. You may have two slices of this type of bread and still have a generous carbohydrate allotment left.

Small, frequent meals are recommended on maintenance, as this will enable you to keep your blood sugar level under control. Also, continue to have a protein entree at least two times a day. Fresh food is always your best choice. If this is not available, frozen foods are better than canned foods, which often contain extra sugar and/or salt. If you must eat canned foods, always drain and wash them prior to serving, and select a brand with no added sugar or fats.

Most people enjoy the maintenance phase because they are allowed so many of their favorite foods, such as popcorn and pasta. You are allowed these foods in moderation, provided you combine them properly. For example, do not combine proteins with carbohydrates or starches. If you want pasta, mix it with another carbohydrate—e.g., assorted vegetables. Pasta primavera is allowed, spaghetti and meatballs is not. I realize that you will occasionally disregard this rule. That's understandable. Just don't make a habit of it or you will experience fatigue, weight gain and other problems.

One rule I do feel it is important to adhere to is the one that applies to fruit: Fruit must always be eaten by itself—and never after 6:00 p.m.

Having learned first-hand the benefits of this diet, you will undoubtedly be encouraged to keep up the good work—to exercise, keep taking your vitamin supplements, refrain from overeating and avoid sugar and refined carbohydrates. Still, old habits die hard—which is why it's so important for you to keep a food diary and monitor your weight.

I am not unrealistic, and I know that you will sneak in a favorite dessert here and there. In fact, let's be honest—you may cheat your socks off. Don't berate yourself and don't panic. Now you know how to flick on your metabolic switch. Just go back to Phase 1 and let the fat fighters go to work.

By the way, a weight gain of three pounds or less is not necessarily cause for concern—a certain amount of fluctuation is to be expected. But if you exceed a five pound gain, or you don't feel quite up to par, then an alarm should go off, and it is time to go back to Phase 1 and/or utilize one of the metabolic triggers discussed in Chapter 27.

Maintenance, even more so than the other phases of the diet, allows you to give full reign to your creativity. Feel free to dine on steak and scampi, veal parmigiana (no breading), veal and peppers, sausage and peppers. Enjoy fruits and salads. Snack on peanuts, almonds and other nuts (except cashews) instead of pretzels and potato chips.

If your sweet tooth acts up, satisfy it with a sugar-free dessert. Eskimo Pie and Klondike both recently introduced sugarless ice cream bars that contain only 11 g. of carbohydrate. They taste great so enjoy them. Most frozen yogurt chains also now offer sugar-free yogurt that has only 3 g. of carbohydrate per ounce. Indulge yourself with sugarless chocolate pudding and sugar-free jello. Visit a chocolate shop—you'll be amazed at the variety of sugarless candy they offer these days. As you know, I am not an advocate of artificial sweeteners, but at least they are not addicting like sugar.

I should make it very clear that sugar is one substance that is not to be reintroduced on this program, even during maintenance. Sugar is addictive, and will lead you straight down the path to weight gain.

Ex-alcoholics, smokers, and drug addicts understand the principle behind abstinence very well. Sugarholics are no different.

The reason this diet makes you feel better is that it corrects your sugar and carbohydrate intolerance, and creates a balance within your body. But sugar will tip the balance and produce an adverse metabolic effect. One decadent dessert can set you back two days. When you eat sugar, you turn your metabolic switch off. Your pancreas will release a long-stored flood of insulin, and you will find yourself restless, exhausted, irritable, depressed—and very possibly several pounds heavier.

Even natural sources of sugar must be approached with caution, if at all. A single eight ounce glass of apple juice contains a whopping 20 g. of carbohydrate. If you want to taste an apple, eat one. If you are thirsty, drink water. Fruit juices are an extremely concentrated form of sugar. I have found that while most sugar or carbohydrate intolerant people can handle small amounts of fruit, they cannot handle fruit juice.

The beauty of this program is that it includes a built-in reward/punishment system. When you remove sugars and refined carbohydrates from your diet, you are rewarded with weight loss (or maintenance), health, and energy. Conversely, reintroducing these substances will lead to punishment in the form of weight gain, fatigue, and health problems. If you are dragging, your regimen is sagging. If you put on weight, don't throw away the program. Remind yourself that weight gain and energy loss are proportionate to carbohydrate intake. Your scale and your state of well-being will let you know when you have overdone it. And if you have gained weight because you have exceeded your carbohydrate level, then you can lose it by reducing your carbohydrate level. It's that simple.

One way to ensure that you don't overindulge is to eat more slowly. I recommend three methods to encourage this habit:

1. Chew your food well. You can't enjoy what you eat if you are practically swallowing it whole. You will find eating much more enjoyable if you allow yourself to experience the subtle tastes in each mouthful. Never take a mouthful of food if you already have food in your mouth. Chew and swallow what is there before going on to the next bite.

2. Take smaller bites. Research has demonstrated that overweight people seem to take larger mouthfuls of food than their thin counterparts. You may not even be aware of the size of your bites, so make it a point to watch how much you put on your fork.

3. Follow the example of thin people; watch their habits and try to imitate them. People who are thin generally have better eating habits than those who are not.

Earlier I encouraged you to "Plan your life and live your plan." This advice is especially relevant for dieters. If you don't prepare to eat as you should, you can be sure that you will soon be eating as you shouldn't. Stock your home with a generous supply of allowable foods. Bring nuts, cheese, and fruit to the office so that you can resist the doughnuts that someone always brings. Be sure to eat protein three or four times a day. And never skip a meal, especially breakfast.

This important meal is unpopular with some people. They oversleep, so breakfast is sacrificed. These missed meals will cause weight gain eventually. Breakfast is your metabolism's wake-up call. If you skip breakfast, you'll be so hungry by lunch that you'll probably eat twice as much, thus overloading your metabolism and making it sluggish. Some of my patients tell me, "I'm not hungry in the morning." My reply to this is, "That's good." What could be better than a dieter without an appetite? You needn't eat a big breakfast; some fresh fruit, a slice of cheese or a natural (no sugar) bran muffin will do. Many of my patients use my vitamin and fiber enriched protein drink as a meal supplement. Although it's effective and nutritious, I don't recommend using it for more than two meals a day, simply because I don't believe that protein formulas should totally replace food. But it makes a fast, easy and nutritious breakfast.

The secret to maintenance is moderation, not starvation. You can eat three to six satisfying meals a day while keeping your energy level up and your weight down. I have not only kept my weight off, my caloric intake is *double* what it was when I was 35 pounds heavier. My wife and friends are amazed at the quantity and quality of my food intake. And

I am far from being a lone success story—my patients are thrilled with their results. The following letters are typical of many others.

"This letter is my expression of thanks for your help in 'reshaping' my life. Being a professional dieter and having tried many diets, in vain, I began your program with a defeatist attitude and was pleasantly surprised. At the end of six weeks, I was nineteen pounds lighter and, most importantly, the experience has been an enjoyable one. I never suffered hunger pangs or ate foods I didn't like. What is more significant is the fact that I could stop taking medication for an acid stomach."

"The diet lends itself to eating out very comfortably, and, as a working, single lady that is important to me. Any restaurant serves 'allowable' entrees and fresh vegetables. Thanks again for you efforts on behalf of your patients."

"I have used Dr. Kaplan's High Energy Weight Loss Diet for over three years and have found it to be the best of all the quick weight loss diets. Lost over 18 pounds in less than one month's time while maintaining a high energy level that enabled me to exercise daily and feel great while losing weight."

"I personally recommend this diet for anyone wanting to lose weight quickly."

I encourage my patients to eat the foods they enjoy. You want ice cream no problem, there are many sugar-free ice creams (do watch your intake of dairy products, though); you want veal parmigiana—no problem, just leave off the breading or use melba toast instead of bread crumbs; you want popcorn—no problem, just go easy on the butter and the salt.

This program is quite simply, "no problem." You can control your metabolic Dow Jones and the rest of your life. You can have a life that is abundant in everything except excess weight.

Maintenance Summary

1. Drink 8, 8 oz. glasses of water a day.

2. Never skip a meal.

3. Eliminate sugar.

4. Monitor your weight daily.

5. Practice moderation.

6. Never let yourself exceed your ideal weight by more than 5 pounds.

7. If you do gain more than 5 pounds, return to Phase 1.

8. Avoid fruits or refined carbohydrates (bread, pasta, etc.) after 6:00 p.m. (Eat them early in the day so your body has ample time to digest them.)

9. Take your vitamins.

10. Continue to exercise.

11. Avoid caffeine.

12. Limit your alcohol intake.

13. Avoid salt and salty products.

14. Don't exceed 60 g. of carbohydrate per day.

15. Don't exceed 60 g. of fat per day.

16. *Remember that you are in control.*

Maintenance is fun, it's easy. There are no secrets to success, just success formulas and principles. Apply them and you will succeed. Let these principles support you—trust them. Let your energy levels, attitude, health, and waistline by your guides. Let these principles be your instruments, for when you combine the guide with the instruments, success will be inevitable and eternal.

It is not the critic who counts; not the man who points out how the strong man stumbled or where the doer of deeds could have done better. The credit belongs to the man who is actually in the arena; whose face is marred by sweat and dust and blood; who strives valiantly; who errs and comes short again and again, who knows the great enthusiasms, the great devotions, and spends himself in a worthy cause; who at best, knows the triumph of high achievement; and who, at the worst, if he fails, at least fails while daring greatly so that his place shall never be with those cold and timid souls who knew neither victory nor defeat.

Theodore Roosevelt

29

Desired Destiny

Thank you for traveling this far with me. The journey is far from over, for it will continue for the rest of your life. But those of you who have read this far have already succeeded. You have learned that the secret to perseverance is to persevere. That success is achieved only by those who try. That the doers of this world—who time and again have put their lives on the line for what they believe—are truly the most successful.

Be a doer. Understand that you must persist. Persist in your quest for persistence; persevere in your quest for perseverance. You can train yourself to become persistent by implementing the following steps: acquire a definite purpose; create the motivation to surmount difficulties; cultivate self-reliance by knowing that you can plan your life and live your plan. You can develop specific success goals through the acquisition of knowledge and the observation of other successful people.

All your endeavors can lead to the acquisition of cooperation, patience, understanding, and discipline. You can accomplish all of this by focusing on your goals and persisting until you have attained them.

Now is the time to practice what you've learned:

Use your affirmations

Make them a daily part of your life, of yourself. You are what you tell yourself you are, so it makes sense to ensure that your self-talk is positive and dynamic. If you tell yourself that you are overweight and unsuccessful, your subconscious will obligingly help you remain in that state. Conversely, if you declare that you are thin, healthy, happy, and successful, your inner self will help you to make these statements a reality.

Take charge of your life

You can either run your life or get run over by it. Yes, it takes effort to persist against obstacles, but it is ultimately more of a struggle to be buried by them. The "Shoulda, Woulda, Coulda Club" has plenty of members, but it's really a lonely organization.

Take risks

Go for it! Tell your friends, family, and neighbors that you are on a diet and you are going to lose weight and keep it off. Once you've informed others that you plan to succeed, it is impossible to quietly retreat. You'll leave yourself with no choice but to forge ahead. Reach out for goals that have seemed beyond your grasp, and don't listen to people who tell you that your dreams are too big. Small dreams produce small results.

Eliminate the word "failure"

If you treat "failure" as a steppingstone to ultimate success, you will lose your fear of temporary setbacks. To a person determined to win, there are no permanent reversals of fortune. Many times a defeat can lead to a sequence of events that will culminate in victory. I'm sure that Abraham Lincoln learned from his failures, grew from them, and ultimately acknowledged their importance in his ultimate success. Ralph Waldo Emerson said it best, "No man ever fails until he fails on the inside."

Accept change

Change is the only constant in the universe. It's useless to resist it and foolish to dread it, for change enables us to grow. Life and love consist of constant change. Through 14 years of marriage, my wife and I have continued to change, as has our love. We have continued to work on living and loving, knowing that each moment will introduce change and that we must meet the challenge it presents. Nothing works for everyone every time. Throughout this book, I have introduced various techniques which I know, from experience and observation, are effective. But as a physician I also know that individuals vary. You must adapt these methods to your own lifestyle, and then readapt them as circumstances change.

Appreciate your uniqueness

Just as a perfume will smell different on two different people, the experience of life will vary from individual to individual. I have always maintained that I am an expert on only one subject—myself. While I can provide you with directions, only you can decide which path to take. Sometimes the road you travel may have so many detours that it seems you will never reach your destination. Only you can decide whether to continue as you are or move in another direction.

Learn to love yourself

It is amazing how hard we can be on ourselves. Few of us would treat a friend the way we sometimes treat ourselves. So why not be your own best friend? Before you can love others—or be loved by them—you must learn to love the person you are. Not the person you would like to be, or will one day become, but the individual you are at this very moment. Self-improvement is really only possible when you have self-acceptance. When you accept yourself, you will find the shackles you have placed on yourself falling away, and health, happiness and success following almost magically.

Be a child again

Children are wonderful. I have two boys, Michael, 12, and Jason, 9. They play with such enthusiasm, energy and joy that they remind me to play again. Children are naturally creative—they are born trusting life. Yet, as they observe adults, they too often lose their creativity and approach life with skepticism. The spontaneity we had as children did not simply disappear after a certain number of birthdays. It is a state of mind which we gradually learned to suppress, but which we can now revive. Robert Lowel said, "The child is the father to the man." What kind of parent are you to your inner child?

Know that you were put here for a purpose

Life is not a random accident, but you'd never know it by the way some people behave. God doesn't make mistakes—you were born for a reason. To simply endure life is a crime against yourself. And the punishment is failure, confusion, and unhappiness. The winners in life are those who believe that they deserve to win, that their lives are too valuable to waste. I believe that the seeds of greatness are within each and every one of us, but they can only blossom if we nurture them.

Stop waiting for conditions to be perfect

I'm going to let you in on a secret—life will never be without problems. To put off doing something until conditions are just right is to put off doing it forever. This principle is beautifully illustrated by a story which I first heard related by Dr. Mark Victor Hanson, a motivational speaker from the self-help capital of the world, California.

"I've got a problem."

The young man had just come up to Dr. Norman Vincent Peale on Fifth Avenue in New York City, grabbed him by the lapels and said, "Dr. Peale, please help me. I can't handle my problems. They're just too much."

Dr. Peale said, "Look I've got to give a talk. If you let go of my lapels, I'll show you a place where there are people with no problems."

The man said, "If you could do that, I'd give anything to go there."

Dr. Peale said, "You may not want to go there, once you see the place. It's just two blocks away."

They walked to Forest Lawn Cemetery and Dr. Peale said, "Look, there are 150,000 people in there. I happen to know that none of them has a problem."

Problems are not an obstacle to living, they are part of living. As soon as you can accept this simple truth, you can move on. Life is a culmination of learning experiences based on obstacles and failures. "It is the rocks in the water that give the stream its music."

Look inside yourself for the answers

The word "guru" simply means teacher. Others can certainly teach us, perhaps help us to avoid certain mistakes, and support us in reaching our goals. But no one else can tell us how to live our lives. I hope that my book has proved a useful resource, but I know it cannot possibly provide all the answers. My purpose has been to guide you, not to lead you. Now, you will continue your journey without me, for today is the first day of the rest of your life.

Remember, "The road to success is always under construction." In life, you are the architect, carpenter, and engineer of your body. You can either create a masterpiece or have to repair a fixer-upper.

How to use the Table of Food Nutritive Values:

> These tables may be used to find the nutritive values of food called for on your daily intake record. The foods are presented in amounts commonly eaten. If you have not eaten the exact amount, say 1 cup of vegetables, divide or multiply to get the approximate value. For, example, if you ate 1/2 cup of vegetables, divide the values in half. The figures are as accurate as analysis can make them. They are intended for estimations, not for exact purposes. For more detailed information, consult the sources listed at the end of the table.

> A note on the "Added Sugar" and "Fiber"categories. Very few analysis of added sugar are available; therefore, with the exception of ready-to-eat cereals, the figures are estimations based on home recipes and other data. Where a useful estimate is not available, the (+) sign indicates that the product usually has a good bit of added sugar.

> The "Fiber" column represents dietary fiber, which is composed of the indigestible part of plant foods and comes in two types—insoluble and soluble fiber (pectins and gums.) Each food contains a mixture of these types, but methods of figuring dietary fiber vary. Some of the figures include just insoluble fiber, others both types. The dietary fiber content for many foods is still unknown. These figures will give you an estimate of your fiber intake, but should not be considered complete.

The highest ideal of cure is the speedy, gentle, and enduring restoration of health by the most trustworthy and least harmful way.
                                                    Dr. Samuel Hahnemann

30

The Alternative Approach

There is a convergence of trends taking place in the health care industry today between eastern and western medicine. It is a trend that is reaching national acclaim with far-reaching implications. As a doctor, I hope it is not too little, too late. This convergence of trends does not take place as a philanthropic approach offered by the medical community but rather, as a convergence warranted by consumer demand. Consumers have witnessed the escalation of health care costs rise to over a trillion dollars annually. This acknowledgment of alternative care within our country was first brought to light by Dr. David Eisenberg from Harvard University. His study was published in the *New England Journal of Medicine* in 1993, and it recognized that 34% of adults in this country had used some form of alternative therapy which cost $13.7 billion dollars ($10 billion dollars of which was paid solely by the consumer). This in a year when $930 billion dollars was spent on conventional health care. While working as an advisor to the President's Council on Sports and Physical Fitness, I had the opportunity to do a project with and was published in the *USA Today* newspaper regarding Dr. Eisenberg's study.

This exciting day provided an opportunity to meet and work with Dr. Jocelyn Elders, who, at that time, was Surgeon General of the United States. I asked her a short, distinct, but far-reaching question: "Dr. Elders, if $930 billion dollars was spent on health care last year and one out of three Americans chose alternative care at a cost of approximately $13 billion dollars, don't you believe we need to analyze the other $917 billion spent and move more Americans toward alternative care?" Dr. Elders smiled and stated, "I like the question. I'll look into it." Dr. Eisenberg's information sent shock waves into the medical and insurance communities.

After the politicians searched for reasons, it was clear that the present model within our system was not effective. A recent article in *USA Today* stated that $30 billion dollars was spent on cancer research, and that we needed to alter our approach. Instead of searching directly for a cure for cancer, we needed to start working on finding the cause. The model that has been utilized by health care within our country has been a sickness-based model. One based on treating symptoms instead of finding the cause. John Lee, M.D., physician/educator, states,

"Most over-the-counter and almost all prescribed drug treatments merely mask the symptoms, or control health problems, or in some way alter the way organs or systems such as the circulatory system work. Drugs almost never deal with the reasons why these problems exist, while they frequently create new health problems as side effects of their activities."[1]

This campaign of alternative medicine is consumer-driven, not physician-driven. Who would have thought 10 years ago that the wall separating East and West Germany would be torn down, or that the power of Russia would become divided and recognized as the Unified States? That Communism as we once knew it would no longer exist in these countries? This transition was not based upon philosophical reasons but rather on personal and consumer need. Last year, 45,000 people died in automobile accidents, but adverse drug affects are responsible for 100,000 deaths.[2] A Harvard study indicated that conventional medical care is now the fourth leading cause of death in this country, right behind the killers of heart disease, cancer, and stroke.[3] What these four leading causes of death have in common is that to some degree they are all preventable. 28% of all hospital admissions in our country are caused by the drugs that were taken to heal the patient, at a cost of $77 billion. It is time that society stop looking for a miracle pill or potion and recognize that healing takes place only within the body. The power that creates the body has the power to heal the body. It is time for us to combine conventional, complementary, alternative, and behavioral medicine; to recognize and encourage the patient to participate and have a pathway to receive a choice of health care. It is time for us to value the psychological and physiological together as components that are associated with health. We must recognize that there are environmental as well as economic factors that are associated with health and illness. Julian Whitaker, M.D., the President of the American Alternative Medical Association states:

"The statistics on the unnecessary harm caused by drugs are enough to make you sick . . . 61,000 people have drug-induced Parkinson's symptoms; 163,000 have drug-induced memory loss or cognitive deficits; 41,000 are hospitalized for ulcers caused by drugs 32,000 hip fractures occur from falls which are due to drugs that make patients sedated or unbalanced; and 16,000 car crashes a year are due to adverse drug reactions. In 1990, the U.S. Government Accounting Office (GAO) reviewed the 198 drugs which were approved from 1976 to 1985. Unbelievably, 102 of them were found to have side effects serious enough to warrant either withdrawal from the market, or marked changes in labeling to warn of their increased dangers."[4]

If the fourth leading cause of death in this country is currently conventional health care, then I, for one, would opt for the alternative.

This past December I was confronted with a personal situation. My wife was diagnosed with colon cancer. Emergency surgery was performed that removed a tumor and left my 45-year-old bride with a colostomy. Further diagnostic testing indicated that my wife had an aggressive form of cancer that exceeded the tumor, the surrounding tissue, and entered her lymph nodes. She was categorized as a grade III Dukes, and basically became a statistic within the system. I will never forget the fear in my wife's eyes, or the pain in the eyes of our medical team, friends, and colleagues, as they told me of my wife's prognosis. On a trip to Sloan-Kettering Hospital, we were further forewarned of the seriousness of my wife's condition and advised not to have her colostomy reversed. We will be forever indebted to our surgeon, Dr. Jefferson Vaughn, for reversing the surgery (at our request) in spite of the risks.

As the President of Complete Wellness Medical Centers it is my job to coordinate conventional and alternative medicine within one office. It is my job is to put medical doctors, chiropractors, acupuncturists, naturopaths, and others working together to create a health paradigm, a wellness model. I felt it was my destiny to utilize this same platform in coordinating the treatment of my wife. I reviewed literature on the Internet, the "information highway" that puts the worlds' library within immediate access, in the comfort of our home. This was a tremendous resource with an infinite amount of material on cancer. I was able to look into the alternative approaches in the treatment of cancer. My cousin, Bruce Garfunkel, Associate Publisher for Penthouse Magazine, informed us about hydrazine sulfate which was utilized by Kathy Keaton, wife of Bob Guccione, founder of Penthouse Magazine. Kathy was told by her physicians that she had six months to live. She went on a successful regimen of hydrazine sulfate that currently is still not approved by the FDA in this country. The research on hydrazine sulfate in Russia was significant. Hydrazine sulfate has been utilized at the Petrov Research Institute of Oncology in St. Petersburg, Russia, for more than 10 years with long-standing success. It received a favorable report in *The Lancet*, one of the most prestigious medical journals in the world. The report concluded, "So the metabolic changes induced by the hydrazine group may prove clinically beneficial."[5]

The reason for the utilization of hydrazine sulfate is as follows: It is estimated that half of all cancer patients experience cachexia (the rapid loss of a large amount of weight along with fatigue, weakness, and loss of appetite). Cachexia is a serious problem among many patients with advanced cancer. Today, researchers are looking for ways to provide supportive care to cancer patients with cachexia. *The Lancet* reported a double-blind study done at UCLA Medical Center clearly defining that hydrazine sulfate assists with cachexia. Hydrazine sulfate is a chemical that interrupts abnormal glucose metabolism. Some studies have suggested the use of this drug helps improve patients appetite and increase their weight.

Work on hydrazine sulfate has been on-going for the last 20 years by Dr. Joseph Gold in Syracuse, N.Y. Although Dr. Gold has demanded that the U.S. Medical establishment give hydrazine sulfate a fair test, he is at least happy that his work is taking place and recognized in Russia. My wife's dramatic improvement has convinced me of hydrazine sulfate's efficacy. It is amazing that even with the research documented by UCLA and Russia, its treatment is still not approved in the U.S. Could cost be a factor? A one month supply of hydrazine sulfate for my wife costs $20. Conversely, chemotherapy and its application for one month costs approximately $1,000 or $12,000 a year, versus $240 (for hydrazine sulfate). The minimum $650 to $700 cancer treatment does not include doctor's visits or tests. Although I in no way disregard the importance of conventional medical care and the possibility that chemotherapy is assisting my wife's recovery, I believe it is the combination of conventional and alternative care that should be utilized. If cancer is the number two cause of death in this country, then it should be a number one priority that we utilize the best research in the world to find a cure. My eyes were opened to hydrazine sulfate by my personal experience. We must not all suffer to learn. It appears that society needs to open its eyes to the numerous forms of research existing in the world today.

My wife was placed on a program that consisted of chemotherapy, hydrazine sulfate, and other associated alternative therapies which we will discuss within this chapter. I am excited to report that in spite of the warnings from the Sloan-Kettering Hospital my wife did have her colostomy reversed, her tumor markers are normal, her cancer is presently in remission, and she has gained back all the weight she lost. If there was ever a walking platform to the combination of eastern and western medicine, and its treatment of cancer, it is my wife. I am grateful to our oncologist, Henry Shapiro, M.D., as well as Danielle Milano, M.D., Jefferson Vaughn, M.D., Sheldon Taub, M.D., and one of my best friends, Dennis Egitto, M.D., who were current on their research and were open to my wife and I on her treatment protocols. Her success to date is a confirmation of the power of "East meets West."

Depak Chopra, one of the best-selling authors on alternative medicine, said, "The past is history; the future is a mystery, but this moment of life is a gift, and that is why we call it 'The Present'." I dedicate every moment of my gift, of My Present, to coordinate conventional and alternative medicine into our system so that a sickness-based model will be the past, and a health-based model will be part of the future. The emergence of alternative medicine is the beginning of a revolution—a health revolution, demanded by a public that is "sick and tired" of being *sick and tired*. We cannot rest on our laurels of being a super-nation if we are not leaders physically, mentally, emotionally, and morally. We cannot rest on our laurels that we won WWII—over 50 years ago. Instead we must look at what the Germans and Japanese have accomplished over the past 50 years. They have exceeded us economically and have developed a health system that many professionals believe is also superior to ours. Much of the scientifically-based knowledge being introduced in this country comes from Germany where the government's attitude towards conventional and alternative medicine is totally different.

In Germany, phytonutrients, or botanical medicines, are approved as over-the-counter drugs by a government body known as Commission-E which is comparable to our Food and Drug Administration. Commission-E provides physicians with strict guidelines on natural remedies: When to prescribe these remedies, for which conditions, the expected effectiveness, and safety precautions. These natural substances are manufactured to pharmaceutical standards, are Government-regulated, and are clearly labeled as to approved dosage, possible side effects, contra-indications, and toxicity. It examines all of the modern scientific evidence available on botanical remedies and has issued over 300 monographs on herbal medicines; 200 of which have been approved as safe and effective. In Germany, Commission-E does double-blind human studies on herbal botanical remedies, whereas the FDA in this country only utilizes these standards for pharmaceutical drugs. I find it ironic that last year over one-billion dollars was spent on vitamins in this country, and these vitamins are often being "prescribed" by a salesperson at a health food store who lacks formal, or even limited training in health care, nutrition, or homeopathy. I am amazed at the number of people who walk in and ask the salesperson what they recommend for ailments such as headaches, and arthritis. It is time our country "stepped up" and "looked up" to Germany's model and invest in creating an alternative protocol. Dr. Lowell Levin, a Professor at Yale University said,

"It sounds like a joke. But the hospital is no place for a sick person to be. The increased use of potent antibiotics is one of the reasons for the ever-present life-threatening hospital infection. As more and more potent antibiotics are developed, increasingly resistant strains of microbes evolve."[6]

According to the *Archives of Internal Medicine* published in October 1995, preventable prescription, drug-related diseases, and death costs us a whopping $77 billion a year.

A study from Harvard Medical School indicated that almost one-third of the 9 million Americans over 65 are taking drugs that should never be taken by the elderly. The Citizen Health Research Group, which is a public-based company in Washington D.C., found that people over the age of 60 take 40% of all prescription drugs. The average number of prescriptions given to people over 60 is 15 per year; 37% of these people are taking five or more drugs at a time, and about 20% are taking seven prescription drugs a day.[7] How do we educate our children about the difference between good and bad drugs? The solution to this problem is that the FDA should follow the precedent set by Commission-E, which allows the public to have confidence in homeopathic remedies for sale. Germans can readily buy these over-the-counter remedies in retail stores. In Germany, all physicians have a level of training of these botanical remedies in medical school. In fact, according to a new survey, 80% of German physicians prescribe phytonutrients or plant medicines which account for 27% of all over-the-counter medicines sold in Germany.[8] A recent report on *20-20* showed that in Germany, the herb, St. John's Wort, was recommend for depression 20:1 over Prozac. Yet in this country, Prozac is the number one prescribed medication for depression, at a cost of approximately $1.7 billion a year, in spite of Prozac's great disfavor by many physicians and consumers because of its sometime fatal side effects. According to Commission-E, there are no known formidable side effects of St. John's Wort in the treatment of depression. Shouldn't we choose the remedy with the least side effects first?

Dr. David Eisenberg's report in the *New England Journal of Medicine* showed that in 1990, Americans made 425 million visits to alternative care providers which was more than visits to all conventional care practitioners. It was this wake-up call that finally moved this country away from ignorance about this issue. In 1978, when I graduated from New York Chiropractic College, I was amazed that our society did not sufficiently recognize the largest natural health care profession in the world. Chapter 25 in this book deals with chiropractic and truly illustrates the literature that has been compiled over the years by medical doctors and practitioners on the efficacy of chiropractic. Unfortunately, this form of treatment and its practitioners, fail to be recognized as the leaders in alternative care.

It is no secret that a crisis exists in modern medicine today. Prior to President Clinton's first term as president of this great country, he issued a mandate as part of his platform that he would call for health care reform. He designated his wife, Hillary, to chair this project. Now in his second term, health care reform is no longer discussed. It is no longer an issue. It was a platform he was not capable of integrating into our present system even though this system is in a terrible state of disarray. There is no doubt that conventional medicine excels in the management of medical emergencies, certain bacterial infections, trauma care, and surgical techniques, but it is easy to say that modern medicine has failed miserably in the areas of disease prevention and the management of new and chronic diseases that are threatening our country. According to Dr. Harold Neu of Columbia University, New York,

"In 1941, a patient could receive 40,000 units of penicillin per day for four days, and be cured of pneumococcal pneumonia. Today, a patient can receive 24 million units of penicillin a day and die of pneumococcal meningitis."[9]

We do not have a health care delivery system in this country—we have a sickness response system. We treat disease but fail to provide an avenue or philosophy of wellness or health. We must change the model to a health-based model. This can be done by educating the public to the avenues of health and implementing and utilizing a natural approach. The treatment of phytonutrients, or herbs, is not new. Digitalis is provided by the herb foxglove, and it is the basis of one of the most prevalent heart medications utilized during the past century. Penicillin, our most powerful antibiotic, was developed by *moldy bread*. Today, treatment of chronic disease accounts for approximately 85% of the national health care bill. As patients, we wait for illness to develop and then spend huge sums of money trying to treat the symptoms rather than recognizing the cause. It is no different than driving down the highway and having the oil light go on. It would be simple to mask the warning sign by removing the bulb because the car will continue to function properly *for a while*. But by not treating the cause and simply removing the symptom, a true correction will never occur. In 1988, former Surgeon General of the United States, C. Everett Koop, M.D., released a report on nutrition and health, which pointed out that dietary imbalances are the leading preventative contributors to premature death in the United States. He recommended the expansion of nutrition and lifestyle modification education to all health care professionals. Doctors are confronted daily with patients suffering from illnesses for which professional medicine offers little or no treatment. Children with chronic ear infections who took amoxicillin experienced two to six times more recurrent ear infections.[10] Last year, an estimated $500 million was spent on the treatment of ear infections in this country. Was this a necessary expense? In 1991, Family Practice News reported that the vast majority of children with recurrent ear infections improved after removing food allergens from their diet. The Canadian Journal of Diagnosis reported in 1989 that up to 60% of all episodes of acute otitis media (ear infections) improved on their own. We must stop using children as guinea pigs and recognize that we *do* have an alternative. This alternative is a natural approach to healing; an approach that allows the powers within to work with elements of nature to heal and repair the sickness and disease that exists within an environment that has been dramatically altered. It is disconcerting to realize how many adults and children suffer from complaints such as headaches, allergies, fatigue, decreased energy, depression, digestive disruptions, and respiratory disorders. This has allowed astute physicians throughout the world to become increasingly aware that something is wrong with the populations' immune system, and that the illnesses are due to decreased immune function. This decline in immune efficiency is something contemporary medical treatment seems unable to do anything about. In this country, doctors and patients alike are perplexed by this failure of drug-based therapies. The philosophies and science of alternative medicine are not new. The philosophies of alternative medicine date back to the father of medicine himself, Hippocrates, for he had insight into which elements were needed to maintain health. These elements were natural and included: hygiene, a balanced mental state, proper nutrition, a sound work and home environment, and exercise. He taught that health depended upon living in harmony with the forces of nature. Dr. Andrew Weil, one of today's most publicized leaders in alternative medicine, said in his best-selling book, *Spontaneous Healing*:

I am uneasy about the suppressive nature of conventional medicine. If you look at the names of the most popular categories of drugs in use today, you will find that most of them begin with the prefix "anti." We use antispasmodics, and antihypertensives, antianxiety agents, antidepressants, antihistamines, antiarrhythmic, antitussives, antipyretics, anti-inflammatories, as well as beta blockers and H2 receptor antagonists. This is truly antimedicine! That is, in essence, counteractive and suppressive.[11]

It is because of leaders like Dr. Andrew Weil, Dr. Julian Whitaker, Dr. Depak Chopra, Dr. Dean Ornish, Dr. Earl Mindell, as well as one of the original founders of alternative medicine who is not living to receive the accolades she truly deserves, Adele Davis, that alternative medicine is becoming mainstream. It was reported in an article in *Town and Country* magazine, January 1997, that 36 medical schools, including Yale and Columbia, now offer courses in alternative therapy, and Harvard Medical School recently held its third conference on the subject in March 1997. In the article, Dr. Eisenberg stated,

"I was very impressed with the open-mindedness of most medical doctors. After all, one of the worst things for someone who went into medicine wanting to help people is to have to say 'I have nothing else to offer you.'"

The article went on to state that more than 33 million Americans suffer from arthritis, 23 million from migraines, and as many as 80% of Americans will at one time or another suffer from back pain. Chiropractic is now recognized for its treatment of back pain, but that is not all it does. These primary natural health care practitioners deserve their due by fighting the American Medical Association in court in the Wilkes Hearing (see Chapter 25), and standing up for their beliefs to offer alternative health care in this country. The purpose of this chapter is to illustrate the dangers that are associated with the blinded use of medical or alternative health care. One form of care that has been greatly over-utilized is the administration of antibiotics. On March 28, 1984, the cover of *Newsweek* featured the headline, "Antibiotics, the End of Miracle Drugs. Warning: No Longer Effective Against Killer Bugs." That was followed by an article in *Time* magazine, September 12, 1994. The cover headline read, "Revenge of the Killer Microbes: Are We Losing the War Against Infectious Diseases?"

In January 1996, in an unprecedented move, 35 medical journals around the world released issues devoted to the same topic: "The Current Crisis in Antibiotic Resistance."[12] In the United States, the American Medical Association spent most of two issues of the *Journal* on this subject. They repeated the message that excessive and inappropriate use of antibiotics is harmful and the cause of many illnesses resurfacing today.

The *Journal of the American Medical Association* reported that doctors wrote 12 million antibiotic prescriptions in a single year for colds, bronchitis, and other respiratory infections, of which the drugs are almost always useless. Researchers noted that more than 90% of these infections are caused by a virus and are impervious to antibiotics.

It was not until the mid 1980s that the active ingredients in the elderberry used in treating influenza viruses were discovered. Dr. Gene Lindenman, the developer of Interferon, first suggested the potential of the elderberry as a research project due to the long history of the plant. In 1992, a team of Israeli scientists formulated a syrup and lozenge containing the active elderberry ingredients combined with other natural compounds. The syrup worked in the laboratory against common strains of flu viruses. The Helsinki Committee, a world-wide organization which approves patient's studies, approved a clinical trial in a double-blind study which was carried out on patients infected with the flu virus during the epidemic in southern Israel. Half of the patients were given four tablespoons of the syrup per day; the other half a placebo. The results were that within 24 hours, the symptoms (fever, cough, and muscle pain) had improved significantly in 20% of the patient's who received the elderberry extract. After the second day, another 75% of this group were clearly much improved, and in three days a complete cure was achieved in 90% of the elderberry patients studied. Among the control group, only 8% of the patients showed an improvement after 24 hours, and for the remaining 92%, improvement was observed within six days or more. Tests were additionally conducted on patients to determine the presence of influenza antibodies. It was found that the level of antibodies was again higher in the patients receiving the elderberry extract versus those receiving a placebo, indicating an enhanced immune response for those patients.[13]

According to research by nationally-recognized virololist Dr. Madeleine Mumcuolglu, 50% of people who receive flu shots according to studies have complications and for a small percentage, these complications are life-threatening. In 1976, the swine flu vaccine caused thousands of cases of Guillain Barre syndrome, a very serious neurological disease, yet the swine flu never even resurfaced.[14]

It is amazing how, with international recognition of a potential cure for the common cold or strain of the influenza virus, so few consumers and/or doctors utilize, prescribe, or recommend alternative treatment.

This treatment has been utilized not only by Complete Wellness Medical Centers but also successfully implemented by my own family. It has been a wonderful experience to be able to offer natural substances to your own children and see the symptoms of their cold virus dissipate naturally within 48 hours of onset. It is time that we changed the model. I present to you an antibiotic time line that was produced in an article by Maya Muir on alternative complimentary therapies.

Antibiotic Time Line

1929	Alexander Fleming discovers penicillin in laboratory experiments
1933	First clinical success with an antibiotic (sulfanilamide)
1938	First clinical success with penicillin
1942	Alexander Fleming warns about the emergence of antibiotic-resistant staphylococci
1950s	Rise of penicillin-resistant staphylococci
1950s	Japanese researchers find new resistance factors in dysentery-causing bacteria
1952	A Japanese researcher isolates the first organism resistant to several different antibiotics
1955	Almost 12% of 474 milk samples from around the United States contain traces of penicillin
1969	Epidemic of antibiotic-resistant dysentery (Shigella) in Guatemala infects 112,000; 12,500 die
1970s	Outbreak of antibiotic-resistant staphylococci sweeps through Europe, United States, Australia, and Greece
1976	Penicillinase-resistant gonorrhea spreads to east and west coasts, responsible for one-third of the cases of sexually transmitted diseases in Los Angeles
1977-79	310 cases of a new antibiotic-resistant salmonellosis in Great Britain; 2 die
1988	The streptococcus resistance for rheumatic heart disease causes an epidemic of the disease in Salt Lake City
1990	Penicillin-resistant gonorrhea rises by 60%
1990s	Penicillin can control only 10% of staphylococci it used to kill[15]

There is a field of knowledge of transcendent significant to mankind which has begun its development. This field deals with the correlation between chemical structure and physiological activity of those substances, manufactured in the body, or ingested in foodstuffs, which are essential for proper growth, and the maintenance of life, as well as many substances which are useful in the treatment of disease.
Nobel Prize Laureate, Linus Pauling, Ph.D.

31

Our Alternative Allies

It is amazing that in a society as intelligent as ours, a health food store is a little out-of-the-way shelter while a super drugstore is next to every supermarket. Drugs are a part of our everyday life, an everyday dilemma. We must recognize that we do have an alternative. As Martin Luther King, Jr. said, "The time is always right to do what is right."

Ayurevidic medicine, Chinese medicine, mind and body medicine, Chiropractic medicine, naturopathy, homeopathy, and aromatherapy (explained later in this chapter), are just the ABCs of alternative therapies that are now being utilized and recognized throughout the world. Homeopathic remedies are generally dilutions of natural substances from plants, minerals, and animals. This is based on the principle of like cures like. Homeopathy was founded in the late 18th century by German physician, Samuel Hahnemann. Dr. Hahnemann came to a breakthrough during an experiment in which two times a day he ingested cinchona, a Peruvian bark well known as a cure for malaria. Soon after Dr. Hahnemann began his experiment, he developed fevers common to malaria. As soon as he stopped taking the cinchona, his symptoms disappeared. He theorized that taking large doses of cinchona created symptoms of malaria in a healthy person, but the same substance taken in a smaller dose by a person suffering from malaria might stimulate the body to fight the disease. His theory was borne out by years of experiments with hundreds of substances that produced similar results. Based on this work, Dr. Hahnemann formulated the principles of homeopathy: 1) Like cures like (law of similars), 2) the more a remedy is diluted the greater its potency (law of infinitesimal dose), 3) an illness is specific to the individual (holistic model).

Dr. Hahnemann believed that each individual case of disease is radically and rapidly annihilated and removed only by a medicine capable of producing within the human body, the most similar and complete manner of the totality of the symptoms. This principle was first recognized by Hippocrates who was also recognized for studying the effects of herbs upon disease. Herbs existed within this universe far sooner than drugs. Digitalis, a major breakthrough in the treatment of heart disease, came from the herb foxglove. Antibiotics were first invented in 1929, so they are not even 100 years old. Prior to antibiotics, medicine was based largely on herbs and natural remedies. It is only over the past 60 years that we have reverted from health care to drug care.

One of the most powerful forms of alternative care utilizes one of nature's most powerful substances: antioxidants. Antioxidants have been recognized as a great disease deterrent and health enhancer. We can live without food for days or weeks, but the primary substance of life is oxygen. In our bodies, we have stable and unstable oxygen molecules.

In 1954, Denham Harmon, M.D., Ph.D., of the University of Nebraska, School of Medicine, founded the free radical theory. It has taken 41 years for the scientific community to embrace this theory and its effect on the aging process. There is a common denominator that causes aging and all of the conditions that occur as we grow older. These damaging agents are called "free radicals." It has been estimated that approximately 10,000 times per day every cell in our body is exposed to free radicals that are destructive. The best way to battle diseases caused by free radicals such as cancer, heart disease, and atherosclerosis is through exercise and a diet filled with antioxidants. Imagine a life free of free radicals. free radicals are simply defined as unstable oxygen molecules (oxidants). Keep in mind that there are both stable and unstable oxygen molecules moving about the body. The stable oxygen molecule is absolutely essential to life. Both stable and unstable oxygen molecules have a purpose. Specialized unstable oxygen molecules (free radicals) are essential in that they enable our bodies to fight inflammation, kill bacteria, and control the tone of smooth muscles. These oxygen molecules regulate the working of internal organs and blood vessels.

The key is the ability to maintain control of free radical balance. If the production of free radicals is exacerbated by exogenous (outside) sources such as stress, poor diet, smoking, drinking, additives, and preservatives, then the body needs free radical scavengers known as "endogenous antioxidants" that gobble up the free radicals preventing them from damaging the body. If the body becomes overwhelmed by free radicals, this shift in balance causes the unstable oxygen molecules to shift from the body's allies into molecular predators. These predators then begin to wreak havoc by attacking both healthy and unhealthy parts of the body. Heart disease, various cancers, cataracts, and many other diseases are the result.

It is essential to maintain a balance between stable and unstable oxygen molecules. Research now clearly indicates that antioxidants can offset many diseases derived from diet, lifestyle, environment, and activity patterns. This breakthrough enhances our ability to control, not only the quantity but the quality of our lives. James Fries, M.D., a professor of preventative medicine at Stanford University Medical School points out that there is a significant difference between chronological age and biological age. Meaning, an individual may be chronologically 60 years old, but biologically have the health of a 45 year old, and vice versa. Imagine having the ability to turn the clock back or even slow down the clock. The public is moving toward antioxidant therapy and away from antibiotic therapy. Is this a radical approach? I don't think so.

The Game of Life

There are 2,598,960 possible five-card poker hands, but you will be dealt only one. In life, we are all dealt different "hands." The beauty of poker (and life) is that you don't have to be dealt the best hand to win. One of the best possible hands in poker is four ACES. This acronym also represents four major antioxidants, the following are the four primary antioxidants I recommend: *Vitamin A* in the form of beta carotene, *Vitamin C* in the form of rose hips and bioflavenoids, *Vitamin E* in the form of mixed tocopherols and *Selenium*. The fourth ACE is now being recognized for its strong antioxidant qualities as well as being a prophylactic against cancer. Dr. Ernest Wynder, President of the American Health Foundation in New York, has done extensive studies on selenium and cancer. In one study done in cooperation with New York's Memorial Sloan-Kettering Cancer Center, men were put on a low fat diet and given supplements of vitamin E, (800 i.u.) selenium, (200 micrograms) as well as soy products. Dr. Wynder reported, "There is evidence all such supplements fight prostate cancer."[16] Dr. Earl Mindell, best-selling author of *The Vitamin Bible*, has also reported success with these supplements. Dr. Larry Clark of the University of Arizona did research on 1,300 older people, giving them 200 mcg of selenium daily and found a 42% reduction in cancer occurrence and cancer deaths by 50% compared with the placebo group.[17] Yet none of these treatments are mainstream. When my wife and I went to Sloan-Kettering, we were not informed about selenium. By arming yourself with these four nutrients, worldwide studies have revealed they are defenses against chronic degenerative diseases. Unfortunately, most people do not eat enough fruits and vegetables to consume the recommended amounts of these vital nutrients. If one does not consume enough of these nutrients, then supplementation is necessary. In April 1994, the *New England Journal of Medicine* reported 34% fewer prostate cancers among men who had taken Vitamin E and 16% fewer colon or rectal cancers. These four ACES antioxidants are probably the most effective insurance policy we can buy. We must insure that we do whatever we can to prevent disease. We must create a personal policy to take a preventative approach. Outside the parameters of health lies disease. Lurking outside of life is death. We are only invincible until we are vincible. If I am going to bet my life on a hand, it would be nice to be holding four ACES. Does it guarantee victory? No, but I like the odds. (For more information on The Four ACES, see Chapter 15.)

Many people ask why we need supplements? In the past, many doctors would say you don't need vitamins, you get them in your diet. Well, if *we are what we eat* then we are in trouble.

Top Ten Foods

According to *The 1992 Top Ten Almanac* by Michael Robbins, (Workman's Publishing) the top ten food items purchased ranked by dollar volume are:

1. Marlboro Cigarettes
2. Coca-cola Classic

3. Pepsi Cola

4. Kraft Processed Cheese

5. Diet Coke

6. Campbell's Soup

7. Budweiser Beer

8. Tide Detergent

9. Folger's Coffee

10. Winston Cigarettes

No wonder we are sick. Our bodies run on caffeine and nicotine and no, Tide detergent does not clean our arteries.

A recent study out of Washington, D.C. demonstrated that men who took 500 mg of vitamin C daily had a 50% less chance of a heart attack and lived six years longer than men taking 100 mg, yet the RDA (recommended daily allowance) is 60 mg.[18] The math just doesn't add up, but the statistics on heart disease do. It is the number one cause of death in this country.

Wouldn't the best insurance policy be to take 500 mg of vitamin C every day? We must create a prevention philosophy, a "wellness model." We must attack symptoms naturally, conservatively at first, and then aggressively. We must follow health models that have been set throughout the world. It was reported that 70% of American men will develop a prostate disorder. One of my top 20 remedies is the herb Saw Palmetto. This is openly recommended in Germany versus the use of the commonly prescribed medication, Proscar, in the United States.

Saw Palmetto Versus Proscar In Treatment of Prostate Enlargement

	Saw Palmetto Extract	Proscar
Urine Flow	38% to 50% improvement	16% to 22% improvement
Residual Volume	42% improvement	No improvement
Overall Symptoms	88% to 92.% improvement	Less than 50%
Decrease in Nocturia	3.12 to 1.69 awakenings	No improvement
Complications	None	Decreased libido
		Ejaculatory disorders
		Impotency
		Urogenital birth defects[19]

The cost for Proscar is $75 per month versus $15 for Saw Palmetto. The key difference is *not* the $60 in savings, but the fact that Saw Palmetto has *no known side effects.*

We must take an active role in our health. We must be educated consumers. Our primary consumption should be Knowledge; its byproduct Prevention. This is one of many natural alternatives available today to treat to diseases.

The following are my 20 favorite herbal therapies and their potential usage. Obviously, prior to participating in any program, consult a doctor with a background in alternative health care.

Kaplan's Top Twenty

1. St. John's Wort—depression, diet, behavioral modification
2. Glucosomine sulfate—arthritis, degenerative joint disease, juvenile rheumatoid arthritis
3. Feverfew—migraines, rheumatoid arthritis
4. Aloe Vera—skin disorders (topical), stomach disorders (internal)
5. Elderberry Extract, Sambucol^tm—colds, cough, flu, viruses
6. Shark Cartilage—cancer inhibitor, osteoarthritis, prostate
7. Saw Palmetto—prostate
8. Garlic—high blood pressure, high cholesterol, heart disease, stomach disorders
9. Ginko Billoba—memory, concentration, Alzheimer's, circulation, cerebral vascular insufficiencies
10. Licorice Root—chronic fatigue syndrome, anti-inflammatory, stomach
11. Ginger—morning sickness, motion sickness, nausea; boosts immune system
12. Dong Quai—premenstrual syndrome, immune function; build muscle, enrich blood
13. Valerian Root—anxiety, insomnia, nervousness, muscle relaxant
14. Fish Oil (Omega 3s)—arrhythmias, attention deficit disorders, triglycerides, inflammatory bowel disease, rheumatoid arthritis
15. Coenzyme Q-10—circulation, heart disease, stamina
16. Grapefruit Fiber—atherosclerosis, cholesterol

17. Milk Thistle—liver disease, toxicity
18. Senna—constipation, irregularity
19. Echinacea—colds, flu, viruses, infections
20. Antioxidants—anti-aging, immunity, general prevention, your best personal insurance policy

Chinese Medicine

China's 5,000-year old medical system is based on the idea that balancing active and passive forces within the body enhances Chi (pronounced Chee), or life force, and leads to healing. The language of Chinese medicine is based on metaphors from nature. Traditional Chinese medicine is a comprehensive system of diagnosis and treatment now established throughout the world. One prime example is that the Chinese treated alcoholism more than 1,300 years ago utilizing kudzu tea. Researchers at Harvard University and the University of North Carolina have furthered this research and confirmed this herb detours the body's desire for alcohol.

For more information:

The American Foundation of Traditional Chinese Medicine
505 Beach Street
San Francisco, CA 94133

Chiropractic

After years of results, chiropractic and chiropractors are finally receiving their due with approximately 50,000 chiropractors treating 15 to 20 million Americans. They are now the third leading health care profession. For more information, please refer to Chapter 25.

Additional sources:

Complete Wellness Centers
725 Independence Avenue
Washington, D.C. 20003
202-543-6800

American Chiropractic Association
1701 Clarendon Blvd.
Arlington, VA 22204

International Chiropractic Association
1110 Glebe Road, Suite 1000
Arlington, VA 22201
1-800-423-4690

Acupuncture

Acupuncture is a component of traditional Chinese medicine. Of all Chinese medicine this is the most accepted in the west. There is compelling scientific evidence for its efficacy as an anesthetic and antidote for chronic pain, migraine, dysmenorrhea, and osteoarthritis.

For more information:

American Academy of Acupuncture
5280 Wilshire Blvd., Suite 500
Los Angeles, CA 90036
1-800-521-2262

Massage

Because of severe injuries to both my shoulders and knee, I am a personal advocate of massage. Although arthritic, massage has a limbering and therapeutic effect on my body. Massage or "body work" comprise traditional massage, shiatsu, Swedish, deep tissue, and deep deep tissue known as rolfing. It can reduce stress, stimulate the lymphatic system, improve circulation, and enhance immune function. Studies show massage can be used as an adjunct in the treatment of cardiovascular disorders, neurological and gynecological problems, and can often be used in place of pharmacological drugs.[20]

For more information:

American Massage Therapy Association
820 Davis Street, Suite 100
Evanston, ILL 60201

Ayurevidic Medicine

One of the most ancient forms of alternative medicines was Ayurevidic Medicine. India's Ayurevidic takes a preventive approach and aims at treating the whole patient. Therapies include diet (tailored to the individual's constitutional type) or dosha, herbs, yoga, breathing exercises, meditation, massages, purges, aromatherapy, and enemas.

Research shows effectiveness with many chronic illnesses including arthritis, rheumatoid arthritis, headaches, sinusitis, and chronic fatigue syndrome.

Ayurevidic medicine holds that in order to restore health one must first understand and correctly diagnose the disease or body imbalance.

For more information:
The Ayurevidic Institute
P.O. Box 23445
Albuquerque, NM 87192

Naturopathy

Naturopathic medicine is not "new age" or a single modality of treatment. It may be defined as an array of healing practices including diet, nutrition, homeopathy, chiropractic, acupuncture, hydrotherapy, aromatherapy, and light therapy. All practices are naturally based and utilize the healing power of nature.

For more information:
American Association of Naturopathic Physicians
2366 Eastlake Avenue, Suite 322
Seattle, WA 98102

The Future—"Back To Basics"

It seems apparent with the onslaught of literature in alternative medicine that if we are to go back to grassroot basics, we need to move from a drug oriented culture to a health oriented culture. If you were not healthy and you wanted to start an alternative regimen, where would you go? Would you go to a hospital, or would a hospital's primary function be to treat disease? Would you go to a medical doctor's office, or again, would their function be to treat symptoms? Would you go to a health club, or are they usually just an exercise studio? In his best-selling book, *Sign Language*, Jerry Seinfeld said, "Everybody wants to be healthy—the amazing thing is nobody knows where to begin."

Presently, I am working with Congressman Tom McMillan, who was appointed by Bill Clinton as the Co-Chairman of the President's Council on Sports and Physical Fitness. As the President of Complete

Wellness Medical Centers, it is our paradigm to bring conventional and alternative health care together. Where the patient (consumer) can find a place that specializes in wellness, and that creates a wellness or health-based model, not a disease-based model. If conventional medical care is the fourth leading cause of death in America, shouldn't *that* be the alternative? And shouldn't conventional care as we know it or the higher risk module of care become the alternative? If we want to reduce the national health care budget, we must go from a sickness-based model to a health care-based model. One that is based upon prevention and locating the cause of disease, not just a model that chases symptoms.

At Complete Wellness Medical Centers, we have the empirical formula that we plan to espouse to the community at large.

Research and documentation shows that alternative care is here to stay. I hope that we follow the research done in Eastern medicine by following the regimens and protocols the Chinese set forth over 5,000 years ago. It is time that we stopped recreating the wheel and realize that the genesis of medicine has really existed within the past hundred years; that penicillin and most medications have evolved in the past 50 years, not a long period of time. Alternative medicine is here to stay, but it should not be secondary care, it should be primary. Our primary choice should be a natural choice; our secondary or alternative choice should be that of drugs. We should consider the words of Thomas Edison who said, "The doctor of the future will give no medicine, instead he will interest patients in the care of the human frame in diet, and in the causes and prevention of disease."

Table of Food Nutritive Values

FOOD	Amount	WEIGHT in grams	CALORIES	PROTEIN (g)	Total FAT (g)	Saturated FAT (g)	Mono FAT(g)	Polyunsaturated FAT (g)	CARBOHYDRATE (g)	Added SUGAR (g)	CHOLESTEROL (mg)	SODIUM (mg)	FIBER (g)
APRICOTS													
raw, 12 / lb	3 apr.	106	50	1	tr	tr	0.2	0.1	12		0	1	
canned, heavy syrup	3 halves	85	70	tr	tr	tr	tr	tr	18	8	0	3	
juice pack	3 halves	84	40	1	tr	tr	tr	tr	10		0	3	
dried (28 lg. or 37 med.)	1 cup	130	310	5	1	tr	0.3	0.1	80		0	13	
APRICOT NECTAR	1 cup	251	140	1	tr	tr	0.1	tr	36		0	8	
ARTICHOKES													
globe, cooked	1 whole	120	55	3	tr	tr	tr	0.1	12		0	79	
hearts	1/2 cup	84	37	2	tr	tr	tr	0.1	9		0	55	
Jerusalem, raw, sliced	1 cup	150	115	3	tr	0	tr	tr	26		0	6	
ASPARAGUS, cooked													
fresh & frozen, 1/2" at base	4 spears	60	15	2	tr	tr	tr	0.1	3		0	2	1
canned, 1/2" at base	4 spears	80	10	1	tr	tr	tr	0.1	2		0	278	
AVOCADOS, raw													
California, 2 / lb	1 avocado	173	305	4	30	4.5	19.4	3.5	12		0	21	6
Florida, 1 / lb	1 avocado	304	340	5	27	5.3	14.8	4.5	27		0	15	
BACON													
regular	3 med. sl.	19	110	6	9	3.3	4.5	1.1	tr		16	303	
Canadian	2 slices	46	85	11	4	1.3	1.9	0.4	1		27	711	
BAGELS, plain, 3 1/2"	1 bagel	68	200	7	2	0.3	0.5	0.7	38		0	245	
BAKING POWDER	1 tsp.	2.9	5	tr	0	0	0	0	1		0	290	
BAMBOO SHOOTS	1 cup	131	25	2	1	0.1	tr	0.2	4		0	105	3.5
BANANAS, 2 1/2 / lb	1 banana	114	105	1	1	0.2	tr	0.1	27		0	1	4
BARBECUE SAUCE, bottled	1 tbsp.	16	10	tr	tr	tr	0.1	0.1	2		0	130	
BEAN SPROUTS, mung, raw	1 cup	104	30	3	tr	tr	tr	0.1	6		0	6	1
BEANS													
black, dry, cooked	1 cup	171	255	15	1	0.1	0.1	0.5	41		0	1	7
great northern, dry, cooked	1 cup	180	210	14	1	0.1	0.1	0.6	38		0	13	6
green or snap													

FOOD	Amount	WEIGHT in grams	CALORIES	PROTEIN (g)	Total FAT (g)	Saturated FAT (g)	Mono FAT(g)	Polyunsaturated FAT (g)	CARBOHYDRATE (g)	Added SUGAR (g)	CHOLESTEROL (mg)	SODIUM (mg)	FIBER (g)
fresh cooked	1 cup	125	45	2	tr	0.1	tr	0.2	10		0	4	3
canned	1 cup	135	25	2	tr	tr	tr	0.1	6		0	339	3
kidney, cooked	1 cup	177	225	15	1	0.1	0.1	0.5	40		0	4	14.5
limas, fresh													
fordhook	1 cup	170	170	10	1	0.1	tr	0.3	32		0	90	9
baby	1 cup	180	190	12	1	0.1	tr	0.3	35		0	52	8
limas, dry, cooked	1 cup	190	260	16	1	0.2	0.1	0.5	49		0	4	9
navy or pea, dry, cooked	1 cup	190	225	15	1	0.1	0.1	0.7	40		0	13	12
pinto, dry, cooked	1 cup	180	265	15	1	0.1	0.1	0.5	49		0	3	10.5
refried, canned	1 cup	290	295	18	3	0.4	0.6	1.4	51		0	1228	
BEANS, baked, canned, vegetarian	1 cup	254	235	12	1	0.3	0.1	0.5	52		0	1008	
BEEF, relatively fat cuts													
Brisket, braised (33% separable fat)													
lean and fat	3 oz.	85	332	20	28	11.2	12.5	1.0	0		79	52	
lean only	3 oz.	85	205	25	11	3.9	4.9	0.3	0		79	61	
Chuck blade, braised as in pot roast (21% separable fat)													
lean and fat	3 oz.	85	330	22	26	11	11.9	1.0	0		87	53	
lean only	3 oz.	85	230	26	13	5.3	5.8	0.4	0		90	60	
Rib, whole, broiled (24% separable fat)													
lean and fat	3 oz.	85	308	18	26	10.8	11.4	0.9	0		73	52	
lean only	3 oz.	85	194	22	11	4.7	4.9	0.3	0		69	50	
Shortribs, braised (33% separable fat)													
lean and fat	3 oz.	85	400	18	36	15.1	16.1	1.3	0		80	43	
T-bone steak, broiled (19% separable fat)													
lean and fat	3 oz.	85	276	20	21	8.7	9.1	0.8	0		71	51	
lean only	3 oz.	85	182	24	9	3.5	3.5	0.3	0		68	56	
Sirloin (20% separable fat)													
lean and fat	3 oz.	85	238	23	15	6.0	6.2	0.6	0		73	52	
lean only	3 oz.	85	177	26	8	3.0	3.3	0.3	0		76	56	

FOOD	Amount	WEIGHT in grams	CALORIES	PROTEIN (g)	Total FAT (g)	Saturated FAT (g)	Mono FAT(g)	Polyunsaturated FAT (g)	CARBOHYDRATE (g)	Added SUGAR (g)	CHOLESTEROL (mg)	SODIUM (mg)	FIBER (g)
BEEF, relatively lean cuts													
Flank (2% seperable fat)													
lean and fat	3 oz.	85	218	23	13	5.6	6.1	0.4	0		61	61	
lean only	3 oz.	85	207	22	13	5.4	5.3	0.4	0		60	61	
Round, full cut, broiled (15% separable fat)													
lean and fat	3 oz.	85	233	22	16	6.2	6.8	0.7	0		71	51	
lean only	3 oz..	85	165	24	7	2.5	2.9	0.3	0		70	54	
Round, eye of, roasted (12% separable fat)													
lean and fat	3 oz.	85	206	23	12	4.9	5.4	0.4	0		62	50	
lean only	3 oz.	85	155	25	6	2.1	2.4	0.2	0		58	52	
Tenderloin (13% separable fat)													
lean and fat	3 oz.	85	226	22	15	6.0	6.2	0.6	0		73	52	
lean only	3 oz.	85	174	24	8	3.1	3.1	0.3	0		72	54	
BEEF BREAKFAST STRIPS	3 slices	34	153	11	12	4.9	5.7	0.5	0		40	766	
BEEF, ground, cooked med.													
lean	3 oz.	85	227	20	16	6.1	6.8	0.6	0		66	47	
regular	3 oz.	85	244	20	18	7.0	7.8	0.7	0		74	51	
BEEF BRAINS, pan fried	3 oz.	85	167	11	14	3.2	3.4	2.0	0		1696	134	
BEEF LIVER, pan fried	3 oz.	85	184	23	7	2.4	1.5	1.5	7		410	90	
BEEF TONGUE, simmered	3 oz.	85	241	19	18	7.6	8.1	0.7	tr		91	51	
BEER													
regular	12 oz.	360	150	1	0	0	0	0	13	13	0	18	
light	12 oz.	355	95	1	0	0	0	0	5	5	0	11	
BEET GREENS, cooked	1 cup	144	40	4	tr	tr	0.1	0.1	8		0	347	1.5
BEETS													
2" fresh	2 beets	100	30	1	tr	tr	tr	tr	7		0	49	3
sliced	1 cup	170	55	2	tr	tr	tr	tr	11		0	83	
canned, sliced	1 cup	170	55	2	tr	tr	tr	0.1	12		0	466	6
BISCUITS, 2"													
home recipe	1 biscuit	28	100	2	5	1.2	2.0	1.3	13		tr	195	
refrigerated	1 biscuit	20	65	1	2	0.6	0.9	0.6	10		1	249	
BLACKBERRIES, raw	1 cup	144	75	1	1	0.2	0.1	0.1	18		0	tr	10.5

FOOD	Amount	WEIGHT in grams	CALORIES	PROTEIN (g)	Total FAT (g)	Saturated FAT (g)	Mono FAT(g)	Polyunsaturated FAT (g)	CARBOHYDRATE (g)	Added SUGAR (g)	CHOLESTEROL (mg)	SODIUM (mg)	FIBER (g)
BLUEBERRIES													
raw	1 cup	145	80	1	1	tr	0.1	0.3	20		0	9	4.5
frozen, sweetened	1 cup	230	185	1	tr	tr	tr	0.1	50	30	0	2	
BLUEFISH, raw	3 oz.	85	105	17	4	0.8	1.5	0.9	0		50	51	
BOK CHOY, cooked (Chinese cabbage)	1 cup	170	20	3	tr	tr	tr	0.1	3		0	58	
BOLOGNA (8 oz. pkg., 8 slices)													
beef	2 slices	56	176	6	16	6.8	7.8	0.6	tr		36	556	
meat	2 slices	57	180	7	16	6.1	7.6	1.4	2		31	581	
BOUILLON, beef, canned, condensed	1 cup	240	15	3	1	0.3	0.2	tr	tr		tr	782	
BRAUNSCHWEIGER, 1 oz. slice	2 slices	57	205	8	18	6.2	8.5	2.1	2		89	652	
BRAZIL NUTS	1 oz.	28	185	4	0	4.6	6.5	6.8	4		0	1	
BREAD CRUMBS, dry	1 cup	100	390	13	5	1.5	1.6	1.0	73		5	736	
BREAD													
cracked wheat	1 slice	25	65	2	1	0.2	0.2	0.3	12		0	106	2
Italian	1 slice	30	85	3	tr	tr	tr	0.1	17		0	176	
mixed grain	1 slice	25	65	2	1	0.2	0.2	0.4	12		0	106	
oatmeal	1 slice	25	65	2	1	0.2	0.4	0.5	12		0	124	
pita, 6 1/2"	1 pita	65	165	6	1	0.1	0.1	0.4	33		0	339	
pumpernickel	1 slice	32	80	3	1	0.2	0.3	0.5	16		0	177	1
raisin	1 slice	25	65	2	1	0.2	0.3	0.4	13		0	92	tr
rye	1 slice	25	65	2	1	0.2	0.3	0.3	12		0	175	1
white	1 slice	25	65	2	1	0.3	0.4	0.2	12		0	129	1
whole wheat	1 slice	28	70	3	1	0.4	0.4	0.3	13		0	180	2
BROCCOLI													
raw	1 spear	151	40	4	1	0.1	tr	0.3	8		0	41	
fresh, cooked	med. spear	180	50	5	1	0.1	tr	0.2	10		0	20	7
frozen, cooked 4 1/2"	1 piece	30	10	1	tr	tr	tr	tr	2		0	7	1
frozen, chopped	1 cup	185	50	6	tr	tr	tr	0.1	10		0	44	7
BROWNIES, frosted 1 1/2" x 1 3/4"	1 brownie	25	100	1	4	1.6	2.0	0.6	16	+	14	59	

FOOD	Amount	WEIGHT in grams	CALORIES	PROTEIN (g)	Total FAT (g)	Saturated FAT (g)	Mono FAT(g)	Polyunsaturated FAT (g)	CARBOHYDRATE (g)	Added SUGAR (g)	CHOLESTEROL (mg)	SODIUM (mg)	FIBER (g)
BRUSSEL SPROUTS, frozen, cooked	1 cup	155	65	6	1	0.1	tr	0.3	13		0	36	5
BULGUR WHEAT, uncooked and unsoaked	1 cup	170	600	19	3	1.2	0.3	1.2	129		0	389	
BUTTER													
stick, 1/4 lb, salted	1/2 cup	113	810	1	92	57.1	26.4	3.4	tr		247	933	
unsalted												12	
tbsp., 1/8 stick, salted	1 tbsp.	14	100	tr	11	7.1	3.3	0.4	tr		11	16	
unsalted												2	
pat (1/3" slice), salted	1 pat	5	35	tr	4	2.5	1.2	0.2	tr		11	41	
unsalted												1	
BUTTERMILK	1 cup	245	100	8	2	1.3	0.6	0.1	12		9	257	
CABBAGE, common and & Chinese varieties													
raw, shredded	1 cup	70	15	1	tr	tr	tr	0.1	4		0	13	3
cooked	1 cup	150	30	1	tr	tr	tr	0.2	7		0	29	3
CAKES, from mixes													
angel food	1/12 cake	53	125	3	tr	tr	tr	0.1	29	25	0	269	
devil's food w/ frosting	1/16 cake	69	235	3	8	3.5	3.2	1.2	40	18	37	181	
" " " "	1 cupcake	35	120	2	4	1.8	1.6	0.6	20	+	19	92	
gingerbread	2 1/2" sq.	63	175	2	4	1.1	1.8	1.2	32	18	1	192	
yellow w/ frosting	1/16 cake	69	235	3	8	3.0	3.0	1.4	40	+	36	157	
CAKES, commercial													
pound loaf	1/2" slice	110	2	5	3.0	1.7	0.2	15	9	64	108		
white layer w/ frosting	1/16 cake	71	260	3	9	2.1	3.8	2.6	42	+	3	176	
CANDY													
caramels	1 oz.	28	115	1	3	2.2	0.3	0.1	22	+	1	64	
chocolate													
milk	1 oz.	28	145	2	9	5.4	3.0	0.3	16	16	6	23	
milk/ almonds	1 oz.	28	150	3	10	4.8	4.1	0.7	15	15	5	23	
milk/ peanuts	1 oz.	28	155	4	11	4.2	3.5	1.5	13	13	5	19	
semisweet	1 cup (6 oz.)	170	860	7	61	36.2	19.9	1.9	98	98	0	24	
sweet dark	1 oz.	28	150	1	10	5.9	3.3	0.3	16	16	0	5	
fondant (mints, candy corn)	1 oz.	28	105	tr	tr	tr	tr	0.1	25	25	0	10	

FOOD	Amount	WEIGHT in grams	CALORIES	PROTEIN (g)	Total FAT (g)	Saturated FAT (g)	Mono FAT (g)	Polyunsaturated FAT (g)	CARBOHYDRATE (g)	Added SUGAR (g)	CHOLESTEROL (mg)	SODIUM (mg)	FIBER (g)
fudge, plain	1 oz.	28	115	1	3	2.1	1.0	0.1	21	21	1	54	
gumdrops	1 oz.	28	100	tr	tr	tr	tr	0.1	25	25	0	10	
hard	1 oz.	28	110	0	0	0	0	0	28	28	0	7	
jellybeans	1 oz.	28	105	tr	tr	tr	tr	0.1	26	26	0	7	
marshmallows	1 oz.	28	90	1	0	0	0	0	23	23	0	25	
CANTALOUPE, 5" diameter	1/2 melon	267	95	2	1	0.1	0.1	0.3	22		0	24	1
CARBONATED DRINKS													
club soda	12 oz.	355	0	0	0	0	0	0	0	0	0	78	
cola	12 oz.	369	160	0	0	0	0	0	41	41	0	18	
ginger ale	12 oz.	366	125	0	0	0	0	0	32	32	0		
lemon-lime	12 oz.	372	155	0	0	0	0	0	46	46	0	48	
root beer	12 oz.	370	165	0	0	0	0	0	42	42	0	48	
CARROTS													
raw, 7 1/2"	1 carrot	72	30	1	tr	tr	tr	0.1	7		0	25	2
sliced, cooked	1 cup	156	70	2	tr	0.1	tr	0.1	16		0	103	4
CARROT JUICE	1 cup	246	98	2	tr	0.1	tr	0.2	23		0	72	
CASHEWS, salted, roasted	1 oz.	28	165	5	14	2.7	8.1	2.3	8		0	177	
CATFISH, breaded, fried	3 oz.	85	194	15	11	2.8	4.8	2.8	7		69	238	
CATSUP	1 tbsp.	15	15	tr	tr	tr	tr	tr	4		0	156	
CAULIFLOWER													
raw	1 cup	100	25	2	tr	tr	tr	0.1	5		0	15	2
cooked	1 cup	125	30	2	tr	tr	tr	0.1	6		0	15	2
CAVIAR, black and red	1 tbsp.	16	40	4	3				1		94	240	
CELERY	1 stalk	40	5	tr	tr	tr	tr	tr	1		0	35	0.5
CEREALS, hot, cooked													
cream of wheat	1 cup	244	140	4	tr	0.1	tr	0.2	29		0	5	
instant, plain	1 pkt.	142	100	3	tr	tr	tr	0.1	21		0	241	
oatmeal	1 cup	234	145	6	2	0.4	0.8	1.0	25		0	2	2
instant, plain	1 pkt.	177	105	4	2	0.3	0.6	0.7	18		0	285	
CEREALS, ready to eat													
All Bran (1/3 cup)	1 oz.	28	70	4	1	0.1	0.1	0.3	21	14	0	320	9
Apple Jacks	1 oz.	28	110	2	0				26	14	0	125	tr
Bran Checks	1 oz.	28	90	3	0					5	0	300	5

FOOD	Amount	WEIGHT in grams	CALORIES	PROTEIN (g)	Total FAT (g)	Saturated FAT (g)	Mono FAT(g)	Polyunsaturated FAT (g)	CARBOHYDRATE (g)	Added SUGAR (g)	CHOLESTEROL (mg)	SODIUM (mg)	FIBER (g)
Bran Flakes–Kellogg's	1 oz.	28	90	4	1	0.1	0.1	0.3	22	5	0	264	4
Bran Flakes–Post	1 oz.	28	90	3	tr	0.1	0.1	0.2	22	5	0	260	4
Cap' n Crunch	1 oz.	28	120	1	3	1.7	0.3	0.4	23	11	0	213	0.3
Cheerios	1 oz.	28	110	4	2	0.3	0.6	0.7	20	1	0	307	1
Corn Chex	1 oz.	28	110	2	0				25	3	0	310	tr
Corn Flakes–Kellogg's	1 oz.	28	110	2	tr	tr	tr	tr	24	2	0	351	tr
Corn Flakes–Post	1 oz.	28	110	2	tr	tr	tr	tr	24	2	0	297	tr
Crispix	1 oz.	28	110	2	0					3	0	220	tr
Fiber One	1 oz.	28	60	4	1				21	2	0	230	12
Fruit Loops	1 oz.	28	110	2	1	0.2	0.1	0.1	25	13	0	145	tr
Frosted Flakes—Kellogg's	1 oz.	28	110	1	tr	tr	tr	tr	26	12	0	230	tr
Fruit & Fibre, harvest medley	1 oz.	28	90	3	1				22	4	0	190	4
Grape Nuts (1/4 cup)	1 oz.	28	100	3	tr	tr	tr	0.1	23	3	0	197	1.3
Honey Nut Cheerios	1 oz.	28	105	3	1	0.1	0.3	0.3	23	10	0	257	tr
Honey Smacks	1 oz.	28	105	2	1	0.1	0.1	0.2	25	16	0	75	tr
Nutri-Grain Wheat	1 oz.	28	110	3	0				24	2	0	195	2
100% Natural Cereal, Quaker	1 oz.	28	125	3	5	3.3	0.7	0.7	19	6	0	58	tr
Product 19	1 oz.	28	110	3	tr	tr	tr	0.1	24	3	0	325	tr
Raisin Bran–Kellogg's	1 oz.	28	90	2	1	0.1	0.1	0.3	21	9	0	150	4
Raisin Bran–Post	1 oz.	28	90	2	1	0.1	0.1	0.3	21	8	0	160	4
Rice Krispies	1 oz.	28	110	2	tr	tr	tr	0.1	25	3	0	280	tr
Shredded Wheat	1 oz.	28	110	3	1	0.1	0.1	0.3	23	0	0	3	3
Special K	1 oz.	28	110	6	tr	tr	tr	tr	21	3	0	230	tr
Super Golded Crisp	1 oz.	28	105	2	tr	tr	tr	0.1	26	14	0	25	tr
Total	1 oz.	28	100	3	1	0.1	0.1	0.3	22	2	0	352	2
Trix	1 oz.	28	110	2	tr	0.2.	0.1	0.1	25	13	0	181	tr
Wheat Chex	1 oz.	28	100	3	0				23	2	0	200	2
Wheaties	1 oz.	28	100	3	tr	0.1	tr	0.2	23	2	0	354	1.8
CHEESE, natural													
blue	1 oz.	28	100	6	8	5.3	2.2	0.2	1		21	396	
brie	1 oz.	28	95	6	8				tr		28	179	
cheddar	1 oz.	28	115	7	9	6.0	2.7	0.3	tr		30	176	
shredded	1 cup	113	455	28	37	23.8	10.6	1.1	1		119	701	

FOOD	Amount	WEIGHT in grams	CALORIES	PROTEIN (g)	Total FAT (g)	Saturated FAT (g)	Mono FAT(g)	Polyunsaturated FAT (g)	CARBOHYDRATE (g)	Added SUGAR (g)	CHOLESTEROL (mg)	SODIUM (mg)	FIBER (g)
cream	1 oz.	28	100	2	10	6.2	2.8	0.4	1		31	84	
feta	1 oz.	28	75	4	6	4.2	1.3	0.2	1		25	316	
mozzarella													
whole milk	1 oz.	28	80	6	6	3.7	1.9	0.2	1		22	106	
skim milk	1 oz.	28	80	8	5	3.1	1.4	0.1	1		15	150	
muenster	1 oz.	28	105	7	9	5.4	2.5	0.2	tr		27	178	
parmesan, grated	1 tbsp.	5	25	2	2	1.0	0.4	tr	tr		4	93	
port du salut	1 oz.	28	100	7	8	4.7	2.3	0.2	tr		35	152	
provolone	1 oz.	28	100	7	8	4.8	2.1	0.2	1		20	248	
ricotta													
whole milk	1 cup	246	430	28	32	20.4	8.9	0.9	7		124	207	
skim milk	1 cup	246	340	28	19	12.1	5.7	0.6	13		76	307	
swiss	1 oz.	28	105	8	8	5.0	2.1	0.3	1		26	240	
CHEESE, pasteurized process													
American	1 oz.	28	105	6	9	5.6	2.5	0.3	tr		27	406	
Swiss	1 oz.	28	95	7	7	4.5	2.0	0.2	1		24	388	
CHEESECAKE 9" diameter	1/12 cake	92	280	5	18	9.9	5.4	1.2	26	+	170	204	
CHERRIES													
sweet, raw	10 cherries	68	50	1	1	0.1	0.2	0.2	11		0	tr	1
sour, canned, water pack	1 cup	244	90	2	tr	0.1	0.1	0.1	22		0	17	
CHESTNUTS, roasted, shelled	1 cup	143	350	5	3	0.6	1.1	1.2	76		0	3	18.5
CHICKEN													
fried w/ skin, batter dipped													
breast	4.9 oz.	140	365	35	18	4.9	7.6	4.3	13		119	385	
drumstick	2.5 oz.	72	195	16	11	3.0	4.6	2.7	6		62	194	
fried w/ skin, flour-coated													
breast	3.5 oz.	98	220	31	9	2.4	3.4	1.9	2		87	74	
drumstick	2.5 oz.	72	195	16	11	3.0	4.6	2.7	6		62	194	
fried w/ skin, flour-coated													
breast	3.5 oz.	98	220	31	9	2.4	3.4	1.9	2		87	74	

FOOD	Amount	WEIGHT in grams	CALORIES	PROTEIN (g)	Total FAT (g)	Saturated FAT (g)	Mono FAT (g)	Poly unsaturated FAT (g)	CARBOHYDRATE (g)	Added SUGAR (g)	CHOLESTEROL (mg)	SODIUM (mg)	FIBER (g)
drumstick	1.7 oz.	49	120	13	7	1.8	2.7	1.6	1		44	44	
roasted, flesh only													
breast	3 oz.	86	140	27	3	0.9	1.1	0.7	0		73	64	
drumstick	1.6 oz.	44	75	12	2	0.7	0.8	0.6	0		41	42	
stewed, light and dark, chopped (as for salad)	1 cup	140	250	38	9	2.6	3.3	2.2	0		116	98	
CHICKEN LIVER, cooked	1 liver	20	30	5	1	0.4	0.3	0.2	tr		126	10	
CHICKEN A LA KING, home recipe	1 cup	245	470	27	34	12.9	13.4	6.2	12		221	760	
CHICKEN CHOW MEIN, canned	1 cup	250	95	7	tr	0.1	0.1	0.8	18		8	725	
CHICKPEAS, cooked	1 cup	163	270	15	4	0.4	0.9	1.9	45		0	11	10
CHILI w/ beans, canned	1 cup	255	340	19	16	5.8	7.2	1.0	31		28	1354	
CHOCOLATE, baking, bitter	1 oz.	28	145	3	15	9.0	4.9	0.5	8		0	1	
CHOCOLATE SYRUP													
thin type	2 tbsp.	38	85	1	tr	0.2	0.1	0.1	22	22	0	36	
fudge type	1 tbsp.	28	125	2	5	3.1	1.7	0.2	21	22	0	42	
CLAM CHOWDER, New England, canned, condensed, prepared	1 cup	248	165	9	7	3.0	2.3	1.1	17		22	992	
CLAMS													
canned	3 oz.	85	85	13	2	0.5	0.5	0.4	2		54	102	
raw	3 oz.	85	63	11	1	0.1	0.1	0.2	2		29	47	
COCOA													
powder, no milk	3/4 oz.	21	75	1	1	0.3	0.2	tr	19		0	56	
prep. w/ 8 oz. milk		265	225	9	9	5.4	2.5	0.3	30		33	176	
powder w/ milk	1 oz.	28	100	3	1	0.6	0.3	tr	22		1	139	
COCONUT													
raw, shredded	1 cup	80	185	3	27	23.8	1.1	0.3	12		0	16	12
dried, sweetened	1 cup	93	470	3	33	29.3	1.4	0.4	44		0	244	
COFFEE CAKE, crumb, piece 2 5/8" sq.	1 piece	72	230	5	7	2.0	2.8	1.6	38		47	310	
COLLARDS, frozen	1 cup	170	60	5	1	0.1	0.1	0.4	12		0	85	
COOKIES													
chocolate chip, 2 1/4"	4 cookies	42	180	2	9	2.9	3.1	2.6	28	+	5	140	

FOOD	Amount	WEIGHT in grams	CALORIES	PROTEIN (g)	Total FAT (g)	Saturated FAT (g)	Mono FAT (g)	Poly unsaturated FAT (g)	CARBOHYDRATE (g)	Added SUGAR (g)	CHOLESTEROL (mg)	SODIUM (mg)	FIBER (g)
fig bar, 1 5/8" sq.	1 cookie	14	53	0.5	1	0.3	0.4	0.3	11	+	7	45	
oatmeal raisin	1 cookie	13	61	1	2.5	0.6	1.1	0.7	9	+	tr	37	
peanut butter	1 cookie	12	61	1	3.5	1.0	1.5	0.7	9	+	6	36	
sandwich type	1 cookie	10	49	0.5	2	0.5	0.9	0.6	7	+	0	47	
shortbread	1 cookie	8	39	0.5	2	0.7	0.8	0.3	5	+	7	31	
sugar, 2 1/2"	1 cookie	12	59	0.5	3	0.6	1.3	0.9	8	+	7	65	
vanilla wafers	10 cookies	40	185	2	7	1.8	3.0	1.8	29	+	25	150	
CORN CHIPS	1 oz. pkg.	28	155	2	9	1.4	2.4	3.7	16		0	233	
CORN													
ear 5" x 1 3/4"	1 ear	77	85	3	1	0.2	0.3	0.5	19		0	13	4
kernals, canned	1 cup	210	165	5	1	0.2	0.3	0.5	41		0	571	11
cream style, canned	1 cup	256	185	4	1	0.2	0.3	0.5	46	often	0	730	
CORNMEAL, enriched, degermed, dry	1 cup	138	500	11	2	0.2	0.4	0.9	108		0	1	
COTTAGE CHEESE													
4% large curd	1 cup	225	235	28	10	6.4	2.9	0.3	6		34	911	
1% low -fat	1 cup	226	180	28	2	1.4	0.6	tr	8		10	840	
nonfat	1 cup	145	125	25	1	0.4	0.2	tr	3		10	19	
CRABMEAT, canned	1 cup	135	135	23	3	0.5	0.8	1.4	1		135	1350	
CRACKERS													
cheese, 1" sq.	10 crackers	10	50	1	3	0.9	1.2	0.3	6		6	112	
cheese/ peanut butter sand.	1 cracker	8	40	1	2	0.4	0.8	0.3	5		1	90	
saltines	4 crackers	12	50	1	1	0.5	0.4	0.2	9		4	165	
snack type	1 round	3	15	tr	1	0.2	0.4	0.1	2		0	30	
wheat, thin	4 crackers	8	35	1	1	0.5	0.5	0.4	5		0	69	
CRANBERRIES	1/2 cup	76	35	tr	tr				8		0	2	
CRANBERRY JUICE COCKTAIL, regular	1 cup	253	145	tr	tr	tr	tr	0.1	38	+	0	10	
CRANBERRY SAUCE, canned	1 cup	277	420	1	tr	tr	0.1	0.2	108	+	0	80	
CREAM													
half & half	1 tbsp.	15	20	tr	2	1.1	0.5	0.1	1		6	6	
" "	1 cup	242	315	7	28	17.3	8.0	1.0	10		89	98	
light cream	1 tbsp.	15	30	tr	3	1.8	0.8	0.1	1		10	6	
" "	1 cup	240	470	6	46	28.8	13.4	1.7	9		159	95	

FOOD	Amount	WEIGHT in grams	CALORIES	PROTEIN (g)	Total FAT (g)	Saturated FAT (g)	Mono FAT (g)	Poly unsaturated FAT (g)	CARBOHYDRATE (g)	Added SUGAR (g)	CHOLESTEROL (mg)	SODIUM (mg)	FIBER (g)
whipping, heavy	1 tbsp.	15	50	tr	6	3.5	1.6	0.2	tr		21	6	
" "	1 cup	238	820	5	88	54.8	25.4	3.3	7		326	89	
CREAM PRODUCTS, imitation													
nondairy creamer, frozen	1 tbsp.	15	20	tr	1	1.4	tr	tr	2		0	12	
powdered	1 tbsp.	2	10	tr	1	0.7	tr	tr	1		0	4	
whipped topping, frozen	1 cup	75	240	1	19	16.3	1.2	0.4	17	+	0	19	
" " "	1 tbsp.	4	15	tr	1	0.9	0.1	tr	1	+	0	1	
powdered, made w/ whole milk	1 cup	80	150	3	10	8.5	0.7	0.2	8	+	13	121	
" " " "	1 tbsp.	4	10	tr	tr	0.4	tr	tr	1	+	tr	3	
pressurized	1 tbsp.	4	10	tr	1	0.6	0.1	tr	1		0	2	
CROISSANTS	1 reg.	57	235	5	12	3.5	6.7	1.4	27		13	452	
CUCUMBER	6 lg. or 8 sm. slices	28	5	tr	tr	tr	tr	tr	1		0	1	tr
CURRENTS, eur, black	1 cup	112	71	2	tr	tr	0.1	0.2	17		0	2	6
CUSTARD, baked	1 cup	265	305	14	15	6.8	5.4	0.7	29	+	278	209	
DANDELION GREENS	1 cup	105	35	2	1	0.1	tr	0.3	7		0	46	
DANISH, pastry w/ fruit	1 pastry	65	235	4	13	3.9	5.2	2.9	28	+	56	233	
DATES, pitted	10 dates	83	230	2	tr	0.1	0.1	tr	61		0	2	7
DOUGHNUTS, cake type, 3 1/4"	1 donut	50	210	3	12	2.8	5.0	3.0	24	+	20	192	
DUCK, roasted, flesh only	1/2 duck	221	445	52	25	9.2	8.2	3.2	0		197	144	
EGGNOG, commercial	1 cup	254	340	10	19	11.3	5.7	0.9	34	+	149	138	
EGGPLANT, steamed	1 cup	96	25	1	tr	tr	tr	0.1	6		0	3	2.5
EGGS													
whole	1 egg	50	80	6	6	1.7	2.2	0.7	1		274	69	
white only	1 white	33	15	3	tr	0	0	0	tr		0	50	
ENCHILADA	1	230	235	20	16	7.7	6.7	0.6	24		19	4451	
ENGLISH MUFFIN	1 plain	50	140	5	1	0.3	0.2	0.3	27		0	378	
FIGS, dried	10	187	475	6	2	0.4	0.5	1.0	122		0	21	30
FILBERTS (hazelnuts)	1 oz.	28	180	4	18	1.3	13.9	1.7	4		0	1	
FISH STICKS, frozen	1 stick	28	70	6	3	0.8	1.4	0.8	4		26	53	
FISH, see name such as flounder, trout, etc.													

FOOD	Amount	WEIGHT in grams	CALORIES	PROTEIN (g)	Total FAT (g)	Saturated FAT (g)	Mono FAT (g)	Poly unsaturated FAT (g)	CARBOHYDRATE (g)	Added SUGAR (g)	CHOLESTEROL (mg)	SODIUM (mg)	FIBER (g)
FLOUNDER, baked without added fat	3 oz.	85	80	17	1	0.3	0.2	0.4	tr		59	111	
FLOUR													
white, all purp., unsifted	1 cup	125	455	13	1	0.2	0.1	0.5	95		0	3	4
whole wheat	1 cup	120	400	16	2	0.3	0.3	1.1	85		0	4	11.5
FRENCH TOAST	1 slice	65	155	6	7	1.6	2.0	1.6	17		112	257	
FRUIT COCKTAIL,													
canned, fruit & juice in heavy syrup	1 cup	255	185	1	tr	tr	tr	0.1tr	48	19	0	15	
juice pack	1 cup	248	115	1	tr	tr	tr	tr	29		0	10	3
FRUIT DRINKS or punch													
fruit punch	6 oz.	190	85	tr	0	0	0	0	22	+	0	15	
grape	6 oz.	187	100	tr	0	0	0	0	26	+	0	11	
pineapple/ grapefruit	6 oz.	187	90	tr	tr	tr	tr	tr	23	+	0	24	
FRUITCAKE, dark	2/3" piece	43	165	2	7	1.5	3.6	1.6	25	+	20	67	
GELATIN, dry	1 pkt.	7	25	6	tr	tr	tr	tr	0		0	6	
GELATIN DESSERT, prepared	1/2 cup	120	70	2	0	0	0	0	17	17	0	55	
GRAHAM CRACKERS, 2 1/2"	2 crkrs.	14	60	1	1	0.4	0.6	0.4	11	+	0	86	
GRAPEFRUIT, 3 3/4"	1/2 fruit	120	40	1	tr	tr	tr	tr	10		0	tr	1.5
GRAPEFRUIT JUICE	1 cup	247	95	1	tr	tr	tr	0.1	23		0	2	
GRAPES	10 grapes	50	35	tr	tr	0.1	tr	0.1	9		0	1	1
GRAPE JUICE, bottle	1 cup	253	155	1	tr	0.1	tr	0.1	38		0	8	
GRAVIES													
canned beef	1 cup	233	125	9	5	2.7	2.3	0.2	11		7	117	
canned chicken	1 cup	238	190	5	14	3.4	6.1	3.6	13		5	1373	
mix, brown	1 cup	261	80	3	2	0.9	0.8	0.1	14		2	1147	
GRITS	1 cup	247	145	3	tr	tr	0.1	0.2	31		0	0	1
GUAVAS	1 fruit	90	45	1	1	0.2	0.1	0.2	11		0	2	
HADDOCK, cooked	3 oz.	85	95	21	1	0.1	0.1	0.3	0		63	74	
HALIBUT, broiled	3 oz.	85	140	20	6	3.3	1.6	0.7	tr		62	103	
HAM													
roasted, lean and fat	3 oz.	85	205	18	14	5.1	6.7	1.5	0		53	1009	
roasted, lean	3 oz.	85	131	21	5	1.6	2.1	0.5	0		46	1128	
luncheon pack 1 oz. slice													

FOOD	Amount	WEIGHT in grams	CALORIES	PROTEIN (g)	Total FAT (g)	Saturated FAT (g)	Mono FAT (g)	Poly unsaturated FAT (g)	CARBOHYDRATE (g)	Added SUGAR (g)	CHOLESTEROL (mg)	SODIUM (mg)	FIBER (g)
reg. cooked	2 slices	57	105	10	6	1.9	2.8	0.7	2		32	751	
lean cooked	2 slices	57	75	11	3	0.9	1.3	0.3	1		27	815	
HERRING, pickled	3 oz.	85	190	17	13	4.3	4.6	3.1	0		85	850	
HOLLANDAISE SAUCE (mix)	1 cup	259	240	5	20	11.6	5.9	0.9	14		52	1564	
HONEY	1 tbsp.	21	65	tr	0	0	0	0	17	17	0	1	
HONEYDEW MELON, 6 1/2"	1/10 melon	129	45	1	tr	tr	tr	0.1	12		0	13	
HOT DOGS (frankfurters) 10 per pound pkg.													
beef	1 dog	45	142	5	13	5.4	6.1	0.6	tr		27	462	
chicken	1 dog	45	115	6	9	2.5	3.8	1.8	3		45	616	
meat	1 dog	45	145	5	13	4.8	6.2	1.2	1		23	504	
ICE CREAM, vanilla													
reg. (11% fat)	1 cup	133	270	5	14	8.9	4.1	0.5	32	+	59	116	
rich (16% fat)	1 cup	148	350	4	24	4.7	6.8	0.9	32	+	88	108	
ICE MILK, vanilla (4% fat)	1 cup	131	185	5	6	3.5	1.6	0.2	29	+	18	105	
JAMS and preserves	1 tbsp.	20	55	tr	tr	0	tr	tr	14	+	0	2	
JELLIES	1 tbsp.	18	50	tr	tr	tr	tr	tr	13	+	0	5	
KALE, chopped	1 cup	130	40	2	1	0.1	tr	0.3	7		0	30	
KIWIFRUIT, peeled	1 fruit	76	45	1	tr	tr	0.1	0.1	11		0	4	tr
KOHLRABI, cooked & diced	1 cup	165	50	3	tr	tr	tr	0.1	11		0	35	2
LAMB													
loin chop, broiled													
lean and fat	2.8 oz.	80	235	22	16	7.3	6.4	1.0	0		78	62	
lean only	2.8 oz.	77	168	23	7	3.1	2.9	0.5	0		72	65	
leg, roasted, lean & fat	3 oz.	85	205	22	13	5.6	4.9	0.8	0		78	57	
rib, roasted													
lean & fat	3 oz.	85	315	18	26	12.1	10.6	1.5	0		77	60	
lean only	3 oz.	85	195	23	11	4.8	4.5	0.8	0		75	69	
LARD	1 tbsp.	13	115	0	13	5.1	5.9	1.5	0		12	0	
LEEKS, cooked	1 leek	124	38	1	tr	tr	tr	0.1	10		0	13	1.5
LEMONADE, fresh frozen	6 oz.	185	80	tr	tr	tr	tr	tr	21	+	0	1	
LEMONS, 4 / lb	1 lemon	58	15	1	tr	tr	tr	0.1	5		0	1	
LEMON JUICE	1 tbsp.	15	5	tr	tr	tr	tr	tr	1		0	tr	

FOOD	Amount	WEIGHT in grams	CALORIES	PROTEIN (g)	Total FAT (g)	Saturated FAT (g)	Mono FAT (g)	Poly unsaturated FAT (g)	CARBOHYDRATE (g)	Added SUGAR (g)	CHOLESTEROL (mg)	SODIUM (mg)	FIBER (g)
LENTILS, dry, cooked	1 cup	200	215	16	1	0.1	0.2	0.5	38		0	26	8
LETTUCE													
iceberg, chopped	1 cup	55	5	1	tr	tr	tr	0.1	1		0	5	1
loose-leaf	1 cup	56	10	1	tr	tr	tr	0.1	2		0	5	1
LIMES (use lemon figures)													
LIVER, beef, fried	3 oz.	85	185	23	7	2.5	3.6	1.3	7		410	90	
LOBSTER, steamed	3 oz.	85	83	17	1	0.1	0.1	0.1	1		61	323	
MACADAMIA NUTS	1 oz.	28	205	2	22	3.2	17.1	0.4	4		0	74	
MACARONI, cooked firm stage	1 cup	130	190	7	1	0.1	0.1	0.3	39		0	1	
MACARONI & CHEESE home recipe	1 cup	200	430	17	22	9.8	7.4	3.6	40		44	1086	
MACKEREL, cooked	3 oz.	85	223	20	15	3.5	6.0	3.7	0		64	71	
MANGOES, 1 1/2 lb	1 mango	207	135	1	1	0.1	0.2	0.1	35		0	4	3
MARGARINE imitation (40% fat)													
soft	1 tbsp.	14	50	tr	5	1.1	2.2	1.9	tr		0	134	
"	1 cup	227	785	1	88	17.5	35.6	31.3	1		0	2178	
regular (80% fat)													
hard, stick	1/2 cup	113	810	1	91	17.9	40.5	28.7	1		0	1066	
hard	1 tbsp.	14	75	tr	9	2.0	3.6	2.5	0		0	139	
hard 1/3" pat	1 pat	5	25	tr	3	0.7	1.3	0.9	0		0	50	
soft	1 cup	114	813	1	91	15.7	32.4	39.3	1		0	1225	
"	1 tbsp.	14	75	tr	9	1.8	4.4	1.9	0		0	139	
spread (60% fat)													
hard, stick	1/2 cup	113	610	1	69	15.9	29.4	20.5	0		0	1123	
hard	1 tbsp.	14	75	tr	9	2.0	3.6	2.5	0		0	139	
hard, 1/3" pat	1 pat	5	25	tr	3	0.7	1.3	0.9	0		0	50	
soft	1/2 cup	114	613	1	69	14.6	35.6	15.7	0		0	1128	
"	1 tbsp.	14	75	tr	9	1.8	4.4	1.9	0		0	139	
MAYONNAISE													
regular	1 tbsp.	14	100	tr	11	1.7	3.2	5.8	tr		8	80	
imitation	1 tbsp.	15	35	tr	3	0.5	0.7	1.6	2		4	75	
MILK, fluid, no millk solids added													

FOOD	Amount	WEIGHT in grams	CALORIES	PROTEIN (g)	Total FAT (g)	Saturated FAT (g)	Mono FAT (g)	Pcly unsaturated FAT (g)	CARBOHYDRATE (g)	Added SUGAR (g)	CHOLESTEROL (mg)	SODIUM (mg)	FIBER (g)
whole (3.3%)	1 cup	244	150	8	8	5.1	2.4	0.3	11		33	120	
low-fat (2%)	1 cup	244	120	8	5	2.9	1.4	0.2	12		18	122	
low-fat (1%)	1 cup	244	100	8	3	1.6	0.7	0.1	12		10	123	
skim, nonfat	1 cup	245	85	8	tr	0.3	0.1	tr	12		4	126	
buttermilk	1 cup	245	100	8	2	1.3	0.6	0.1	12		9	257	
MILK, canned													
condensed, sweetened	1 cup	306	980	24	27	16.8	7.4	1.0	166	+	104	389	
evaporated, whole	1 cup	252	340	17	19	11.6	5.9	0.6	25		74	267	
evaporated, skim	1 cup	255	200	19	1	0.3	0.2	tr	29		9	293	
MILK, dried, nonfat, unmixed	1 cup	68	245	24	tr	0.3	0.1	tr	35	12	373		
MILK, chocolate, commercial													
regular	1 cup	250	210	8	8	5.3	2.5	0.3	26	15	31	149	
low-fat (1%)	1 cup	250	160	8	3	1.5	0.8	0.1	26	14	7	152	
MISO	1 cup	276	470	29	13	1.8	2.6	7.3	65		0	8142	8
MIXED NUTS w/ peanuts, salted	1 oz.	28	175	5	16	2.5	9.0	3.8	6		0	185	
MOLASSES	2 tbsp.	40	85	0	0	0	0	0	22	22	0	38	
MUFFINS, commercial mix (use to estimate home recipe)													
blueberry	1 muffin	45	140	3	5	1.4	2.0	1.2	22		45	225	1
bran	1 muffin	45	140	3	4	1.3	1.6	1.0	24		28	385	4
corn	1 muffin	45	145	3	6	1.7	2.3	1.4	22		42	291	
MUSHROOMS													
raw, sliced	1 cup	70	20	1	tr	tr	tr	0.1	3		0	3	2
canned, drained	1 cup	35	35	3	tr	0.1	tr	0.2	8		0	663	
MUSSELS, steamed	3 oz.	85	147	20	4	0.7	0.9	1.0	6		48	313	
MUSTARD, prepared	1 tsp.	5	5	tr	tr	tr	0.2	tr	tr		0	63	
MUSTARD GREENS	1 cup	140	20	3	tr	tr	0.2	0.1	3		0	22	1
NECTARINES, 3 / lb	1 fruit	136	65	1	1	0.1	0.2	0.3	16		0	tr	
NOODLES (egg type) cooked	1 cup	160	200	7	2	0.5	0.6	0.6	37		57	3	
NOODLES, chow mein	1 cup	45	220	6	11	2.1	7.3	0.4	26		5	450	
OILS, salad or cooking													
corn	1 tbsp.	14	125	0	14	1.8	3.4	8.2	0		0	0	
olive	1 tbsp.	14	125	0	14	1.9	10.3	1.2	0		0	0	

FOOD	Amount	WEIGHT in grams	CALORIES	PROTEIN (g)	Total FAT (g)	Saturated FAT (g)	Mono FAT (g)	Poly unsaturated FAT (g)	CARBOHYDRATE (g)	Added SUGAR (g)	CHOLESTEROL (mg)	SODIUM (mg)	FIBER (g)
peanut	1 tbsp.	14	125	0	14	2.4	6.5	4.5	0		0	0	
safflower	1 tbsp.	14	125	0	14	1.3	1.7	10.4	0		0	0	
soybean	1 tbsp.	14	125	0	14	2	3.1	7.8	0		0	0	
soybean, hydrogenated	1 tbsp.	14	125	0	14	2.1	6.0	5.3	0		0	0	
soybean-cottonseed blend, hydrogenated	1 tbsp.	14	125	0	14	2.5	4.1	6.7	0		0	0	
sunflower	1 tbsp.	14	125	0	14	1.4	2.7	9.2	0		0	0	
OKRA, 3", cooked	8 pods	85	25	2	tr	tr	tr	tr	6		0	274	2.5
OLIVES, canned													
green	4 med. or 3 Xlg.	13	15	tr	2	0.2	1.2	0.1	tr		0	312	0.5
black (U.S.)	3 med. or 2 lg.	9	15	tr	2	0.3	1.3	0.2	tr		0	68	tr
Greek black, salt cure	2 med.	5	16	tr	2	0.2	1.4	0.4	tr		0	85	tr
ONIONS													
raw, chopped	1 cup	160	55	2	tr	0.1	0.1	0.2	12		0	3	1.5
cooked	1 cup	210	60	2	tr	0.1	tr	0.1	13		0	17	2.5
ONION RINGS, frozen, breaded, panfried	2 rings	20	80	1	5	1.7	2.2	1.0	8		0	75	
ORANGES, 2 1/2"/lb	1 orange	131	60	1	tr	tr	tr	tr	15		0	tr	2.5
ORANGE JUICE	1 cup	248	110	2	tr	0.1	0.1	0.1	26		0	2	
OYSTERS													
raw, meat only (13-19 selects)	1 cup	240	160	20	4	1.4	0.5	1.4	8		120	175	
breaded, fried	1 oyster	45	90	5	5	1.4	2.1	1.4	5		35	70	
PANCAKES, 4" diameter	1 pancake	27	60	2	2	0.5	0.9	0.5	8		16	160	
PAPAYAS, 1/2" cubes	1 cup	140	65	1	tr	0.1	0.1	tr	17		0	9	1.5
PARSLEY, dried	1 tbsp.	0.4	tr	tr	tr	tr	tr	tr	tr		0	2	
PARSNIPS, diced	1 cup	156	125	2	tr	0.1	0.2	0.1	30		0	16	5
PASTRAMI	1 oz.	28	99	5	8	3.0	4.1	0.3	1		26	348	
PEACHES													
fresh, raw, 4 / lb	1 peach	87	35	1	tr	tr	tr	tr	10		0	tr	2
juice pack	1 half	77	35	tr	tr	tr	tr	tr	9		0	3	
dried, uncooked	1 cup	160	380	6	1	0.1	0.4	0.6	98		0	11	

FOOD	Amount	WEIGHT in grams	CALORIES	PROTEIN (g)	Total FAT (g)	Saturated FAT (g)	Mono FAT (g)	Poly unsaturated FAT (g)	CARBOHYDRATE (g)	Added SUGAR (g)	CHOLESTEROL (mg)	SODIUM (mg)	FIBER (g)
canned fruit & liquid heavy syrup	1 half	81	60	tr	tr	tr	tr	tr	16	/	0	5	
frozen, sweetened	1 cup	250	235	2	tr	tr	0.1	0.2	60	+	0	15	
PEANUTS, roasted, salted	1 oz.	28	165	8	14	1.9	6.9	4.4	5		0	122	
PEANUTBUTTER	1 tbsp.	16	95	5	8	1.4	4.0	2.5	3		0	75	0.5
PEARS													
fresh, w/ skin 2 1/2 /lb	1 pear	166	100	1	1	tr	0.1	0.2	25		0	tr	4
canned, fruit & liquid heavy syrup	1 half	79	60	tr	tr	tr	tr	tr	15	5	0	4	
juice pack	1 half	77	40	tr	tr	tr	tr	tr	10		0	3	
PEAS													
black-eyed fresh	1 cup	165	180	13	1	0.3	0.1	0.6	30		0	7	4.5
dried, cooked	1 cup	250	190	13	1	0.2	tr	0.3	35		0	20	
green, frozen	1 cup	160	125	8	tr	0.1	tr	0.2	23		0	139	8
snow pea (edible pod)	1 cup	160	65	5	tr	0.1	tr	0.2	11		0	6	2.5
split, dry, cooked	1 cup	200	230	16	1	0.1	0.1	9.3	42		0	26	4.5
PECANS, halves	1 oz.	28	190	2	19	1.5	12.0	4.7	5		0	tr	
PEPPERS													
hot chili	1 pepper	45	20	1	tr	tr	tr	tr	4		0	3	
sweet, 5 / lb	1 pepper	74	20	1	tr	tr	tr	0.2	4		0	2	1
PERCH, ocean													
broiled	3 oz.	85	103	20	2	0.3	0.7	0.5	0			82	
fried, breaded	1 fillet	85	185	16	11	2.6	4.6	2.8	7		66	138	
PICKLES CUCUMBER													
dill, whole, 3–3 1/4"	1 pickle	65	5	tr	tr	tr	tr	0.1	1		0	928	
fresh pack, 1/4"	2 slices	15	10	tr	tr	tr	tr	tr	3		0	101	
sweet gherkin, 2 1/2"	1 pickle	15	20	tr	tr	tr	tr	tr	5		0	107	
PICKLE RELISH, sweet	1 tbsp.	15	20	tr	tr	tr	tr	tr	5		0	107	
PIE CRUST, 9" diameter	1 shell	180	900	11	60	14.8	25.9	15.7	79		0	1100	
PIES, piece is 1/6 of 9" pie													
apple	1 piece	158	405	3	18	4.6	7.4	4.4	60	17	0	476	
cherry	1 piece	158	410	4	18	4.7	7.7	4.6	61	33	0	480	

FOOD	Amount	WEIGHT in grams	CALORIES	PROTEIN (g)	Total FAT (g)	Saturated FAT (g)	Mono FAT (g)	Poly unsaturated FAT (g)	CARBOHYDRATE (g)	Added SUGAR (g)	CHOLESTEROL (mg)	SODIUM (mg)	FIBER (g)
creme	1 piece	152	455	3	23	15.0	4.0	1.1	59	33	8	369	
custard	1 piece	152	330	9	17	5.6	6.7	3.2	36	17	169	436	
lemon meringue	1 piece	140	355	5	14	4.3	5.7	2.9	53	35	143	395	
pecan	1 piece	138	575	7	32	4.7	17	7.9	71	60	95	305	
pumpkin	1 piece	152	320	6	17	6.4	6.7	3.0	37	23	109	325	
PIES, fried													
apple (or cherry)	1 pie	85	255	2	14	5.8	6.6	0.6	31	+	14	326	
PINEAPPLE													
fresh, diced	1 cup	155	75	1	1	tr	0.1	0.2	19		0	2	2.5
canned, crushed or pieces, heavy syrup	1 cup	255	200	1	tr	tr	tr	0.1	52	13	0	3	
juice pack	1 cup	250	150	1	tr	tr	tr	0.1	39		0	3	
PINEAPPLE JUICE	1 cup	250	140	1	tr	tr	tr	0.1	34		0	3	
PINE NUTS (piñones)	1 oz.	28	160	3	17	2.7	6.5	7.3	5		0	2	
PISTACHIO NUTS, shelled	1 oz.	28	165	6	14	1.7	9.3	2.1	7		0	2	
PIZZA, cheese (slice is 1/8 of 15")	1 slice	120	290	15	9	4.1	2.6	1.3	39		56	699	
PLANTAINS	1 fruit	179	220	2	1	0.3	0.1	0.1	57		0	7	
PLUMS													
fresh, 6 1/2 / lb	1 plum	66	35	1	tr	tr	0.3	0.1	9		0	tr	1.5
canned, fruit & liquid, heavy syrup	3 plums	133	120	tr	tr	tr	0.1	tr	31	17	0	25	
juice pack	3 plums	95	55	tr	tr	tr	tr	tr	14		0	1	
POPCORN, unbuttered													
air-popped, unsalted	1 cup	8	30	1	tr	tr	0.1	0.2	6		0	tr	2.5
oil-popped, salted	1 cup	11	55	1	3	0.5	1.4	1.2	6		0	86	
POPSICLE, 3 fl oz.	1 pop	95	70	0	0	0	0	0	18		0	11	
PORK, fresh, not cured													
loin, broiled													
lean & fat	3 oz.	85	294	20	23	8.4	10.6	2.6	0		80	56	
lean only	3 oz.	85	218	24	13	4.5	5.8	1.6	0		81	64	
loin, center rib, broiled													
lean & fat	3 oz.	85	291	21	22	8.1	10.3	2.5	0		79	52	
lean only	3 oz.	85	219	25	13	4.4	5.7	1.5	0		80	57	

FOOD	Amount	WEIGHT in grams	CALORIES	PROTEIN (g)	Total FAT (g)	Saturated FAT (g)	Mono FAT (g)	Poly unsaturated FAT (g)	CARBOHYDRATE (g)	Added SUGAR (g)	CHOLESTEROL (mg)	SODIUM (mg)	FIBER (g)
loin, center rib, pan-fried (as a chop)													
lean & fat	3 oz.	85	331	18	28	10.1	12.9	3.2	0		71	38	
lean only	3 oz.	85	219	24	13	4.8	5.8	1.6	0		69	43	
shoulder, roasted													
lean & fat	3 oz.	85	277	19	22	7.9	10.0	2.5	0		81	58	
lean only	3 oz.	85	207	22	13	4.4	5.7	1.5	0		82	65	
POTATO CHIPS	10 chips	20	105	1	7	1.8	1.2	3.6	10		0	94	
POTATOES, cooked													
baked, 2 / lb													
w/ skin	1 potato	202	220	5	tr	0.1	tr	0.1	51		0	16	4
flesh only	1 potato	156	145	3	tr	tr	tr	0.1	34		0	8	
boiled, peeled before boil													
3 / lb unpeeled	1 potato	135	115	2	tr	tr	tr	0.1	27		0	7	1.5
french fries, frozen, strips 2"–3 1/2"													
heat in oven	10 strips	50	110	2	4	2.1	1.8	0.3	17		0	16	
fry in oil	10 strips	50	160	2	8	2.5	1.6	3.8	20		0	108	
hash browns	1 cup	156	340	5	18	7.0	8.0	2.1	44		0	53	
mashed w/ milk only	1 cup	210	160	4	1	0.7	0.3	0.1	37		4	636	
scalloped, from dry mix	1 cup	245	230	5	11	6.5	3.0	0.5	31		27	835	
PRETZELS													
stick, 2 1/4" long, thin	10 sticks	3	10	tr	tr	tr	tr	tr	2		0	48	
twisted, 2 3/4"	1 pretzel	16	65	2	1	0.1	0.2	0.2	13		0	258	
PRUNES, dried	5 lg. or 4 Xlg.	49	115	1	tr	tr	0.2	0.1	31		0	2	8
PRUNE JUICE	1 cup	256	180	2	tr	tr	0.1	tr	45		0	10	
PUDDINGS													
canned													
chocolate	5-oz. can	142	205	3	11	9.5	0.5	0.1	30	+	1	285	
vanilla	5-oz. can	142	220	2	10	9.5	0.2	0.1	33	+	1	305	
dry mix made w/ whole milk	1/2 cup	130	155	4	4	2.3	1.1	0.2	27	+	14	440	
PUMPKIN													
fresh, mashed	1 cup	245	50	2	tr	0.1	tr	tr	12		0	2	

FOOD	Amount	WEIGHT in grams	CALORIES	PROTEIN (g)	Total FAT (g)	Saturated FAT (g)	Mono FAT (g)	Poly unsaturated FAT (g)	CARBOHYDRATE (g)	Added SUGAR (g)	CHOLESTEROL (mg)	SODIUM (mg)	FIBER (g)
canned	1 cup	245	85	3	1	0.4	0.1	tr	20		0	12	
PUMPKINSEED KERNEL	1 oz.	28	155	7	13	2.5	4.0	5.9	5		0	5	
QUICHE LORRAINE 1/8 of 8"	1 piece	176	600	13	48	23.2	17.8	4.1	29		285	653	
RADISHES	4 rad	18	5	tr	tr	tr	tr	tr	1		0	4	tr
RAISINS, seedless													
not pressed down	1 cup	145	435	5	1	0.2	tr	0.2	115		0	17	10
1/2 oz. packet	1 pkt.	14	40	tr	tr	tr	tr	tr	11		0	2	1
RASPBERRIES													
fresh	1 cup	123	60	1	1	tr	0.1	0.4	14		0	tr	9
frozen, sweetened	1 cup	250	255	2	tr	tr	tr	0.2	65		0	3	
RHUBARB, cooked w/ sugar	1 cup	240	280	1	tr	tr	tr	0.1	75		0	2	4.5
RICE, cooked, no butter/ margarine added													
brown	1 cup	195	230	5	1	0.3	0.3	0.4	50		0	0	
white	1 cup	205	225	4	tr	0.1	0.1	0.1	50		0	0	
ROLLS, commercial													
dinner, 2 1/2"	1 roll	28	85	2	2	0.5	0.8	0.6	14		tr	155	
hot dog or hamburger bun, 8 to pkg.	1 roll	40	115	3	2	0.5	0.8	0.6			tr	241	
hard, 3 3/4"	1 roll	50	155	5	2	0.4	0.5	0.6	30		tr	313	
submarine, 11 1/2"	1 roll	135	400	11	8	1.8	3.0	2.2	72		tr	683	
SALAD DRESSINGS, commercial, regular													
blue cheese	1 tbsp.	15	75	1	8	1.5	1.8	4.2	1		3	164	
French	1 tbsp.	16	85	tr	9	1.4	4.0	3.5	1		0	188	
Italian	1 tbsp.	15	80	tr	9	1.3	3.7	3.2	1		0	162	
thousand island	1 tbsp.	16	60	tr	6	1.0	1.3	3.2	2		4	112	
SALAD DRESSINGS, commercial, low calorie													
French	1 tbsp.	16	25	tr	2	0.2	0.3	1.0	2		0	306	
Italian	1 tbsp.	15	10	tr	tr	tr	tr	tr	2		0	136	
SALAD DRESSING, vinegar & oil													
vinaigrette	1 tbsp.	16	70	0	8	1.5	2.4	3.9	tr		0	tr	

FOOD	Amount	WEIGHT in grams	CALORIES	PROTEIN (g)	Total FAT (g)	Saturated FAT (g)	Mono FAT (g)	Poly unsaturated FAT (g)	CARBOHYDRATE (g)	Added SUGAR (g)	CHOLESTEROL (mg)	SODIUM (mg)	FIBER (g)
SALAMI													
beef beer	1 slice	23	76	3	7	3.0	3.2	0.3	tr		14	236	
cooked type, 1-oz slice	2 slices	57	145	8	11	4.6	5.2	1.2	1		37	607	
dry type, (hard) 12 slices / 4 oz.	2 slices	20	85	5	7	2.4	3.4	0.6	1		16	372	
SALMON													
canned (pink)	3 oz.	85	140	17	5	0.9	1.5	2.1	0		34	443	
baked	3 oz.	85	140	21	5	1.2	2.4	1.4	0		60	55	
smoked	3 oz.	85	150	18	8	2.6	3.9	0.7	0		51	1700	
SARDINES, oil pack	3 oz.	85	175	29	9	2.1	3.7	2.9	0		85	425	
SAUERKRAUT	1 cup	236	45	2	tr	0.1	tr	0.1	10		0	1560	
SAUSAGES													
brown & serve	1 link	13	50	2	5	1.7	2.2	0.5	tr		9	105	
Italian	1 link	67	217	13	17	6.1	8.0	2.2	1		52	618	
pork link 16 / lb	1 link	13	50	3	4	1.4	1.8	0.5	tr		11	168	
patties	1 patty	27	100	5	8	2.9	3.8	1.0	tr		22	349	
Vienna	1 sausage	16	45	2	4	1.5	2.0	0.3	tr		8	152	
SCALLOPS breaded, frozen	6 scallops	90	195	15	10	2.5	4.1	2.5	10		70	298	
SESAME SEEDS	1 tbsp.	8	45	2	4	0.6	1.7	1.9	1		0	3	
SHERBERT	1 cup	193	270	2	4	2.4	1.1	0.1	59	+	14	88	
SHORTENING, vegetable	1 cup	205	1810	0	205	51.3	91.2	53.5	0		0	0	0
"	1 tbsp.	13	115	0	13	3.3	5.8	3.4	0		0	0	0
SHRIMP													
fresh, steamed	3 oz.	85	84	18	1	0.2	0.2	0.4	0			190	
fried	3 oz.	85	200	16	10	2.5	4.1	2.6	11		168	384	
SNAPPER, broiled	3 oz.	85	109	22	2	0.3	0.3	0.5	0		40	48	
SOLE, see flounder													
SOUPS, condensed, prepared w/ equal vol. of milk													
cream of chicken	1 cup	248	190	7	11	4.6	4.5	1.6	15		27	1047	
cream of mushroom	1 cup	248	205	6	14	5.1	3.0	4.6	15		20	1076	
tomato	1 cup	248	160	6	6	2.9	1.6	1.1	22		17	932	
SOUPS, condensed, prepared w/ equal volume of water													

FOOD	Amount	WEIGHT in grams	CALORIES	PROTEIN (g)	Total FAT (g)	Saturated FAT (g)	Mono FAT (g)	Poly unsaturated FAT (g)	CARBOHYDRATE (g)	Added SUGAR (g)	CHOLESTEROL (mg)	SODIUM (mg)	FIBER (g)
bean w/ bacon	1 cup	253	170	8	6	1.5	2.2	1.8	23		3	951	
chicken noodle	1 cup	24 i	75	4	2	0.7	1.1	0.6	9		7	1106	
chicken rice	1 cup	241	60	4	2	0.5	0.9	0.4	7		7	815	
minestrone	1 cup	241	80	4	3	0.6	0.7	1.1	11		2	911	
pea, green	1 cup	250	165	9	3	1.4	1.0	0.4	27		0	988	
tomato	1 cup	244	85	2	2	0.4	0.4	1.0	17		0	690	
vegetable beef	1 cup	244	80	6	2	0.9	0.8	0.1	10		5	1890	
vegetarian	1 cup	241	70	2	2	0.3	0.8	0.7	12		0	822	
SOUPS, dehydrated, prepared w/ water, 1 pkt. makes 6 fl oz.													
chicken noodle	1 pkt.	188	40	2	1	0.2	0.4	0.3	6		2	957	
onion	1 pkt.	184	20	1	tr	0.1	0.2	0.1	4		0	635	
tomato vegetable	1 pkt.	189	40	1	1	0.3	0.2	0.1	8		0	856	
SOUR CREAM	1 cup	230	495	7	48	30.0	13.9	1.8	10		102	123	
" "	1 tbsp.	12	25	tr	3	1.6	0.7	0.1	1		5	6	
SOYBEANS, dry, cooked	1 cup	180	135	20	10	1.3	1.9	5.3	19		0	4	
SOY SAUCE	1 tbsp.	18	10	2	0	0	0	0	2		0	1029	
SPAGHETTI, al dente	1 cup	130	190	7	1	0.1	0.1	0.3	39		0	1	
SPINACH													
raw, chopped	1 cup	55	10	2	tr	tr	tr	0.1	2		0	43	1
cooked, leaf	1 cup	190	55	6	tr	0.1	tr	0.2	10		0	163	5
SPINACH SOUFFLE	1 cup	136	220	11	18	7.1	6.8	3.1	3		184	763	
SQUASH, cooked													
summer, sliced	1 cup	180	35	2	1	0.1	tr	0.2	.8		0	2	3
winter, baked	1 cup	205	80	2	1	0.3	0.1	0.5	18		0	2	2.5
STRAWBERRIES													
fresh, whole	1 cup	149	45	1	1	tr	0.1	0.3	10		0	1	3
frozen, sweetened	1 cup	225	245	1	tr	tr	tr	0.2	66		0	8	
STUFFING, bread, dry type	1 cup	140	500	9	31	6.1	13.3	9.6	50		0	1254	
SUGAR													
brown, packed	1 cup	220	820	0	0	0	0	0	212	212	0	97	
powdered, white	1 cup	100	385	0	0	0	0	0	100	100	0	2	

FOOD	Amount	WEIGHT in grams	CALORIES	PROTEIN (g)	Total FAT (g)	Saturated FAT (g)	Mono FAT (g)	Poly unsaturated FAT (g)	CARBOHYDRATE (g)	Added SUGAR (g)	CHOLESTEROL (mg)	SODIUM (mg)	FIBER (g)
white, granulated	1 cup	200	770	0	0	0	0	0	199	199	0	5	
white, granulated	1 tbsp.	12	45	0	0	0	0	0	12	12	0	tr	
" "	1 pkt.	6	25	0	0	0	0	0	6	6	0	tr	
SUNFLOWER SEEDS	1 oz.	28	160	6	14	1.5	2.7	9.3	5		0	1	
SWEET POTATOES, 2 1/2 / lb													
baked, peeled	1 potato	114	115	2	tr	tr	tr	0.1	28		0	11	3
boiled, peeled	1 potato	151	160	2	tr	0.1	tr	0.2	37		0	20	
candied, 2 1/2"	1 piece	105	145	1	3	1.4	0.7	0.2	29		8	74	
SYRUP (corn or maple)	2 tbsp.	42	122	0	0	0	0	0	32	32	0	19	
TACO	1 taco	81	195	9	11	4.1	5.5	0.8	15		21	456	
TAHINI	1 tbsp.	15	90	3	8	1.1	3.0	3.5	3		0	5	
TANGERINES	1 tan.	84	35	1	tr	tr	tr	tr	9		0	1	1.5
TANGERINE JUICE, canned sweetened	1 cup	252	155	1	tr	tr	tr	0.1	41		0	15	
TARTAR SAUCE	1 tbsp.	14	75	tr	8	1.2	2.6	3.9	1		4	182	
TOASTER PASTRIES	1 pastry	54	210	2	6	1.7	3.6	0.4	38	+	0	248	
TOFU (bean curd)	2 1/2" sq.	120	85	9	5	0.7	1.0	2.9	3		0	8	0.5
TOMATOES													
fresh, 4 / lb	1 tomato	123	25	1	tr	tr	tr	0.1	5		0	10	2.5
canned	1 cup	240	50	2	1	0.1	0.1	0.2	10		0	391	
TOMATO JUICE	1 cup	244	40	2	tr	tr	tr	0.1	10		0	881	
TOMATO PASTE	1 tbsp.	16	14	1	tr	tr	tr	tr	3		0	11	
TOMATO PUREE	1 cup	250	105	4	tr	tr	tr	0.1	25		0	50	
TOMATO SAUCE	1 cup	245	75	3	tr	0.1	0.1	0.2	18		0	1482	
TORTILLAS, corn	1 tortilla	30	65	2	1	0.1	0.3	0.6	13		0	1	
TROUT, rainbow, broiled	3 oz.	85	129	22	4	0.7	1.1	1.3	0		62	29	
TUNA, canned													
oil pack	3 oz.	85	165	24	7	1.4	1.9	3.1	0		55	303	
water pack	3 oz.	85	135	30	1	0.3	0.2	0.3	0		48	468	
TUNA SALAD, made with relish and mayonnaise	1 cup	205	375	33	19	3.3	4.9	9.2	19		80	877	
TURKEY, roasted													
light meat	3 oz.	85	135	25	3	0.9	0.5	0.7	0		59	54	
dark meat	3 oz.	85	160	24	6	2.1	1.4	1.8	0		72	67	

FOOD	Amount	WEIGHT in grams	CALORIES	PROTEIN (g)	Total FAT (g)	Saturated FAT (g)	Mono FAT (g)	Poly unsaturated FAT (g)	CARBOHYDRATE (g)	Added SUGAR (g)	CHOLESTEROL (mg)	SODIUM (mg)	FIBER (g)
chopped light and dark meat	1 cup	140	240	41	7	2.3	1.4	2.0	0		106	98	
TURNIP GREENS	1 cup	164	50	5	1	0.2	tr	0.3	8		0	25	
TURNIPS, diced	1 cup	156	30	1	tr	tr	tr	0.1	8		0	78	6
VEAL													
cutlet, broiled	3 oz.	85	185	23	9	4.1	4.1	0.6	0		108	56	
rib, roasted	3 oz.	85	230	23	14	6.0	6.0	1.0	0		109	57	
VEGETABLE JUICE cocktail	1 cup	242	45	2	tr	1	tr	0.1	11		0	883	
VEGETABLES, mixed	1 cup	163	75	4	tr	0.1	tr	0.2	15		0	243	3.5
VINEGAR, cider	1 tbsp.	15	tr	tr	0	0	0	0	1		0	tr	
WAFFLES, 7" diameter	1 waffle	75	245	7	13	4.0	4.9	2.6	26		102	445	
WALNUTS													
black, chopped	1 oz.	28	170	7	16	1.0	3.6	10.6	3		0	1	
English	1 oz.	28	180	4	18	1.6	4.0	11.1	5		0	3	
WATER CHESTNUTS	1 cup	140	70	1	tr	tr	tr	tr	17		0	11	
WATERCRESS	1 cup	160	52	tr	tr				2		0	1	
WATERMELON, diced	1 cup	160	50	1	1	0.1	0.1	0.3	11		0	3	tr
WHITE SAUCE	1 cup	250	395	10	30	9.1	11.9	7.2	24		32	888	
WINE, table	3 1/2 oz.	102	80	tr	0	0	0	0	3	0	5		

Sources:

Gebhardt, Susan E. and Ruth H. Matthews, *Nutritive Value of Foods*, Human Nutrition Information Service, Home and Garden Bulletin, No. 72, 1981.

Leveille, Gilbert A., Mary Ellen Zabik, and Karen J. Morgan, *Nutrients in Foods*, Cambridge, Massachusetts, The Nutrition Guild, 1983.

Ready to Eat Cereals, Consumer Reports, October 1986, pp. 628–637.

The National Cancer Institute, *Diet, Nutrition, & Cancer Prevention: The Good News*, U.S. Department of Health and Human Service, NIH Publication No. 87–2878, 1986.

U.S. Department of Agriculture, Human Nutrition Information Service, *Composition of Foods: Raw, Processed, Prepared*, Agriculture Handbook No. 8, Vol. 1–16.

Reference Notes

Chapter One
1. Mendelson, Robert S., M.D. *How To Raise a Happy and Healthy Child in Spite of Your Doctor.*
2. Hill, Napoleon. *Think And Grow Rich.*

Chapter Two
1. Williams, Art. *All You Can Do Is All You Can Do.*
2. Dean, David. *Now Is Your Time To Win.*

Chapter Three
1. Trump, Donald. *The Art Of The Deal.*
2. Williams, Art. *All You Can Do Is All You Can Do.*
3. Markson, Larry, D.C. *Text, Markson Management Service.*

Chapter Four
1. Dean, David. *Now Is Your Time To Win.*
2. Ibid.
3. Hill, Napolean. *Think And Grow Rich.*

Chapter Five
1. Atkins, Robert C., M.D. *Dr. Atkins' Diet Revolution.*
2. Ibid.
3. Atkins, Robert C., M.D. *Dr. Atkins' Super Energy Diet.*
4. Ibid.
5. Ibid.
6. Friend, Tim. USA Today. *Protein Gives Chemotherapy Patients Relief.*
7. Yudkin, John, M.D. Lipids. *Dietary Factors in Arteriosclerosis Sucrose.*
8. Atkins, Robert C., M.D. *Dr. Atkins' Super Energy Diet.*
9. Ibid.

Chapter Six
1. Atkins, Robert C., M.D. *Super Energy Diet.*
2. Duffy, William. *Sugar Blues.*
3. Ibid.
4. Atkins.
5. Duffy.
6. Ibid.
7. Ibid.
8. Ibid.
9. Ibid.

Chapter Seven
1. Duffy, William. *Sugar Blues.*
2. Ibid.
3. Ibid.
4. Ibid.
5. Atkins, Robert C., M.D. *Dr. Atkins' Super Energy Diet.*
6. Atkins, Robert C., M.D. *Dr. Atkins' Diet Revolution.*

7. Atkins, Robert C., M.D. *Dr. Atkins' Super Energy Diet.*

8. Duffy.

9. Atkins.

10. Duffy.

11. Diamond, Harvey and Marilyn. *Fit For Life.*

12. Mendelson, Robert S. *How To Raise a Happy and Healthy Child in Spite of Your Doctor.*

Chapter Eight

1. Atkins, Robert C., M.D. *Dr. Atkins' Diet Revolution.*

2. Ibid.

3. Atkins, Robert C., M.D. *Dr. Atkins' Super Energy Diet.*

4. Haas, Robert. *Eat To Win.*

Chapter Nine

1. Atkins, Robert C., M.D. *Dr. Atkins' Diet Revolution.*

2. Ibid.

3. Ibid.

Chapter Ten

1. Duffy, William. *Sugar Blues.*

2. Ibid.

3. Ibid.

Chapter Eleven

1. Atkins, Robert C., M.D. *Dr. Atkins' Nutritional Breakthrough.*

Chapter Twelve — No End Notes

Chapter Thirteen

1. Hill, Napolean. *Think And Grow Rich.*

Chapter Fourteen

1. Fredericks, Carlton, Ph.D. *Carlton Fredericks' Cookbook.*

2. Giller, Robert M., M.D. *Medical Makeover.*

Chapter Fifteen

1. Editors of Prevention magazine; Rodale Press. *The Complete Book of Vitamins And Minerals For Health.*

2. Ibid.

3. Ibid.

4. Ibid.

5. Ibid.

6. Editors of Prevention. and *Thorsons Complete Guide to Vitamins and Minerals-* Mervyn.

7. Editors of *Prevention.*

8. Ibid.

9. Editors of Prevention, Mervyn.

10. Creedman, Michael. *The NFL All Pro Workout.*

11. Mervyn, Atkins.

12. Editors.

13. Mariani, John F. USA Today, 4-5-89, *Mediterranean Cuisine: Feast For Health.*

14. Editors of Prevention.

15. Ibid.

Chapter Sixteen

1. Atkins, Robert C., M.D. *Dr. Atkins' Super Energy Diet.*
2. Ibid.
3. Editors of Prevention magazine. *The Complete Book of Vitamins and Minerals For Health.*
4. Mervyn, Leonard, Ph.D. *Thorson's Complete Guide to Vitamins and Minerals.* Mindell, Earl. *New and Revised Vitamin Bible.*
5. Atkins.
6. Ibid.
7. Ibid.
8. Mervyn.
9. Ibid.
10. Editors of Prevention.
11. Ibid.
12. Mervyn.
13. Mindell, Mervyn.
14. Ibid.
15. Ibid.
16. Ibid.
17. Editors of Prevention.
18. Mindell, Mervyn.
19. Ibid.
20. Editors of Prevention.
21. Atkins.
22. Ibid.
23. Mindell, Mervyn.
24. Atkins.
25. Mindell.
26. Editors of Prevention.
27. Mervyn, Atkins, Mindell.
28. Mindell, Mervyn, Editors of Prevention.
29. Mindell, Mervyn.
30. Editors of Prevention.
31. Atkins.
32. Mervyn, Mindell.
33. Ibid.
34. Mervyn.
35. Mindell, Mervyn.
36. Editors of Prevention.
37. Ibid.
39. Editors of Prevention.
40. Mervyn, Mindell.
41. Editors of Prevention.
42. Ibid.
43. Mervyn, Mindell.
44. Mervyn, Mindell.

Chapter Seventeen
1. Diamond, Harvey and Marilyn. *Fit For Life.*
2. Mervyn, Leonard, Ph.D. *Thorson's Complete Guide To Vitamins and Minerals.*
3. Mervyn.
4. Mervyn.
5. Mindell, Earl. *New and Revised Vitamin Bible.*
6. Editors of Prevention magazine. *The Complete Book of Vitamins and Minerals For Health.*
7. Ibid.
8. Ibid.
9. Mindell.
10. Mervyn.
11. Mervyn, Mindell.
12. Editors of Prevention.
13. Ibid.
14. Ibid.
15. Ibid.
16. Ibid.
17. Mervyn, Mindell
18. Mervyn
19. Editors of Prevention.
20. Ibid.
21. Editors of Prevention, Mindell.
22. Editors of Prevention.
23. Ibid.
24. Ibid.
25. Mervyn.

Chapter Eighteen
1. Editors of Prevention magazine. *The Complete Book of Vitamins and Minerals For Health.*
2. Ibid.
3. Ibid.
4. Atkins, Robert C., M.D. *Dr. Atkins' Nutritional Breakthrough.*

Chapter Nineteen
1. Pearson, Derk and Shaw, Sandy. *Life Extension Weight Loss Program.*
2. Pearson, Derk and Shaw, Sandy. *Life Extension—A Practical Scientific Approach.*
3. Pearson, Derk and Shaw, Sandy. *Life Extension Companion.*
4. Pearson, Derk and Shaw, Sandy. *Life Extension—A Practical Scientific Approach.*
5. Ibid.
6. Pearson, Derk and Shaw, Sandy. *Life Extension Weight Loss Program.*

Chapter Twenty
1. Mendelson, Robert S., M.D. *How to Raise A Happy and Healthy Child in Spite of Your Doctor.*
2. Ibid.
3. Ibid.
4. Ibid.
5. Airola, Paavo, Ph.D. M.D. *Rejuvenation Secrets From Around The World.*

6. Diamond, Harvey and Marilyn. *Fit For Life.*
7. Ibid.
8. Diamond, Harvey and Marilyn. *Fit For Life II.*
9. Ibid.
10. Mendelson.
11. Diamond, Harvey and Marilyn. *Fit For Life.*
12. *Encyclopedia Britanica.*
13. Diamond, Harvey and Marilyn. *Fit For Life.*
14. Atkins, Robert C., M.D. *Dr. Atkins' Super Energy Diet.*
15. Ibid.
16. Ibid.
17. Ibid.
18. Ibid.
19. Ibid.
20. Ibid.
21. Ibid.
22. Berger, Stuart M. *How To Be Your Own Nutritionist.*
23. Atkins.
24. Ibid.

Chapter Twenty-one — No End Notes

Chapter Twenty-two — No End Notes

Chapter Twenty-three
1. Airola, Paavo, Ph.D., M.D. *Rejuvenation Secrets From Around The World.*
2. Diamond, Harvey and Marilyn. *Fit For Life.*
3. Ibid.
4. Mindell, Earl. *New and Revised Vitamin Bible.*

Chapter Twenty-four
1. Giller, Robert M., M.D. *Medical Makeover.*
2. Diamond, Harvey and Marilyn. *Fit For Life.*
3. Duffy, William. *Sugar Blues.*
4. Ibid.
5. Yudkin, John M.D. *Lipids.*
6. Allman, Fred L. Jr. M.D. *The Fitness Diary For Executives.*
7. Giller.
8. Ibid.
9. Ibid.
10. Ibid.

Chapter Twenty-five
1. *Chiropractic Acclaimed Worldwide.*
2. Leach, Robert, D.C. *The Chiropractic Theories—A Synopsis of Scientific Research.*
3. Nelson, William. *The Real Truth About Health.*
4. Spinal Column Newsletter.
5. Diamond, Harvey and Marilyn. *Fit For Life.*
6. *Chiropractic Acclaimed Worldwide.*
7. Rubin, Herman, M.D. Fellow of the American Association for the Advancement of Science in Eugenics.
8. Gutzeit, K., M.D. *The Spine as Causative Factor of Disease.*

9. Hyman, Harold T. *American Journal of Medical Science.*
10. Brailsford, James, M.D. *Journal of Surgery.*
11. Gotten, H.B., M.D. *Journal of Tennessee Medical Association.*
12. Mennell, John, M.D. "The Science and Art of Joint Manipulation."
13. King, M.E., M.D. *Therapeutic Review.*
14. Allendy, R.F., M.D. "Orientation Des Idees Medicales."
15. Cyria, James, M.D. *Medicine et Hygiene.*
16. Rocher, Charles M., M.D. *Bordeaux Chirurgical.*
17. Zillinger, G., M.D. *Hippocrates.*
18. Cramer, Albert, M.D. *Hippocrates.*
19. Melvin, W.J.S., M.D. President of Ontario Medical Association.
20. Warbassee, James P., M.D. *Surgical Treatment,* Vol. 1.
21. Tennis magazine
22. Today's Chiropractic magazine.
23. American Chiropractic Journal.
24. *Hippocrates.*
25. Cramer, Albert, M.D.
26. DeBrunner, H., M.D.
27. Berry, R.J., M.D. *Brain and Mind.*
28. Leeman, R.A., M.D. *Canadian Medical Association Journal.*
29. Millar, T. *The Clinical Journal.*
30 Speransky, A.D.
31. Capper-Johnson, L. *British Journal of Physical Medicine.*
32. Boje.
33. Rocher, Charles M., M.D. *Bordeaux Chirurgical.*
34. Ministry of Public Health and Welfare.
35. Hochfeld, A.A.
36. Chiropractic Report.
37. Chiropractic Report.

Chapter Twenty-six — No End Notes

Chapter Twenty-seven

1. Atkins, Robert C., M.D. *Super Energy Diet.*
2. Ibid.
3. Ibid.
4. Mendelson, Robert S., M.D. *Dissent In Medicine.*
5. Ibid.
6. Hellmich, Nanci. USA Today. *Liquid Diets Regain Their Popularity.*
7. Ibid.

Chapter Twenty-eight — No End Notes

Chapter Twenty-nine — No End Notes

Chapter Thirty

1. *Alternative Medicine, The Definitive Guide*, The Burton Goldberg Group, FutureMedicine Publishing, Inc.
2. Whitaker, Julian M.D., *Health and Healing*, January 1996, vol. 6, no.1.
3. Ibid.
4. Whitaker, Julian M.D., *Health and Healing*, January 1996, vol. 6, no.1.
5. *The Lancet*, Saturday August 11, vol. II, 1987, no. 8553.

6. *Health Alert*, Volume Three, no. 1.

7. Whitaker, Julian M.D., *Health and Healing*, January 1996, vol. 6, no. 1.

8. *Health and Healing*.

9. Neu, H.C., *Science*, 1992, p. 257, 1064-1073.

10. *The Journal of the American Medical Association*, 1991; Cantekin, E.L., McGuire, T.W., 3309-3317.

11. Weil, Andrew, *Spontaneous Healing*, Fawcett Columbine, May 1996.

12. Muir, Maya, *Alternative Complementary Therapies*, vol. II, no. 3, May/June 1996.

13. Mumcuolglu, Madeleine, *Sambucus*, Black Elderberry Extract, RSS Publishing, Inc.

14. Ibid.

15. Muir, Maya, *Antibiotic Resistance, Alternative Complimentary Therapies*, vol. 2, no. 3, May/June 1996, p. 141.

16. Carper, Jean, *Miracle Cures*, Harper Collins.

17. Ibid.

18. Enstrom, J.E., et al, *Vitamin C Intake and Mortality Among A Sample Of U.S. Population*. Epedemiol 3 (3) pp. 194-202, 1994.

19. *Whitman's Guide to Natural Healing*, Prima Publishing, p. 22.

20. *Alternative Medicine*, The Burton Goldberg Group, FutureMedicine Publishing, Inc.

Bibliography

Airola, Paavo, Ph.D., M.D. *Rejuvenation Secrets From Around The World.* Phoenix, Arizona: Health Plus Publications, 1974.

Allman, Fred L., Jr., M.D. *The Fitness Diary For Executives.* Atlanta, Georgia: Aurora Publishing Co., 1983.

American Chiropractic Journal, 1988.

American Journal of Clinical Nutrition, Vol. 20, 1967, Vol. 26, 1973.

Associated Press, *50% of lower back disc surgery unneeded, specialist says.*

Atkins, Robert C., M.D. *Dr. Atkins' Diet Revolution.* New York: Bantam Books, Inc., 1972.

Atkins, Robert C. M.D. *Dr. Atkins' Nutritional Breakthrough.* New York: Bantam Books, Inc., 1981.

Atkins, Robert C. M.D. *Dr. Atkins' Super Energy Diet.* New York: Bantam Books, Inc., 1977.

Bach, Marcus. *The Chiropractic Story.* Austell, Georgia: Si-Nell Publishing Co., 1968.

Bach, Richard. *Illusions.* New York: Dell Publishing Co., 1977.

Berger, Stuart M. *How To Be Your Own Nutritionist.* New York: Avon Books, 1987.

Boyd, William. *Textbook of Pathology,* 8th Ed. Philadelphia, Pennsylvania: Lea & Febiger, 1970.

Cecil Textbook of Medicine, 15th Ed. Philadelphia, Pennsylvania: Cylinders 1969–1989.

Celebrities Choose Chiropractic!—Pamphlet, 1981, Form #182.

Chiropractic Acclaimed Worldwide—Pamphlet, 1981, Form #201.

Chiropractic Report, January 1988, Vol. 2, No. 2; March 1988, Vol. 2, No. 3. Toronto, Canada: Editor, David Chapman Smith.

Creedman, Michael. *The NFL All Pro Workout.* New York: St. Martins Press, 1987.

Darden, Ellington, Ph.D. *The Athlete's Guide To Sports Medicine.* Chicago, Illinois: Contemporary Books, Inc., 1981.

Davis, Adelle. *Let's Eat Right To Keep Fit.* New York: Harcourt-Brace Jovanovich, Inc., 1954.

Davis, Francine. *Low Blood Sugar Cookbook.* New York: Bantam Books, 1973.

Dean, David. *Now Is Your Time To Win.* Wheaton, Illinois: Tyndale House Publications, Inc., 1983.

Diamond, Harvey and Marilyn. *Fit For Life.* New York: Warner Books, 1987.

Diamond, Harvey and Marilyn. *Fit For Life II.* New York: Warner Books, 1988.

Dorland's Medical Dictionary.

Duffy, William. *Sugar Blues.* New York: Warner Books, Inc., 1975.

Encyclopedia Britanica, Vol. 19. Chicago, Illinois: Encyclopedia Britanica, Inc., 1980.

The Facts Are In: Chiropractic Care is Cost Effective in Treatment of Work-Related Back Injuries—Pamphlet, 1981, Form #261.

Farley, Christopher. *Health Has Become A Laughing Matter, USA Today,* January 19, 1988.

Fredericks, Carlton, Ph.D. *Carlton Fredericks' Cookbook.* New York: Berkley Publishing Group, 1986.

Fredricks, Carlton, Ph.D. *New Low Blood Sugar and You.* New York: Putnam Publishing Group, 1985.

Fredericks, Carlton, Ph.D., and Goodman, Herman, M.D. *Low Blood Sugar and You,* New York: Berkley Publishing Group, 1987.

Friend, Tim. *USA Today, Protein Gives Chemotherapy Patients Relief; Blame Dark Days For Winter Blues; Dense Cholesterol: New Heart Warning; Low Level of 'Good' Cholesterol is Bad.*

Galton, Lawrence. *The Silent Disease—Hypertension.* New York: Signet Books, 1973.

Giller, Robert M., M.D. *Medical Makeover.* New York, Derri h Tipp Books, 1986.

Haas, Robert. *Eat To Win.* New York: Signet Books, 1983.

Hansen, Mark Victor. *Be Fit.* Newport Beach, California: Mark Victor Hansen Publishers, 1988.

Hansen, Mark Victor. *Dare To Win.* Newport Beach, California: Mark Victor Hansen Publications, 1988.

Hauser, Gaylord. *Be Happier and Healthier.* Greenwich, Connecticut: Fawcett Publications, 1952.

Healy, Michelle. USA Today, 4-6-88. *Are You An Exercise Addict?*

Hellmich, Nanci. USA Today, 6-9-88. *Liquid Diets Regain Their Popularity.*

Hill, Napolean. *Think and Grow Rich.* New York: Ballantine Books, 1960.

Jones, Charles "T". *Life is Tremendous.* Harrisburg, Pennsylvania: Executive Books Publications, 1968.

Kirschmann, John D., Director. *Nutrition Almanac.* New York: McGraw-Hill, 1973.

Leach, Robert, D.C. *The Chiropractic Theories—A Synopsis of Scientific Research,* New York: Williams and Wilkins, 1986.

M.D.'s Comment On Chiropractic—Pamphlet, 1972, Form #119.

Maltz, Maxwell, M.D. *Psychocybernetics.* Hollywood, California: Wilshire Book Company, 1960.

Mariani, John F. *USA Today, 4-5-89. Mediterranean Cuisine: Feast For Health.*

Markson, Larry, M.D. *Text, Markson Management Service.* New York: Markson Management Service, Inc., 1983.

McDougall, John A. and McDougall, Mary. *The McDougall Plan.* Picataway,New Jersey: New Century Publications, Inc., 1983.

Medical Journal of Australia.

Mendelson, Robert S., M.D. *Confessions of a Medical Heretic.* Chicago Illinois: Contemporary Books, Inc., 1979.

Mendelson, Robert S., M.D. *How to Raise A Happy and Healthy Child in Spite of Your Doctor.* Chicago, Illinois: Contemporary Books, Inc., 1984.

Mendelson, Robert S., M.D.; Crile, George, M.D.; Epstein, Samuel, M.D.; Heimlich, Henry, M.D., Levin, Alan Scott, M.D.; Pinckney, Edward R., M.D.; Spodick, David, M.D.; Moskowitz, Richard, M.D.; White, Gregory, M.D. *Dissent In Medicine.* Chicago, Illinois: Contemporary Books, Inc., 1985.

Mervyn, Leonard, Ph.D. *Thorson's Complete Guide to Vitamins and Minerals.* Rochester, Vermont: Thorson Publications, Inc., 1987.

Mindell, Earl. *New and Revised Vitamin Bible.* New York: Warner Books, 1985.

Mirkin, Gabe, M.D., and Hoffman, Marshall. *The Sports Medicine Book.* Boston, Massachusetts: Little, Brown & Co., 1978.

Nelson, William. *The Real Truth About Health.* Costa Mesa, California: Katpur Press, 1987.

New York Magazine, March 31, 1975.

Orenstein, Neil S., Ph.D. *Nutritional Biochemistry.* Douglas Labs, Draft 8/30/88.

Painter, Kim. USA Today, 4-19-88. *Personality Is Your Best Cancer Defense.*

Palmer, B. J., DC. *Innate.* Romulus, Michigan: Inner Winners Seminars, 1988.

Panter, James. *Today's Chiropractic Magazine.* "She Serves To Conquer: Billie Jean King's Quest For Excellence."

Passwater, Richard A., Ph.D. *L-Glutamine: The Surprising Brain Fuel.* Solgar Brand, 1986.

Pearson, Derk and Shaw, Sandy. *Life Extension—A Practical Scientific Approach,* New York: Warner Books, 1982.

Pearson, Derk and Shaw, Sandy. *Life Extension Companion.* New York: Warner Books, 1984.

Pearson, Derk and Shaw, Sandy. *Life Extension Weight Loss Program.* Garden City, New York: Doubleday Co., 1987.

Peterson, Roger. *USA Today,* 4-6-88. "It's A Slow Steady Race To Fitness."

Editors of Prevention magazine, *The Complete Book of Vitamins and Minerals For Health,* Rodale Press, Emmaus, Pennsylvania., 1988.

Pritikin, Nathan, M.D. *The Pritikin Program for Diet and Exercise.* New York, New York: Bantam Books, 1979.

Pritikin, Nathan, M.D. *The Pritikin Permanent Weight-Loss Manual.* New York: Bantam Books, 1981.

Prochnow, Herbert V., and Prochnow, Herbert V., Jr. *The Public Speaker's Treasure Chest.* New York: Harper & Row Publications, 1986.

Reader's Digest. April 1988.

Reilly, Harold J., M.D., and Brod, Ruth. *The Edgar Casey Handbook For Health Through Drugless Therapy.* New York: Jove Publishers, 1975.

Robertson, Donald S., M.D. "Water." Body Shop.

Roth, June. *The Food Depression Connection.* Chicago, Illinois: Contemporary Books, Inc., 1978.

Sperling, Dan. USA Today. *A Health Food for Blood Fat and More. We're Slacking Off on Good Nutrition,* 5-12-88; *Health and Happiness Go Hand and Hand,* 6-8-88.

Spinal Column Newsletter, Clearwater, Florida: D.C. International, July/Aug.1986, vol. 4, no. 3; Nov./Dec. 1986, vol. 4, no. 5; March/April 1987, vol. 5; Jan./Feb. 1987, vol. 5, no. 1.

Steen, Edwin B., Ph.D, and Montagu, Ashley, Ph.D. *Anatomy and Physiology,* New York: Barnes and Noble, 1959.

Stern, Bert. *The Food Book.* New York: Dell Books, 1987.

Sutton, Remar. *Body Worry.* "The Walking Test." New York: Penguin Books, 1987.

Today's Doctors of Chiropractic Have Six or More Years of College, Parker Chiropractic Research Foundation—Pamphlet, 1981, Form #224.

Trump, Donald J. *The Art Of The Deal.* New York: Random House, 1987.

Williams, Art. *All You Can Do Is All You Can Do.* Nashville, Tennessee: Thomas Nelson Publishers, 1988.

Yudkin, John, M.D. *Lancet,* 10-29-60; *Nature,* vol. 239, 1972; *Lipids,* vol. 13. *Dietary Factors in Arteriosclerosis Sucrose,* 1978.

Addendum To Bibliography:

The following sources were used for the charts in chapters 16 and 17.

Bowes and Church's Food Values of Portions Commonly Used, Jean A.T. Pennington and Helen Nichols Church (New York: Harper & Row, 1980).

Composition of Foods, Agriculture Handbook No. 8, by Bernice K. Watt and Annabel L. Merrill (Washington, D.C.: Agricultural Research Service, U.S. Department of Agriculture, 1975).

Composition of Foods: Beef Products, Agriculture Handbook No. 8-13, by Nutrition Monitoring Division (Washington, D.C.: Human Nutrition Information Service, U.S. Department of Agriculture, 1986).

Composition of Foods: Breakfast Cereals, Agriculture Handbook No. 8-8, by Consumer Nutrition Center (Washington, D.C.: Human Nutrition Information Service, U.S. Department of Agriculture, 1982).

Composition of Foods: Dairy and Egg Products, Agriculture Handbook No. 8-1, by Consumer and Food Economics Institute (Washington, D.C.: Agriculture Research Service, U.S. Department of Agriculture, 1976).

Composition of Foods: Fats and Oils, Agriculture Handbook No. 8-4, by Consumer and Food Economics Institute (Washington, D.C.: Science and Education Administration, U.S. Department of Agriculture, 1979).

Composition of Foods: Fruits and Fruit Juices, Agriculture Handbook No. 8-9, by Consumer Nutrition Center (Washington, D.C.: Human Nutrition Information Service, U.S. Department of Agriculture, 1982).

Composition of Foods: Legumes and Legume Products, Agricultural Handbook No. 8-16,-by Nutrition Monitoring Division (Washington, D.C.: Human Nutrition Information Service, U.S. Department of Agriculture, 1986).

Composition of Foods: Nut and Seed Products, Agriculture Handbook No. 8-12, by Nutrition Monitoring Division (Washington D.C.: Human Nutrition Information Service, U.S. Department of Agriculture, 1984).

Composition of Foods: Poultry Products, Agriculture Handbook No. 8-5, by Consumer and Food Economics Institute (Washington, D.C.: Science and Education Administration, U.S. Department of Agriculture, 1979).

Composition of Foods: Vegetables and Vegetable Products, Agricultural Handbook No. 8-11, by Nutrition Monitoring Division (Washington, D.C.: Human Nutrition Information Service, U.S. Department of Agriculture, 1984).

DeLuca, Hector F., *Handbook of Lipid Research: The Fat-Soluble Vitamins,* New York: Plenum Press, 1978.

Journal of the American Dietetic Association, April, 1975.

McCance and Widdowson's The Composition of Foods, A.A. Paul and D.A.T. Southgate (New York: Elsevier/North-Holland Biomedical, 1978).

McLaughlin, P.J. and John L. Weihrauch, *Vitamin E Content of Foods,* Journal of the American Dietetic Association, December, 1979.

Nutritive Value of American Foods in Common Units, Agriculture Handbook No. 456, by Catherine F. Adams (Washington, D.C.: Agricultural Research Service, U.S. Department of Agriculture, 1975).

Nutrient Data Research Branch, U.S. Department of Agriculture, Washington, D.C.

Pennington, Jean T. and Doris Howes, *Copper Content of Foods,* Calloway, Research, August, 1973.

Perloff, P. Perloff and R.R. Butrum, *Folacin in Selected Foods,* Journal of the American Dietetic Association, February 1977.

Pantothenic Acid, Vitamin B6 and Vitamin B12, Home Economics Research Report No. 36, by Martha Louise Orr (Washington, D.C.: Agricultural Research Service, U.S. Department of Agriculture, 1969).

Index

Books by Starburst Publishers
www.starburstpublishers.com

Dr. Kaplan's Lifestyle of the Fit & Famous
—Eric Scott Kaplan

Subtitled: *A Wellness Approach to "Thinning and Winning."* This newly expanded guide is more than a health book—it is a lifestyle based on the empirical formulas of healthy living and wellness that now incorporates two chapters on alternative medicine. Dr. Kaplan's food-combined principles take into account all the major sources, so that you can dine on omelets for breakfast, scampi for lunch, steak for dinner and still lose weight. Learn to incorporate exercise, vitamins, and nutrition and delicious meals for a happier healthier life.

(trade paper) ISBN 0914984993 **$16.95**

Allergy Cooking With Ease
—Nicolette M. Dumke

Subtitled: *The No Wheat, Milk, Eggs, Corn, Soy, Yeast, Sugar, Grain, and Gluten Cookbook.* A book designed to provide a wide variety of recipes to meet many different types of dietary and social needs and, whenever possible, save you time in food preparation. Includes: Recipes for those special foods that most food allergy patients think they will never eat again; Timesaving tricks; and Allergen Avoidance Index.

(trade paper) ISBN 091498442X **$14.95**

Migraine –Winning the Fight of Your Life
—Charles Theisler

This book describes the hurt, loneliness and agony that migraine sufferers experience and the difficulty they must live with. It explains to the reader the different types of migraines and their symptoms, as well as explaining the related health hazards. Gives 200 ways to help fight off migraines, and shows how to experience fewer headaches, reduce their duration, and decrease the agony and pain involved.

(trade paper) ISBN 0914984632 **$10.95**

The Crystal Clear Guide to Sight for Life
—Gayton & Ledford

Subtitled: *A Complete Manual of Eye Care for Those Over 40. The Crystal Clear Guide to Sight For Life* makes eye care easy-to-understand by giving clear knowledge of how the eye works with the most up-to-date information available from the experts. Contains more than 40 illustrations, a detailed index for cross-referencing, a concise glossary, and answers to often-asked questions.

(trade paper) ISBN 0914984683 **$15.95**

The World's Oldest Health Plan
—Kathleen O'Bannon Baldinger

Subtitled: *Health, Nutrition and Healing from the Bible.* Offers a complete health plan for body, mind and spirit, just as Jesus did. It includes programs for diet, exercise and mental health. Contains foods and recipes to lower cholesterol and blood pressure, improve the immune system and other bodily functions, reduce stress, reduce or cure constipation, eliminate insomnia, reduce forgetfulness, confusion and anger, increase circulation and thinking ability, eliminate "yeast" problems, improve digestion, and much more.

(trade paper) ISBN 0914984578 **$14.95**

Eat for the Health of It
—Erickson & Dempsey

A back-to-basics approach to eating and learning how to maintain and preserve your body: Tells why some people gain weight on six grams of fat. Tells how to improve your health with or without medicine. Gives 21 reasons why blood cholesterol rises. Contains hundreds of anecdotes, meal plans, resources and recipes. *Eat for the Health of It* will have you eating towards a better life!

(trade paper) ISBN 0914984780 **$15.95**

The Low-Fat Supermarket
—Judith & Scott Smith

A comprehensive reference of over 4,500 brand name products that derive less than 30% of their calories from fat. Information provided includes total calories, fat, cholesterol and sodium content. Organized according to the sections of a supermarket. Your answer to a healthier you.

(trade paper) ISBN 0914984438 **$10.95**

Books by Starburst Publishers—cont'd.

Health, Happiness & Hormones
—Arlene Swaney

Subtitled: *One Woman's Journey Toward Health After a Hysterectomy.* A frightening and candid look into one woman's struggle to find a cure for her medical condition. In 1990, when her story was first published in *Prevention* magazine, author Arlene Swaney received an overwhelming response from women who also were plagued by mysterious, but familiar, symptoms leading to continuous misdiagnoses. Starting with a hysterectomy Swaney details the years of lost health that followed as she searched for an accurate diagnosis. Her story is told with warmth and compassion.

(trade paper) ISBN 0914984721 **$9.95**

Stay Well Without Going Broke
—Gulling, Renner, & Vargas

Subtitled: *Winning the War Over Medical Bills.* Provides a blueprint for how health care consumers can take more responsibility for monitoring their own health and the cost of its care—a crucial cornerstone of the health care reform movement today. Contains inside information from doctors, pharmacists and hospital personnel on how to get cost-effective care without sacrificing quality. Offers legal strategies to protect your rights when illness is terminal.

(hardcover) ISBN 0914984527 **$22.95**

The Frazzled Working Woman's Practical Guide to Motherhood
—Mary Lyon

It's Emma Bombeck meets Martha Stewart meets cartoonist Cathy Guisewite. The author's extensive original cartoon illustrations further enliven a sparklingly humorous narrative, making her a new James Thurber! *Frazzled* is an essential companion for any working woman who thinks she wants a baby, or is currently expecting one. Especially if she could use a good laugh to lighten her load and her worries. This book also offers an innovative update on effective working mom strategies to women who are already off and running on the "Mommy Track."

(trade paper) ISBN 0914984756 **$11.95**

Parenting With Respect and Peacefulness
—Louise A. Dietzel

Subtitled: *The Most Difficult Job in the World.* Parents who love and respect themselves parent with respect and peacefulness. Yet, parenting with respect is the most difficult job in the world. This book informs parents that respect and peace communicate love—creating an atmosphere for children to maximize their development as they feel loved, valued, and safe. Parents can learn authority and control by commonsense, interpersonal, and practical approaches to day-to-day issues and situations in parenting.

(trade paper) ISBN 0914984667 **$10.95**

Lease–Purchase America!
—John Ross

A first-of-its-kind book that provides a simple "nuts and bolts" approach to acquiring real estate. Explains how the lease-purchase technique pioneered by John Ross can now be used in real estate to more easily buy and sell a home. Details the value of John's technique from the perspective of each participant in the real estate transaction. Illustrates how the reader can use lease-purchase successfully as a tool to achieve his or her real estate goals.

(trade paper) ISBN 0914984454 **$9.95**

Baby Steps to Happiness
—John Q. Baucom

Subtitled: *52 Inspiring Ways to Make Your Life Happy.* This unique 52-step approach will enable the reader to focus on small steps that bring practical and proven change. The author encourages the reader to take responsibility for the Happiness that only he can find. Chapter titles, such as, *Have a Reason to Get Out of Bed, Deal with Your Feelings or Become Them, Would You Rather Be Right or Happy?,* and *Love To Win More Than You Hate to Lose* give insight and encouragement on the road to happiness.

(trade paper) ISBN 0914984861 **$12.95**

Books by Starburst Publishers—cont'd.

Little Baby Steps to Happiness
—John Q. Baucom

Inspiring, witty and insightful, this portable collection of quotes and affirmations from *Baby Steps to Happiness* will encourage Happiness one little footstep at a time. This book is the perfect personal "cheerleader."

(trade paper) ISBN 091498487X **$6.95**

Baby Steps to Success
—Vince Lombardi Jr. & John Q. Baucom

Subtitled: *52 Vince Lombardi-Inspired Ways to Make Your Life Successful.* Vince Lombardi's is one of the most quoted success stories in the history of the world. From corporate boardrooms to athletic locker rooms, his wisdom is studied, read, and posted on walls. The same skills that Coach Lombardi used to turn the Green Bay Packers from cellar dwellers to world champions is now available to you in *Baby Steps To Success*. This book can help you be more successful in your career, personal or family life. The same principles that made the Packers Super Bowl champions can make you a "Super Bowl" employee, parent or spouse. These principles are broken down into 52 unique and achievable "Baby Steps."

(trade paper) ISBN: 0914984950 **$12.95**

Little Baby Steps to Success
—Vince Lombardi Jr. & John Q. Baucom

Subtitled: *Vince Lombardi-Inspired Motivational Wisdom & Insight to Make Your Life Successful.* Motivational, inspiring and filled with insight that will get you off the bench and into the game of success. This wisdom-filled, pocket-sized collection of the best of Lombardi will help you one small step at a time to reach the goals you have imagined.

(trade paper) ISBN: 0914984969 **$6.95**

The Miracle of the Sacred Scroll
—Johan Christian

In this poignant book, Johan Christian masterfully weaves historical and biblical reality together with a touching fictional story to bring to life this marvelous work—a story that takes its main character, Simon of Cyrene, on a journey which transforms his life, and that of the reader, from one of despair and defeat to success and triumph!

(hardcover) ISBN 091498473X **$14.95**

From Grandma With Love
—Ann Tuites

Subtitled: *Thoughts for Her Children Everywhere.* People are taught all kinds of things from preschool to graduate school, but they are expected to know instinctively how to get along with their families. Harmony within the home is especially difficult when an aging relative is involved. The author presents personal anecdotes to encourage caregivers and those in need of care. Practical, emotional and spiritual support is given so that all generations can learn to live together in harmony.

(hardcover) ISBN 0914984616 **$14.95**

Purchasing Information:
www.starburstpublishers.com

Books are available from your favorite bookstore, either from current stock or special order. To assist bookstore in locating your selection be sure to give title, author, and ISBN #. If unable to purchase from the bookstore you may order direct from STARBURST PUBLISHERS. When ordering enclose full payment plus $3.00 for shipping and handling ($4.00 if Canada or Overseas). Payment in US Funds only. Please allow two to three weeks minimum (longer overseas) for delivery. Make checks payable to and mail to STARBURST PUBLISHERS, P.O. Box 4123, LANCASTER, PA 17604. Credit card orders may also be placed by calling 1-800-441-1456 (credit card orders only), Mon-Fri, 8:30 a.m. – 5:30 p.m. Eastern Time. **Prices subject to change without notice.** Catalog available for a 9 x 12 self-addressed envelope with 4 first-class stamps.   2-98